Immunopsychiatry

Immunopsychiatry

An Introduction

Edited by

Neil Harrison
Professor of Psychiatry, Cardiff University

Golam Khandaker
Wellcome Trust Intermediate Clinical Fellow, University of Cambridge

Edward Bullmore
Professor of Psychiatry, University of Cambridge

Robert Dantzer
Professor and Deputy Chair, MD Anderson Cancer Center

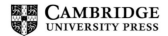
CAMBRIDGE
UNIVERSITY PRESS

CAMBRIDGE
UNIVERSITY PRESS

University Printing House, Cambridge CB2 8BS, United Kingdom

One Liberty Plaza, 20th Floor, New York, NY 10006, USA

477 Williamstown Road, Port Melbourne, VIC 3207, Australia

314–321, 3rd Floor, Plot 3, Splendor Forum, Jasola District Centre, New Delhi – 110025, India

103 Penang Road, #05–06/07, Visioncrest Commercial, Singapore 238467

Cambridge University Press is part of the University of Cambridge.

It furthers the University's mission by disseminating knowledge in the pursuit of education, learning, and research at the highest international levels of excellence.

www.cambridge.org
Information on this title: www.cambridge.org/9781108424042
DOI: 10.1017/9781108539623

© Cambridge University Press 2021

First published 2021

A catalogue record for this publication is available from the British Library.

ISBN 978-1-108-42404-2 Hardback

Contents

Colour plates can be found between pages 182 and 183

Foreword

John H. Krystal, M.D.
Robert L. McNeil Jr Professor of Translational Research
Professor of Psychiatry, Neuroscience, and Psychology
Chair, Department of Psychiatry
Co-Director Yale Center for Clinical Investigation
Yale School of Medicine
300 George St. Suite #901
New Haven, CT 06511 USA
T: 203-785-6396
F: 203-785-6916
E: john.krystal@yale.edu

June 7, 2021

The *Textbook of Immunopsychiatry* is very timely. The field of psychiatry is surely the most rapidly evolving of all areas of medicine. The very notion of a biology of psychiatric disorder is a relatively recent concept. As our understanding of the biology of psychiatric disorders advanced, the complexity of the phenomena that we were studying similarly increased. The initial psychiatric focus on monoamines led to an appreciation of the profusion of neural signaling mechanisms. An initial focus on the interplay of neuronal types led to the understanding of the role of astroglia and oligodendrocytes in neural signaling. The emergence of immunopsychiatry represents an extradimensional shift in our thinking about the brain and its relationship with the rest of the body. Rather than viewing the brain as distinct from the body, immunopsychiatry highlights the fundamental importance of immunoregulation of brain function and, likewise, the role of the brain in regulating peripheral immune processes.

The scope of immunopsychiatry is both broad and deep. In reviewing this book, I was reminded of a quote from George Engel from the 1950's, "we repeatedly affirm our belief that all diseases are "psycho-somatic," in the sense that psychological processes are always involved [1]." Similarly, the *Textbook of Immunopsychiatry* makes the case that most aspects of brain function and psychiatric pathophysiology have an immunologic component. This view has profound implications. First, immunologic mechanisms are implicated increasingly in specific ways in the neurodevelopmental emergence of psychiatric pathophysiology. This view is exemplified by the implication of activated microglia in the enhanced synaptic elimination associated with the development of schizophrenia [2]. Second, the brain is affected in profound ways by inflammatory processes that affect the entire body, even when the brain's inflammatory response opposes the changes in the periphery [3]. Thus, psychological and cognitive symptoms may predict medical outcomes, like heart disease, because of their organ-specific responses to common inflammatory processes. Further, the first two points imply that a deep understanding of neuroimmunology could inform the development of immunosuppressant treatments or prevention strategies; particularly within a precision medicine framework. Third, as elegantly reviewed in this book, the brain is affecting the peripheral immune processes.

One unanticipated consequence of the emergence of immunopsychiatry is that it has built new collaborative bridges between psychiatry and other areas of medicine. We are now studying common pathophysiologic mechanisms with our colleagues in cardiology, rheumatology, neurology, and other areas of medicine. This shared platform enabled us, as a field, to contribute to studying neural, psychosocial and other medical outcomes during the COVID pandemic.

I think the *Textbook of Immunopsychiatry* is a wonderful way to learn about this important and rapidly emerging area. Its fifteen chapters provide a historical context and then build a framework for understanding the complex interplay of brain and immune function, setting the stage for understanding neuroimmune illnesses and treatments.

1. Engel, G.L., *Selection of clinical material in psychosomatic medicine: the need for a new physiology.* Psychosom Med, 1954. **16**(5): p. 368–73.

2. Sekar, A., et al., *Schizophrenia risk from complex variation of complement component 4.* Nature, 2016. **530**(7589): p. 177–83.

3. Bhatt, S., et al., *PTSD is associated with neuroimmune suppression: evidence from PET imaging and postmortem transcriptomic studies.* Nat Commun, 2020. **11**(1): p. 2360.

Contributors

Esha Abrol
University College London Division of Psychiatry, UK

Carly Apar
New York State Psychiatric Institute, Columbia University Medical Center, New York, USA

Bernhard T. Baune
Department of Psychiatry, Melbourne Medical School, The University of Melbourne, Melbourne, Australia

Julie-Myrtille Bourgognon
Institute of Health & Wellbeing, University of Glasgow, Scotland, UK

Alan S. Brown
New York State Psychiatric Institute, Columbia University Medical Center, New York, USA

Edward Bullmore
Department of Psychiatry, University of Cambridge, UK

Jonathan Cavanagh
Institute of Health & Wellbeing, University of Glasgow, Scotland, UK

Alessandro Colasanti
Department of Neuroscience, Brighton & Sussex Medical School, Brighton, UK

Fiona Conway
New York State Psychiatric Institute, Columbia University Medical Center, New York, USA

Colm Cunningham
Trinity Biomedical Sciences Institute and Trinity College Institute of Neuroscience, Trinity College Dublin

John F. Cryan
APC Microbiome Ireland, University College Cork, Cork, Ireland. Department of Anatomy and Neuroscience, University College Cork, Cork, Ireland

Robert Dantzer
MD Anderson Cancer Center, University of Texas, USA

Bill Deakin
Division of Neuroscience and Experimental Psychology, University of Manchester, UK

Ted Dinan
APC Microbiome Ireland, University College Cork, Cork, Ireland. Department of Psychiatry & Neurobehavioural Science, University College Cork, Cork, Ireland

Genevieve Falabella
New York State Psychiatric Institute, Columbia University Medical Center, New York, USA

Célia Fourrier
Discipline of Psychiatry, University of Adelaide, Adelaide, Australia

Neil Harrison
Clinical Professor in Neuroimaging, University of Cardiff

Clive Holmes
Clinical and Experimental Sciences, Faculty of Medicine, University of Southampton, UK Memory Assessment and Research Centre, Moorgreen Hospital, Southern Health Foundation Trust, Southampton, UK

Tanja Jovanovic
Department of Psychiatry and Behavioral Sciences, Emory University School of Medicine, Atlanta, Georgia, USA

Nils Kappelmann
Max Planck Institute of Psychiatry, Munich, Germany

Keith W. Kelley
Department of Pathology, College of Medicine and Department of Animal Sciences, College of ACES, University of Illinois at Urbana-Champaign, 212 Edward R. Madigan Laboratory, 1201 West Gregory Drive, Urbana, Il 61801, USA

Golam Khandaker
Clinical Fellow, Department of Psychiatry, University of Cambridge, UK

Rajeev Krishnadas
Institute of Neuroscience & Psychology, University of Glasgow, Scotland, UK

Alison McColl
Institute of Health & Wellbeing, University of Glasgow, Scotland, UK

Vasiliki Michopoulos
Department of Psychiatry and Behavioral Sciences, Emory University School of Medicine, Atlanta, Georgia, USA
Yerkes National Primate Research Center, Atlanta, Georgia, USA

John T. O'Brien
Department of Psychiatry, University of Cambridge, Cambridge, UK

Kiran V. Sandhu
APC Microbiome Ireland, University College Cork, Cork, Ireland

Eoin Sherwin
APC Microbiome Ireland, University College Cork, Cork, Ireland

Donal T. Skelly
Nuffield Department of Clinical Neurosciences, University of Oxford, UK

Maria Suessmilch
Institute of Health & Wellbeing, University of Glasgow, Scotland, UK

Ajenthan Surendranathan
Department of Psychiatry, University of Cambridge, Cambridge, UK

Catherine Toben
Discipline of Psychiatry, University of Adelaide, Adelaide, Australia

Lorinda Turner
Department of Medicine, University of Cambridge, Addenbrookes Hospital, Hills Road, Cambridge, UK

Rachel Upthegrove
Institute for Mental Health, University of Birmingham, UK

Michael S. Zandi
University College London Queen Square Institute of Neurology and National Hospital for Neurology and Neurosurgery

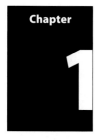

Chapter 1

Basic Concepts in Immunobiology

Lorinda Turner and Neil Harrison

1.1 Introduction

Once thought to be an immune-privileged site, we now know that there is a complex and essential bidirectional interplay between the central nervous system (CNS) and the immune system (1). Technological advances in imaging, genomic medicine and immunology have resulted in major revisions to some of the most fundamental and long-held assumptions in neuroscience, and we now understand that the immune system is critically involved not only in brain pathology, but also in the normal processes of brain development and homeostasis.

'Immunopsychiatry', namely the study of the interactions between neuroscience, mental health and the immune system, has rapidly become a major priority for psychiatric research. Accumulating evidence indicates roles for the immune system in the pathophysiology of many neurodegenerative and psychiatric disorders including Alzheimer's disease (AD), schizophrenia, major depressive disorder (MDD), multiple sclerosis (MS) and others. In particular, pro-inflammatory cytokines associated with inflammation, which is common to many of these disorders, can influence the brain to bring about a host of physiological as well as behavioural alterations such as changes in mood and cognition. Raised pro-inflammatory cytokines are consistently reported in MDD (2) and schizophrenia (3). Moreover, systemic inflammation brought about by acute infection, diabetes, obesity and atherosclerosis can accelerate cognitive decline in the elderly and present significant risk for the development or acceleration of AD and delirium (4). With this new knowledge come new targets to be exploited as biomarkers for diagnosis or informing treatment. A number of immune-modulating therapeutics are currently being trialled for the treatment of MDD, schizophrenia, AD and others.

In this chapter we aim to provide an overview of the key concepts in immunology and lay the foundations for understanding the role of the immune system in normal CNS homeostasis, and its contribution to neurodegeneration and psychiatric illness.

1.2 Overview of the Immune System

The most fundamental function of the immune system is to prevent and eradicate threats to bodily integrity. Frequently these threats are exogenous, invading microbes for example; but can also be endogenous in the form of damaged or dying tissue and malignancy.

The immune system can be broadly classified into two arms: the innate immune system and the adaptive immune system. Innate or natural immunity is always present in the individual. It consists of barriers that physically prevent entry of invading microbes, and a range of cells and non-cellular products that recognize and respond to threat. The innate immune system is critical for conveying messages to the brain warning of infection, resulting in the fever response. Additionally, components of the innate immune system enhance the adaptive immune response to pathogens. The adaptive immune system consists of T and B cells and their products. Where the innate immune system recognizes structures that are shared by many classes of microbes, and mounts the same response on repeated exposure, the adaptive immune system recognizes a wide variety of molecules with exquisite specificity, generates memory, and mounts a stronger response with each subsequent exposure. The innate and adaptive arms of the immune system work co-operatively to respond to threats and preserve bodily integrity. Failure can result in overwhelming infection, autoimmunity, or tissue damage, such as occurs in neurodegeneration. The immune system is increasingly recognized for its additional non-immune functions: wound healing, organ development and maintenance of homeostasis. The innate and adaptive immune systems and their contributions to immunopsychiatry will be discussed in this chapter.

1.3 Innate Immune System: Barriers

The first line of defence against invading microbes are the skin and mucosal epithelium, including the digestive tract, lungs and urogenital tract, which together provide a continuous physical barrier preventing the entry of microbes into the bloodstream. Within the healthy CNS, the blood-brain-barrier (BBB) and the blood-cerebrospinal fluid barrier (BCSFB) play analogous roles, blocking entry of microbes and selectively restricting the entry of immune cells. However, it is important to recognize that they are highly dynamic interfaces that communicate with the adjacent environments and serve the needs of the CNS (5). The BBB is a complex system comprising highly specialized endothelial cells that are joined by tight junctions, an underlying basement membrane embedded with pericytes, perivascular antigen presenting cells (APCs) and astrocytic endfeet (6). The BCSFB on the other hand consists of the choroid plexus, which provides a physical interface between the blood and the cerebrospinal fluid (CSF). The choroid plexus epithelial cells generate approximately two-thirds of the CSF and help to control its composition by regulating the passage of ions, metabolites and molecules between the blood and the CSF (7). Tight junctions between the cells of the BBB and BCSFB inhibit the unrestricted diffusion of water soluble molecules, and both interfaces express active and passive cellular transporters that allow passage of select molecules, such as cytokines, hormones, amino acids and peptides between the blood and the CNS (5) (Figure 1.1).

The BBB should not be thought of as an uninterrupted physical barrier. Certain regions of the brain, such as the circumventricular organs (CVOs) and the nucleus tractus solitarius have a specialized BBB with fenestrated capillary walls that enhance sensing of circulating molecules. Others, like the large vessels of the pial and subarachnoid space, and the sensory ganglia of the spinal and cranial nerves, contain 'functional leaks', allowing passage of molecules and substances into the Virchow–Robin spaces and participation in glymphatic flow. While the amounts of material entering the CNS through these pathways is small, it is probably the route through which natural and therapeutic antibodies gain access to the brain, such as anti-amyloid-β antibodies currently in trials for the treatment of AD (8).

1.4 Innate Immune System: Cells

In the periphery, a range of innate immune cells interact to prevent or limit the spread of infection. These cells include phagocytic neutrophils and monocytes, dendritic cells (DCs),

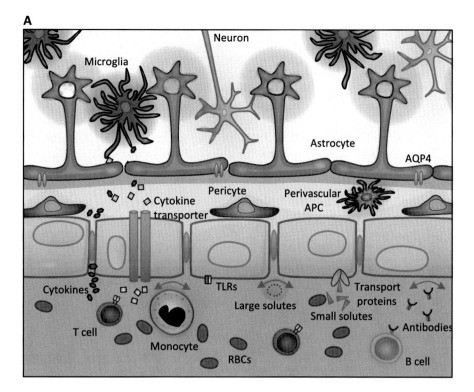

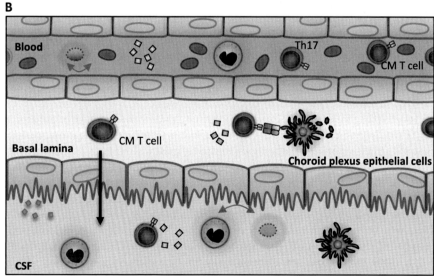

Figure 1.1 Schematic representation of the Blood Brain Barrier and the blood cerebrospinal fluid barrier (BCSFB).

A. The BBB consists of highly specialized endothelial cells joined by tight junctions. They deposit an endothelial basement membrane (yellow) in which pericytes are embedded. The parenchymal basement membrane (orange) is deposited by astrocytes and together with astrocytic endfeet forms the glia limitans perivascularis. The endothelial layer prevents the unrestricted movement of large solutes, antibodies and immune cells while allowing the passage of smaller solutes, cytokines and other proteins through dedicated transport systems.

B. The BCSFB is made up by the choroid plexus epithelial cells which similarly prevent the unrestricted passage of molecules between the blood and the CSF. Central memory T cells are the predominant immune population in the CSF, and it is thought that they may cross the BCSFB, although the molecular mechanisms behind this are still unclear. (A black and white version of this figure will appear in some formats. For the colour version, please refer to the plate section.)

mast cells and eosinophils, as well as specific subsets of lymphocytes such as innate lymphoid cells (ILCs), natural killer (NK) cells and NK-T cells. Within the CNS the range of innate immune cells is more limited, the most prevalent being the tissue-resident macrophage population known as microglia, which make up 10–15% of all brain cells (9). These cells populate the CNS early in embryonic development, performing typical phagocytic functions such as clearance of apoptotic cell debris and sensing local tissue damage, as well as tissue-specific functions including synapse elimination, regulation of neurogenesis and remodelling of neural circuits (10). While microglia are the resident immune population of the brain parenchyma, they are not the only innate cells to populate the CNS. Macrophages, NK cells, mast cells and DCs also reside within the choroid plexus, perivascular spaces of the CNS and its meningeal coverings, sampling local debris and communicating with surrounding cells (11). Within the body, histamine released from mast cells plays an important role in dilating postcapillary venules and increasing blood vessel permeability leading to the oedema, warmth and redness associated with classical inflammation. Within the CNS, mast cells also play a critical role in regulating BBB permeability and have been implicated in increases in BBB permeability associated with stress (12).

While the innate immune system comprises a diverse array of cells with specific functions in host defence, this discussion will focus on selected cell types and their contributions to immunopsychiatry.

1.4.1 Macrophages/Microglia

Macrophages and monocytes are closely related professional phagocytes that engulf and digest microbes and dead and dying host cells. During an inflammatory reaction, circulating blood monocytes can extravasate into tissues where they differentiate into specialized macrophages. The majority of tissues in the body contain phenotypically distinct tissue-resident macrophage populations which act as immune sentinels and perform additional tissue-specific functions. Langerhans cells (skin), Kupffer cells (liver), alveolar macrophages (lungs) and microglia (brain) are examples of tissue-resident macrophage populations. Fate mapping studies indicate that most tissue-resident macrophage populations derive from yolk sac or foetal liver origins, with blood monocytes existing in tissues only transiently (13). The microglia of the brain are established in their niche prenatally, and derive from cells in the yolk sac (14). Experimental evidence suggests that microglia undergo self-renewal via local proliferation; however under certain circumstances infiltrating blood monocytes can differentiate into a microglial-like phenotype within the brain parenchyma (15,16).

Macrophages are a highly dynamic cell population which undergo significant structural and functional changes depending on their local environment. They are critically important not only in the innate immune recognition of foreign and self-antigens, but also in the presentation of antigen to T cells and in guiding the outcome of the adaptive immune response through the secretion of specific cytokines.

Several studies have associated peripheral monocyte/macrophage numbers or activation status with psychiatric disorders. Monocytes/macrophages in both the blood and CSF may be increased in patients with schizophrenia or during acute psychotic episodes (17,18). While the number of monocytes does not appear to be altered in bipolar disorder, gene expression studies suggest that monocytes may be shifted towards a pro-inflammatory phenotype (19).

Traditionally, microglia have been thought of as existing in two states: 'resting' or 'activated', a misleadingly simplistic classification. Imaging studies have shown that 'resting' microglia are in fact highly active, continuously sampling the local environment with extremely motile processes (20). Microglia express an array of receptors including: purinergic, neurotransmitter, cytokine, complement and Fc receptors, as well as pattern recognition receptors (PRRs), that allow them to detect subtle changes in their microenvironment (20). In this 'resting' state microglia can secrete many neurotrophic factors including brain-derived neurotrophic factor (BDNF), transforming growth factor (TGF)-β, insulin-like growth factor 1 (IGF1), as well as pro- and anti-inflammatory cytokines (20). In response to homeostatic disruption such as injury, infection or increased neuronal activity, microglia become activated and switch from undirected monitoring to targeted movement of microglial processes towards the site of insult (20,21). Additional changes to morphology, motility, cell number, phagocytic capacity and cytokine secretion can also occur. Importantly, the shift from 'resting' (M1) to 'activated' (M2) phenotypes is accompanied by increased expression of the translocator protein (TSPO) which can be detected with positron emission tomography (PET) tracers such PK11195, FEPPA and DTA714 (22). Microglial dysregulation is associated with a number of psychiatric and neurodegenerative disorders including amyotrophic lateral sclerosis (ALS), AD, Parkinson's disease, MDD and schizophrenia (10,23).

A range of cytokines are secreted by microglia in both the healthy and the diseased brain. Microglial-derived IL-1β appears to be critical for normal hippocampus-dependent cognition, learning and memory formation (24), whereas abnormally high levels of IL-1β and tumour necrosis factor (TNF)-α profoundly impair memory and are associated with the development of AD and other neurodegenerative disorders (25,26).

Microglia are critically dependent on colony stimulating factor 1 receptor (CSF1R) signalling for survival (27,28). Congenital absence of CSF1R in mice results in abnormal postnatal brain development, with enlarged ventricles, increased neuronal density in the cortex, elevated numbers of astrocytes and reduced oligodendrocytes, with these animals rarely surviving to adulthood (27). Whereas adult mice briefly depleted of microglia using CSF1R inhibitors show no readily apparent behavioural abnormalities or cognitive deficits, suggesting that microglia may not be essential for these functions in the fully developed brain (28). Pharmacological inhibition of CSF1R in mice with AD-like pathology halts microglial proliferation, prevents synaptic degeneration and improves cognitive performance (29). Interestingly, microglial activation as a result of cranial irradiation for the treatment of brain cancer is associated with progressive and severe cognitive dysfunction. Experimental evidence suggests that elimination of microglia prior to cranial irradiation of mice ameliorates these cognitive defects (30). Therapies designed to deplete microglia using CSF1R inhibitors or similar in the human brain could have efficacy for disorders associated with microglial activation and cognitive decline.

1.4.2 NK Cells

NK cells detect the absence of major histocompatibility complex (MHC) Class I proteins on infected, damaged or malignant cells and respond by inducing apoptosis of the target cell, independent of the adaptive immune system. Reduced NK cell numbers have been repeatedly found in patients with MDD, with some studies suggesting that reduced NK cell number or activity is associated with treatment resistance (31–33). Abnormal NK cell activity has also been associated with schizophrenia; however, the direction of association is less consistent, possibly owing to clinical heterogeneity in the patient cohorts and small sample sizes (34). Of general relevance to psychiatry is the concept that psychological stress, a common feature across psychiatric disorders, is often accompanied by reduced NK cell activity (35–37).

1.5 Innate Immune System: Molecules

The innate immune system employs a network of soluble and cell surface associated molecules to detect and combat invading microbial pathogens, remove potentially damaging dead and dying cells, and promote tissue repair. Like much of the immune system, these molecules are understood to also play roles in the maintenance of homeostasis, during development and in various aspects of normal and pathological mental function.

Innate immune cells express PRRs that recognize distinct microbial molecules known as pathogen-associate molecular patterns (PAMPs), or molecules released from damaged or dying host cells known as damage-associated molecular patterns (DAMPs). PAMPs are generally microbial structures that are essential for the survival or infectivity of the microbe, making this feature of innate immune recognition highly effective.

1.5.1 Toll-Like Receptors

TLRs are expressed on the cell surface or endosomal membranes of innate immune cells, including macrophages, NK cells, and DCs, as well as some non-immune cells such as endothelial cells. Importantly, TLRs are expressed by microglia, astrocytes, oligodendrocytes, neurons, neural progenitor cells and the BBB endothelium (38). They are recognized for their importance in innate immune defence, and more recently they have been acknowledged for their roles in CNS plasticity and regulation of cognitive function in the absence of pathogen-derived ligands.

Individual TLRs recognize PAMPs that are shared across various classes of pathogen, and host-derived DAMPs. For example, TLR4 recognizes bacterial lipopolysaccharide (LPS) that is common to the outer membrane of all Gram-negative bacteria, as well as endogenous proteins such as heat shock protein-70 (HSP-70). In the CNS, TLR2 and TLR4 are expressed predominantly by glial cells including microglia, and both have been implicated in neuropathic pain (39,40). Interestingly, opioids such as morphine are capable of activating microglia by binding to the TLR4 accessory protein MD2 (41), and by stimulating the release of HSP-70 from neurons which in turn potentiates the TLR4 mediated inflammatory response (42). Furthermore, activation of TLR4 signalling by opioids is thought to contribute to the development of opioid tolerance and dependence, supporting a role for immune signalling in drug reward and opening up new possibilities for the treatment of addictions (43). TLR2, TLR3 and TLR4 are expressed by human neural progenitor cells and influence cell proliferation and differentiation (38). Increased gene expression of TLRs has been found in the brains of depressed suicide victims (44), and peripheral blood of patients with MDD (45).

1.5.2 NOD-Like Receptors and the Inflammasome

The innate immune system utilizes a number of other PRRs in addition to TLRs. The nucleotide-binding oligomerization domain (NOD)-like receptors (NLRs) are a family of cytosolic receptors that sense both PAMPs and DAMPs in the cytoplasm of host cells. Engagement of NLRs by their ligand results in activation of the nuclear factor κ-light-chain-enhancer of activated B cells (NFκB) transcription factor and upregulation of pro-inflammatory cytokine gene expression. The NLRs form an important component of most inflammasomes. These are multimeric protein complexes that consist of an inflammasome sensor (often an NLR), the adaptor protein ASC, and caspase 1. Activation of the inflammasome generally results in cleavage of the inactive cytokine precursors, pro-IL-1β and pro-IL-18 and the subsequent release of their active forms, IL-1β and IL-18, respectively (46).

Of particular importance for immunopsychiatry is the NLR family pyrin domain containing 3 (NLRP3) inflammasome, a cytosolic inflammasome complex that responds to a diverse range of PAMPs and DAMPs by enhancing production of the pro-inflammatory cytokines IL-1β and IL-18 and has been implicated in the pathophysiology of MDD (47,48), bipolar disorder (49) and AD (50). Psychological stress can activate the NLRP3 inflammasome via adenosine triphosphate (ATP) stimulation of the P2X7 receptor in the mouse hippocampus, ultimately leading to an increase in IL-1β secretion and increased neuroinflammation (51). Interestingly, deletion of the NLRP3 gene from mice renders them resistant to the depressive behaviour normally induced by chronic unpredictable stress, possibly implicating the NLRP3 inflammasome in the well-established links between stress and increased risk of MDD (51). Together, these studies identify potential therapeutic targets for the treatment of depressive and neuroinflammatory disorders.

The final group of PRRs of importance to immunopsychiatry are the secreted forms, particularly C-reactive protein (CRP). CRP is an acute-phase protein synthesized in the liver with the primary function of activating the complement cascade. CRP is commonly measured in the clinic as an indicator of inflammation, and has consistently been shown to be raised in a proportion of patients with MDD (52–54). CRP shows promise as a peripherally accessible biomarker to predict the development of depression (55) and for predicting therapeutic response to serotonergic and noradrenergic antidepressants (56). CRP has additionally been implicated in schizophrenia (57,58); bipolar disorder, where it appears to be particularly increased during periods of mania (59); and autism (60).

1.5.3 The Complement System

The complement system is a network of more than 30 circulating and membrane-associated proteins responsible for induction of the complement cascade and inflammatory response. While complement components are synthesized predominantly by the liver, they can also be produced selectively by various other cell types including monocytes, fibroblasts, epithelial cells and, notably, all brain cell populations (61). Initially recognized for its role in innate immune defence against pathogens, the complement system is now also known for its importance in the maintenance of brain homeostasis, synaptic plasticity and regeneration. Over-activation of the complement system has been implicated in the pathology of stroke, traumatic brain injury, AD, Parkinson's disease and ALS (61). More recently, excessive complement activity in the brain has been functionally linked to genetic risk for schizophrenia (62). Sekar et al. found that gene expression of complement component 4 (C4A) is elevated in the brains of individuals with schizophrenia and that higher levels of C4A expression are associated with a greater risk of schizophrenia. In addition to its critical role in innate immunity, many complement components including C4 are involved in synaptic pruning. Frequently documented pathological finding in the brains of individuals with schizophrenia include cortical grey matter loss and reduced numbers of synaptic structures (63,64). Given that microglia express the majority of complement receptors in the brain and are critically important in synaptic pruning, Sekar and colleagues offer an intriguing mechanistic explanation: that excessive synaptic pruning by microglia, driven by C4 deposition at the synapses, contributes to the pathology of schizophrenia (62). While C4 and other complement components have potential as diagnostic biomarkers or therapeutic treatment targets, much work still needs to be done before complement therapies reach the clinic.

1.6 Linking Innate and Adaptive Immunity: Cytokines and Chemokines

Cytokines are small proteins secreted by immune and non-immune cells that are responsible for intercellular communication, mediating many of the cellular responses of both innate and adaptive immunity. In innate immunity, most cytokines are produced by mast cells, DCs and macrophages, whereas the main cytokine producers of the adaptive immune system are T helper cells. Chemokines are a class of cytokines that act as chemoattractants for immune cells. Together, the cytokine network includes the interleukins, interferons, tumour necrosis factors, TGFs, colony stimulating factors and chemokines (CCL and CXCL nomenclature). Under steady-state conditions these molecules circulate in very low (pico-molar) concentrations, but during infection or trauma blood concentrations can increase up to 1,000-fold. Cytokines can be pro- or anti-inflammatory, and can act in an autocrine, paracrine or endocrine manner. Examples of the latter include the systemic fever response triggered by IL-1β and TNF-α acting on the hypothalamus, a component of sickness behaviours (65) (covered in detail in Chapter 8), and IL-6 acting on the liver to stimulate production of acute-phase proteins such as CRP. Cytokines typically display a high degree of redundancy and pleiotropy and can enhance or inhibit the action of other cytokines in complex interactions, impeding simple functional classification. Nevertheless, one clinically useful division is between pro-inflammatory cytokines such as IL-1β, TNF-α, IL-6, IFN-γ and IL-12 – which share the common function of promoting inflammation; and anti-inflammatory cytokines – such as IL-4 and IL-10 that reduce inflammation and promote healing and tissue regeneration. Classification of cytokines can also be based on their roles in T helper cell polarization and function. IFN-γ and IL-12 are typically considered Th1 cytokines; IL-4, IL-5 and IL-13 are regarded as Th2 cytokines; and IL-17 and IL-22 as Th17 cytokines.

Some cytokines may cross the BBB through dedicated transporter systems or when barrier function is disrupted (66). Within the CNS, microglial activation results in the production of a number of pro-inflammatory cytokines and chemokines such as IL-1β, TNF-α, IL-6 and CCL2. Like many features of the immune system, cytokines are now known to play additional non-immunological roles, such as in regulation of complex cognitive processes like sleep (67) and hippocampus-dependent learning and memory formation (68). There is also extensive evidence that some CNS cytokines, IL-1β in particular, are directly involved in the pathogenesis of neurodegenerative disorders (69).

CCL2, also known as monocyte chemoattractant protein 1 (MCP1) controls monocyte and macrophage migration. CCR2, the receptor that binds CCL2, is constitutively expressed by immune cells and can also be expressed by microglia, astrocytes, and dopaminergic and cholinergic neurons (70). Increased CCL2 gene expression by monocytes or astrocytes has been linked to a number of neuroinflammatory disorders including MS, stroke, AD, epilepsy, traumatic brain injury and schizophrenia (70). Elevated peripheral CCL2 has been consistently found in MDD and schizophrenia (71–73).

Numerous studies show increased levels of circulating pro-inflammatory cytokines, particularly IL-6 and TNF-α, and the acute-phase protein CRP, in MDD and schizophrenia (2,74,75). Importantly, peripheral levels of IL-6 are thought to precede depressive episodes (55,76) and are often higher in individuals with a history of childhood adversity (77). There is considerable interest in exploiting IL-6 as a therapeutic target, with a number of humanized monoclonal antibodies targeting IL-6 or the IL-6 receptor currently in clinical trials. Evidence linking pro-inflammatory cytokines and depression will be covered in detail in Chapter 10. Another group of cytokines important to immunopsychiatry are the interferons, key players in the antiviral response that have been used therapeutically for the treatment of certain cancers and the chronic viral infection hepatitis C. Although it has been an effective treatment for hepatitis C, sustained therapeutic use of IFN-α precipitates major depressive episodes in approximately one-third of patients, although the risk can be minimized through pretreatment with the antidepressant paroxetine (78).

1.7 Adaptive Immune System

In contrast to the innate immune system, which functions through the recognition of shared microbial structures and does not possess any form of memory, the adaptive immune system is characterized by the generation of memory responses by lymphocytes that recognize microbes with exquisite specificity. The adaptive immune system can be broadly classified into two functional arms: cellular immunity which is mediated by T cells, and humoral immunity which is mediated by B cells and their secreted antibodies. Key features of the adaptive immune system are the antigen receptors: namely, membrane-bound antibodies in the case of B cells, and the T cell receptor (TCR) complex on T cells. These receptors recognize antigens with a high degree of specificity. The ability of the immune system to discriminate self from non-self, and thereby avoid mounting a pathological response to self antigens, is known as tolerance and is achieved through two processes, termed central and peripheral tolerance. Central tolerance largely occurs in the primary lymphoid organs (thymus and bone marrow) and is a process whereby lymphocytes that strongly recognize self-antigens presented by MHC molecules are removed before they enter the circulation. Additionally, some of the immature CD4$^+$ T cells that do recognize self-antigen develop into T regulatory cells (Treg) that are important for peripheral tolerance (discussed in Section 1.8.1 below). If self-reactive T cells do leave the primary lymphoid organs, they can be further controlled by peripheral tolerance mechanisms through which mature self-reactive T cells are rendered functionally inactive (anergic) or their response is controlled by Tregs. Autoimmunity occurs when immune tolerance breaks down, causing the adaptive immune system to mount a pathogenic response against self-antigens. While the precise aetiology of the inflammatory demyelinating disorder MS is incompletely understood, breakdown of immune tolerance leading to auto-reactive T and B cells plays a major role.

1.7.1 Major Histocompatibility Complex (MHC)

All nucleated cells express MHC Class I, while professional APCs such as DCs and B cells express MHC Class II. CD4$^+$ and CD8$^+$ T cells can only recognize antigen bound to MHC Class I or Class II, respectively. The MHC locus contains more than 200 genes and includes those that encode the MHC Class I and Class II molecules themselves, and other genes collectively known as the Class III genes which include complement components, cytokines, and some genes with no known immune function. The MHC genes are highly polymorphic, with over 10,000 Class I alleles and 3,000 Class II alleles estimated in the human population. The polymorphic gene variants are inherited and determine which peptides can be presented by the MHC molecules. Given their crucial role in immunity it is unsurprising that single nucleotide polymorphisms (SNPs) in the MHC region have been linked to a diverse range of diseases. Over the last decade, several independent genome wide association studies (GWAS) have revealed persuasive evidence for involvement of MHC genes in schizophrenia susceptibility (79,80).

1.7.2 Adaptive Immunity: T Cells

Microbial antigens that enter the body are transported to and concentrated within peripheral lymphoid organs where they are most likely to come into contact with lymphocytes bearing antigen receptors that can recognize and respond to them. Lymphocytes continuously circulate between the bloodstream and the peripheral lymphoid organs with perhaps only 2% present in the blood. T cells are functionally classified into three main subsets; CD4$^+$ T helper cells (Th), CD4$^+$ Tregs and CD8$^+$ cytotoxic T cells (Tc).

Th cells do not kill infected cells or microbes directly, but as their name implies, help other cell types to eliminate microbes. They are the primary source of cytokines in the adaptive immune system. Following antigen recognition, naïve Th cells rapidly proliferate (a process known as clonal expansion) and differentiate into effector cells of various subtypes that perform distinct and targeted functions in host defence. The three main subsets of Th cells are Th1, Th2 and Th17 cells, each distinguished by their cytokine profiles, chemokine receptor expression and targeted functions. There is considerable plasticity in the cytokine profile of T cells, allowing one subset to convert to another given the right conditions (See Figure 1.2).

The differentiation of Th effector cells into Th1 cells occurs in the presence of IL-12 and IFN-γ. Th1 cells secrete an abundance of IFN-γ and enhance the efficiency of macrophage killing of ingested microbes. In contrast, Th2 cells are induced during parasitic worm infections and allergy, and are characterized by the secretion of IL-4, IL-5 and IL-13. Th17 cells are important for the control of extracellular bacteria and fungi, but also play a detrimental role in many chronic inflammatory disorders. They are induced by IL-6, IL1-β, IL-23 and TGF-β and characterized by their secretion of IL-17 and IL-22.

Autoimmune Th cells of both the Th1 and Th17 subsets have been well described in MS, where they cross the BBB and accumulate in inflammatory lesions (81,82). Notably, the ratio of Th1:Th17 cells appears to determine where in the CNS the inflammation will occur. Myelin-specific Th cells infiltrate the meninges regardless of lineage; however, inflammation of the brain parenchyma only occurs when the balance is shifted towards Th17 cells, resulting in an increase in IL-17 in the brain (83). While each of the Th subsets has been variously implicated in psychiatric disorders (31,84,85), their roles are still unclear and many studies regarding Th17 cells in schizophrenia report contradictory findings (86–88). The discrepancies in these studies could be attributed to a number of factors such as inadequate sample size, ill-defined disease status (e.g., chronic versus recent onset psychosis), age, sex, body mass index (BMI) and treatment history. Moreover, antipsychotics may well have an effect on the inflammatory profile of immune

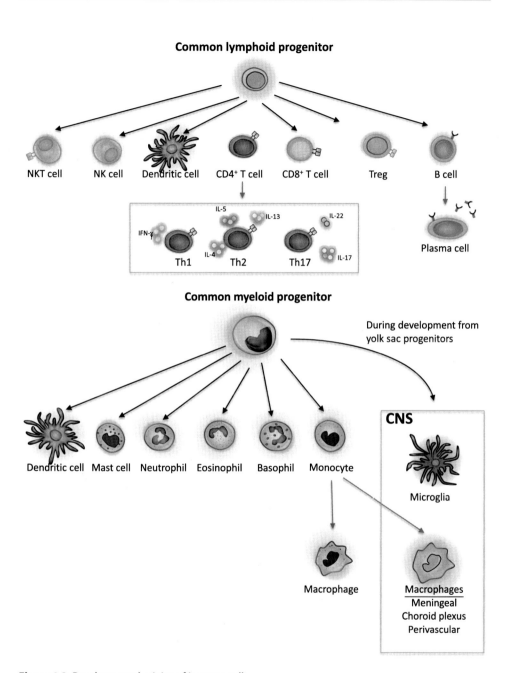

Figure 1.2 Developmental origins of immune cells.
Lymphocytes and some dendritic cells derive from the common lymphoid progenitor cell line. CD4+ T cells can differentiate into T helper cells with specific functions, defined by their cytokine profiles. Activated B cells give rise to antibody secreting plasma cells. Granulocytes (mast cells, neutrophils, eosinophils and basophils), monocytes, some dendritic cells and microglia derive from the common myeloid progenitor cell line. However, microglia are established in the brain prenatally during development from yolk sac progenitors and are transcriptionally distinct from other myeloid cells. Monocytes give rise to macrophages, some in peripheral tissues and others in the CNS. (A black and white version of this figure will appear in some formats. For the colour version, please refer to the plate section.)

cells (89–91). Risperidone and clozapine, two antipsychotics commonly used for the treatment of schizophrenia, have shown therapeutic potential in ameliorating experimental autoimmune encephalitis (EAE), an experimental mouse model of MS (92). The immunomodulatory activity of these antipsychotics occurs primarily in the CNS, significantly reducing microglial activation in EAE mice. Although the precise molecular mode of action of most antipsychotics is incompletely understood, they are generally thought to exert their therapeutic effects through the blockade of dopamine and serotonin receptors, both of which have immunomodulatory properties themselves. It is thus conceivable that antipsychotics may have therapeutic potential in non-psychotic inflammatory disorders.

In contrast to Th cells, Tc cells recognize antigen bound to MHC Class I, present on all nucleated cells including neurons (93). Following activation, naïve Tc cells differentiate into cytotoxic T lymphocytes (CTLs) that are adept at killing infected cells, thereby eliminating the reservoir of infection. Tc cells have been less well-studied in immunopsychiatry, although there is some evidence that increased proportions of Tc cells may predict non-responsiveness to antidepressant treatment (33).

Following resolution of infection, a fraction of Th and Tc cells persist as long-lived memory cells. These cells circulate throughout the lymphoid organs, mucosa, peripheral tissues and the blood stream, and upon exposure to their antigen they rapidly and vigorously respond. Memory cells are defined by the lack of CD45RA and by the expression of CD45RO. While the numbers of lymphocytes and leukocytes in the CSF of normal healthy humans are low, there is a predominance of central memory CD45RO$^+$ Th cells (94). Few studies have investigated the phenotype of immune cells in the CSF of patients with psychiatric disorders. However, there is some evidence that these populations differ from those found in healthy CSF (17,95). The question of whether or not these cells are detrimental in the CNS is an interesting one. Early studies showed that in response to CNS injury, effector T cells and Treg cells become activated, with autoimmune brain-reactive T cells playing a protective role and preventing further neurodegeneration, and Tregs playing a detrimental role by dampening the effector response (96–98). However, subsequent studies have shown that both depletion and administration of Tregs is associated with impaired neuronal survival (99). While this seems paradoxical, alterations in Treg numbers correlate with macrophage phenotype at the injury site. The broader relevance of this is yet to be defined. In addition to their preventative or pathologic roles in neurodegeneration, T cells also appear to be important in cognition and learning behaviour, as mice lacking T cells exhibit abnormal cognitive function. In the absence of T cells, meningeal myeloid cells acquire a pro-inflammatory phenotype which is associated with impaired learning behaviour (100). Taken together these studies suggest an important role for CNS T cells in maintaining homeostasis, that may have pathological implications when disrupted.

1.7.3 Adaptive Immunity: B Cells

B cells are able to recognize macromolecules of many types including proteins, lipids, carbohydrates and nucleic acids, without the requirement for MHC presentation. Activation of naïve B cells upon antigen exposure results in their clonal expansion and differentiation into antibody secreting plasma cells. The antibodies that are secreted have the same antigen specificity as the surface antibody receptor of the naïve B cell that initiated the response. Th cells are critical for the activation of B cells and the maturation of the humoral immune response. B cells can also have specificity for self-antigen, secreting antibodies that recognize self-antigens (autoantibodies) and mounting an unwanted immune response. In 2007, the first cases of antibody-mediated encephalitis and associated psychosis were reported by Josep Dalmau and colleagues (101) and since this seminal publication, autoantibodies to multiple neuronal antigens or synaptic proteins have been described (102). Psychiatric or behavioural manifestations are often seen in patients with these autoantibodies. However, they have also frequently been detected in healthy control patients without psychiatric symptomology. A recent study estimates approximately 9% of patients presenting with first episode psychosis have serum anti-neuronal antibodies, which may be treatable with immunotherapy (102). This will be discussed in further detail in Chapter 5. Some preliminary evidence suggests that maternal brain-reactive antibodies may contribute to the development of autism in the child (103). Autoantibodies are also associated with Parkinson's disease, where the presence of anti-α-synuclein antibodies is reduced compared with healthy controls (104). While the function of these autoantibodies in the healthy CNS is currently unknown, it is possible that they help to clear pathological α-synuclein, a key characteristic of Parkinson's disease. Thus, like CNS T cells, CNS autoantibodies may serve both protective and pathologic functions which could be exploited for therapeutic or diagnostic benefit.

1.8 Glymphatics

Until recently the CNS was thought to be devoid of lymphatic vasculature, despite scattered reports over the years indicating its presence. With the 2012 demonstration of the 'glymphatic system' which functions as a fluid and solute clearance pathway (105), and the subsequent 2015 discovery of meningeal lymphatic vasculature lining the dural sinuses and meningeal arteries to drain lymphatic fluid, immune cells and other solutes (106,107), our mechanistic understanding of CNS drainage has undergone major revision. These two systems are now believed to work in concert to maintain homeostasis and contribute to CNS function and health (108).

In the periphery, toxic metabolites, cell debris, infiltrating microbes, DCs carrying microbial antigens, lymphocytes and interstitial fluid (IF) are drained from tissues via the lymphatic system. Located strategically along the lymphatic vessels are the lymph nodes through which the draining fluid passes before its return to the blood circulation. As lymphatic fluid passes through the lymph nodes its contents are sampled by B cells which can respond by producing antibodies, and APCs which internalize, process and present antigen to T cells, initiating the cell-mediated immune response. However, the CNS parenchyma lacks a classical lymphatic drainage system. Nedergard and colleagues demonstrated that CSF enters the brain within the periarterial spaces and then exchanges with IF, facilitated by aquaporin-4 (AQP4) water channels positioned within perivascular astrocyte endfoot processes. This fluid collects within perivenous spaces and drains to the subarachnoid CSF, which subsequently drains either to the venous circulation, extracranial lymphatic vessels or lymph nodes. Named the glial-associated lymphatic system, or 'glymphatic system', due to the dependence on AQP4 on astrocytes and the lymphatic function it serves. The glymphatic system allows nutrients such as glucose to diffuse through the brain parenchyma and functions to clear extracellular metabolites, waste products such as lactate, and protein aggregates such as amyloid-β from the brain parenchyma and into the CSF.

Interestingly, glymphatic clearance of amyloid-β declines with age, and amyloid-β in turn suppresses glymphatic influx in a detrimental feedback loop. The drainage of amyloid-β is further impeded by APOE4, the most important genetic risk factor for late-onset AD, demonstrating the importance of the glymphatic system in the pathology of AD and highlighting its potential as a therapeutic target (105).

The meninges that surround the brain and spinal cord are composed of three layers: the pia, arachnoid and dura maters. Despite scattered reports of the presence of lymphatic vessels within the meninges, it was not until 2015 that their presence gained wider attention thanks to work from Kipnis and Alitalo (106,107). These two studies, published simultaneously, used advanced imaging techniques and fluorescent tracer experiments to demonstrate draining lymphatic vessels adjacent to arteries, major venous sinuses and cranial nerves (Figure 1.3).

Though still in the early stages, intensive research is underway to exploit these systems therapeutically for the treatment of disorders with CNS involvement.

1.9 Central and Peripheral Communication

Bidirectional crosstalk between the CNS and the peripheral immune system is now well established. An important example of immune-brain communication is the inflammatory reflex which consists of two arcs. The afferent or sensory arc involves visceral sensory neurons which detect and respond to inflammatory stimuli, such as changes in pro-inflammatory cytokines, by relaying information to the brain stem via the vagus nerve. Inflammation detected in the periphery can have profound effects on the brain, resulting in impaired learning and memory, cognitive abnormalities and altered mood (110,111) and this pathway is important in the generation of sickness behaviours (see Section 1.10 below). The efferent arc in which immunomodulatory signals are delivered from the brain stem to immune cells via the vagus nerve, is also known as the anti-inflammatory cholinergic pathway and signals through acetylcholine receptors expressed by immune cells, leading to NFκB activation and modulation of immune response (112). Additionally, all primary and secondary lymphoid organs, including the thymus, bone marrow and spleen, receive direct sympathetic innervation (113). These sympathetic nerve fibres release the catecholamine norepinephrine (NE) in response to stress and other stimuli, which binds to β-adrenergic receptors on immune cells and modulates diverse immunological processes including lymphocyte activation, cytokine production and cell trafficking (114).

It is clear that some classical neurotransmitters, like acetylcholine in the inflammatory reflex, are not only expressed by immune cells but also functionally important for immune system signalling. Dopamine signalling, in particular, has been linked to modulation of the immune synapse that forms between an APC, typically a DC and a naïve T cell (115). This interaction determines the fate of the T cell and is conditioned by dopamine released presynaptically from DCs activating dopamine receptors (DR) postsynaptically expressed by T cells. For example, activation of D3DR inhibits the suppressive capability of Tregs (98) which may be important for dysregulated cognition. Dysregulated dopaminergic neurotransmission has been implicated in the pathogenesis of Parkinson's disease, schizophrenia, dementia with Lewy bodies and attention deficit hyperactivity disorder. In addition to these central defects in dopamine function, Parkinson's disease has been replicably associated with increased (86,116,117) and schizophrenia with decreased (118) peripheral expression of the gene coding the *D3DR* gene. Collectively

A

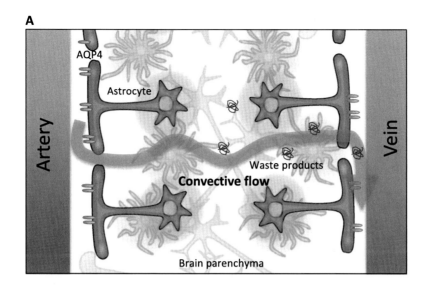

B

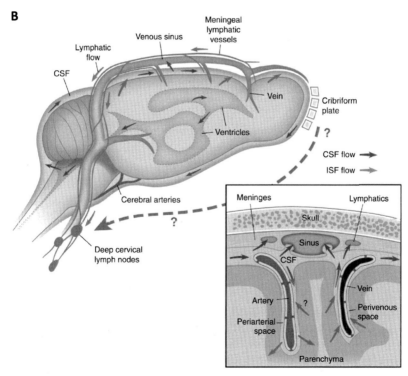

Figure 1.3 CNS lymphatic and glymphatic systems. A. Schematic of the glymphatic system. CSF enters the brain parenchyma along paraarterial routes, exchanges with interstitial fluid and is cleared along paravenous routes. Convective flow is facilitated by AQP4 pores which are abundantly expressed on astrocytic endfeet. Clearance of solutes, proteins and waste products such as amyloid-β occur along this pathway. Draining fluid may be dispersed into the subarachnoid CSF, venous circulation or lymphatics.

B. Schematic representation of lymphatic drainage of the brain. Meningeal lymphatic vessels (green) adjacent to the venous sinuses and arteries drain molecules and meningeal immune cells in the CSF into the deep cervical lymph nodes. Adapted with permission from Louveau et al. *Neuron.* 2016; 91:957–73 (109). (A black and white version of this figure will appear in some formats. For the colour version, please refer to the plate section.)

these studies indicate that the peripheral immune system is capable of interacting with the nervous system through the secretion and recognition of neurotransmitters. With further research, the peripheral expression of neurotransmitter-related genes may prove useful as biomarkers for dopaminergic disorders such as schizophrenia and Parkinson's disease.

1.10 Sickness Behaviour

In addition to immune activation, the physiological response to infection is accompanied by behavioural changes such as lethargy, malaise, irritability, impaired concentration, behavioural depression, decreased social activity, anhedonia and somnolence. Collectively these symptoms are known as 'sickness behaviours', notable for their remarkable similarity to common symptoms of depression. The main pro-inflammatory cytokines responsible for sickness behaviour are IL-1β and TNF-α, both of which are increased in the brain following peripheral infection or experimental administration of LPS in the absence of infection (65,119). Conversely, anti-inflammatory cytokines such as IL-10 limit sickness behaviour and attenuate the behavioural effects induced by LPS stimulation (65). Pro-inflammatory cytokines act on the brain to reorient motivation towards prioritizing wound healing and fighting infection. The behavioural phenotypes of social avoidance and anhedonia help to protect from further insult and pathogen exposure (120). When inflammation is severe or prolonged, as in chronic inflammatory conditions, major depressive episodes frequently arise. Roughly one-third of patients receiving recombinant IL-2 or IFN-α develop major depression, even previously euthymic individuals (78), and similar patterns of brain dysfunction are seen in both IFN-α induced depression and idiopathic MDD (121). See Chapter 8 for an in-depth review of sickness behaviour.

1.10.1 Kynurenine Pathway

Cytokine immunotherapy in cancer patients is accompanied by a marked reduction in plasma tryptophan concentration that is positively correlated with depression scores (120,123). Actively transported into the brain, tryptophan is an essential precursor for the synthesis of serotonin, a neurotransmitter well known for its involvement in mood regulation. Decreased plasma tryptophan in patients undergoing immunotherapy could be due to the action of the tryptophan metabolizing enzymes tryptophan dioxygenase (TDO) or indoleamine 2,3 dioxygenase (IDO), both of which divert tryptophan metabolism away from serotonin synthesis and towards kynurenine synthesis. Under normal circumstances TDO is the dominant enzyme, however the enzymatic activity of IDO is enhanced during inflammation and is potently induced by several pro-inflammatory cytokines including IFN-γ and TNF-α (Figure 1.4). Kynurenine is readily transported across the BBB into the CNS where its metabolites can be either neuroprotective or neurotoxic (65). Kynurenine metabolites may prove useful as biomarkers; for example, a high kynurenine/tryptophan ratio predicted remission in a recent trial of the anti-inflammatory COX-2 inhibitor celecoxib (124). Interestingly, previous clinical trials suggest that the antidepressant effects of celecoxib are linked to its capacity to reduce serum IL-6 (125). While the causative role of IDO activation in MDD still needs to be thoroughly investigated in humans, there is convincing evidence from rodent studies that therapeutic targeting of IDO may help to alleviate inflammation-associated depression (126).

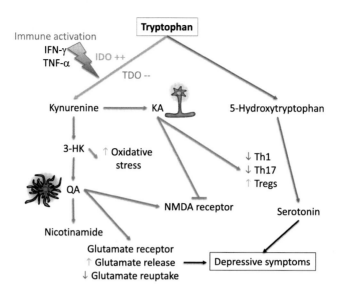

Figure 1.4 **The enzymatic activity of IDO is enhanced during inflammation and diverts tryptophan metabolism away from serotonin synthesis and towards the kynurenine pathway.** Kynurenine is readily transported across the BBB where it can be metabolized to 3-hydroxykynurenine (3-HK), quinolinic acid (QA) or kynurenic acid (KA). 3-HK can increase oxidative stress and may be neurotoxic. QA is preferentially produced by microglia and is an NMDA-receptor agonist which may be neurotoxic, whereas KA is produced by astrocytes and is an NMDA-receptor antagonist which may be neuroprotective. In the periphery KA is thought to modulate immune cell phenotypes. Impaired glutamatergic and serotonergic neurotransmission are both associated with the development of depressive behaviour.

1.11 Conclusion

This chapter serves as a broad introduction to some of the immunological concepts relevant to the study of neurodegenerative and psychiatric disorders. A greater understanding of the causative role of the immune system in these disorders could generate novel immunotherapeutic targets for diagnosis and treatment. Convincing evidence from preclinical studies indicate that inflammation is a key contributor to MDD; several clinical trials using anti-inflammatory immunotherapies to treat MDD are in various stages of completion and are showing promising results. Recent advances in our understanding of how the immune system interacts with the brain to cause pathology offer a range of new therapeutic targets for researchers and clinicians to utilize. Although the field of immunopsychiatry is still relatively young, close collaborations between researchers, clinicians and industry will deliver high quality research and therapeutic targets for tackling what are currently some of the most common and debilitating human illnesses.

References

1. Savitz J, Harrison NA. Interoception and Inflammation in Psychiatric Disorders. *Biol Psychiatry Cogn Neurosci Neuroimaging*. 2018 Jun;3(6): 514–24.

2. Dowlati Y, Herrmann N, Swardfager W, et al. A meta-analysis of cytokines in major depression. *Biological Psychiatry*. 2010 Mar 1;67(5):446–57.

3. Miller BJ, Buckley P, Seabolt W, Mellor A, Kirkpatrick B. Meta-analysis of cytokine

alterations in schizophrenia: clinical status and antipsychotic effects. *Biological Psychiatry*. 2011 Oct 1;70(7):663–71.

4. Cunningham C, Hennessy E. Co-morbidity and systemic inflammation as drivers of cognitive decline: new experimental models adopting a broader paradigm in dementia research. *Alzheimers Res Ther*. BioMed Central Ltd. 2015;7(1):33.

5. Banks WA. From blood-brain barrier to blood-brain interface: new opportunities for CNS drug delivery. *Nature Publishing Group*. 2016 Apr;15(4):275–92.

6. Engelhardt B, Sorokin L. The blood-brain and the blood-cerebrospinal fluid barriers: function and dysfunction. *Semin Immunopathol*. 2009 Nov;31(4):497–511.

7. Liddelow SA. Development of the choroid plexus and blood-CSF barrier. *Front Neurosci*. Frontiers. 2015 Mar 3;9 (154):319–13.

8. Sevigny J, Chiao P, Bussière T, et al. The antibody aducanumab reduces Aβ plaques in Alzheimer's disease. *Nature*. 2016 Sep 1;537(7618):50–6.

9. Ransohoff RM, Cardona AE. The myeloid cells of the central nervous system parenchyma. *Nature*. 2010 Nov 11;468 (7321):253–62.

10. Li Q, Barres BA. Microglia and macrophages in brain homeostasis and disease. *Nat Rev Immunol*. 2017 Nov 20.

11. Ransohoff RM, Engelhardt B. The anatomical and cellular basis of immune surveillance in the central nervous system. *Nat Rev Immunol*. 2012 Sep;12(9):623–35.

12. Esposito P, Gheorghe D, Kandere K, et al. Acute stress increases permeability of the blood-brain-barrier through activation of brain mast cells. *Brain Res*. 2001 Jan 5;888 (1):117–27.

13. Davies LC, Jenkins SJ, Allen JE, Taylor PR. Tissue-resident macrophages. *Nat Immunol*. 2013 Oct;14(10):986–95.

14. Ginhoux F, Greter M, Leboeuf M, et al. Fate mapping analysis reveals that adult microglia derive from primitive macrophages. *Science*. 2010 Nov 5;330 (6005):841–5.

15. Ajami B, Bennett JL, Krieger C, Tetzlaff W, Rossi FMV. Local self-renewal can sustain CNS microglia maintenance and function throughout adult life. *Nat Neurosci*. 2007 Dec;10(12):1538–43.

16. Mildner A, Schmidt H, Nitsche M, et al. Microglia in the adult brain arise from Ly-6ChiCCR2+ monocytes only under defined host conditions. *Nat Neurosci*. 2007 Dec;10(12):1544–53.

17. Nikkilä HV, Müller K, Ahokas A, et al. Accumulation of macrophages in the CSF of schizophrenic patients during acute psychotic episodes. *Am J Psychiatry*. 1999 Nov;156(11):1725–9.

18. Jackson AJ, Miller BJ. Meta-analysis of total and differential white blood cell counts in schizophrenia. *Acta Psychiatr Scand*. 2020 Jul;142(1):18–26.

19. Padmos RC, Hillegers MHJ, Knijff EM, et al. A discriminating messenger RNA signature for bipolar disorder formed by an aberrant expression of inflammatory genes in monocytes. *Arch Gen Psychiatry*. American Medical Association; 2008 Apr; 65(4):395–407.

20. Nimmerjahn A, Kirchhoff F, Helmchen F. Resting microglial cells are highly dynamic surveillants of brain parenchyma in vivo. *Science*. 2005 May 27;308(5726): 1314–8.

21. Davalos D, Grutzendler J, Yang G, et al. ATP mediates rapid microglial response to local brain injury in vivo. *Nat Neurosci*. 2005 Jun;8(6):752–8.

22. Setiawan E, Wilson AA, Mizrahi R, et al. Role of translocator protein density, a marker of neuroinflammation, in the brain during major depressive episodes. *JAMA Psychiatry*. 2015 Mar;72(3): 268–75.

23. Tay TL, Béchade C, D'Andrea I, et al. Microglia gone rogue: impacts on psychiatric disorders across the lifespan. *Front Mol Neurosci*. 2017;10:421.

24. Williamson LL, Sholar PW, Mistry RS, Smith SH, Bilbo SD. Microglia and memory: modulation by early-life infection. *J Neurosci*. 2011 Oct 26;31 (43):15511–21.

25. Marin I, Kipnis J. Learning and memory . . . and the immune system. *Learn Mem.* 2013 Sep 19;20(10):601–6.

26. Holmes C, Cunningham C, Zotova E, et al. Systemic inflammation and disease progression in Alzheimer disease. *Neurology.* 2009 Sep 8;73(10): 768–74.

27. Erblich B, Zhu L, Etgen AM, Dobrenis K, Pollard JW. Absence of colony stimulation factor-1 receptor results in loss of microglia, disrupted brain development and olfactory deficits. *PLoS ONE.* 2011;6 (10):e26317.

28. Elmore MRP, Najafi AR, Koike MA, et al. Colony-stimulating factor 1 receptor signaling is necessary for microglia viability, unmasking a microglia progenitor cell in the adult brain. *Neuron.* 2014 Apr 16;82(2):380–97.

29. Olmos-Alonso A, Schetters STT, Sri S, et al. Pharmacological targeting of CSF1R inhibits microglial proliferation and prevents the progression of Alzheimer's-like pathology. *Brain.* 2016 Mar;139(Pt 3):891–907.

30. Acharya MM, Green KN, Allen BD, et al. Elimination of microglia improves cognitive function following cranial irradiation. *Sci Rep.* 2016 Aug 12;6 (1):31545.

31. Grosse L, Hoogenboezem T, Ambrée O, et al. Deficiencies of the T and natural killer cell system in major depressive disorder: T regulatory cell defects are associated with inflammatory monocyte activation. *Brain Behavior and Immunity.* 2016 May;54:38–44.

32. Suzuki H, Savitz J, Teague TK, et al. Altered populations of natural killer cells, cytotoxic T lymphocytes, and regulatory T cells in major depressive disorder: Association with sleep disturbance. *Brain Behavior and Immunity.* 2017 Nov 1;66:193–200.

33. Grosse L, Carvalho LA, Birkenhager TK, et al. Circulating cytotoxic T cells and natural killer cells as potential predictors for antidepressant response in melancholic depression. Restoration of T regulatory cell populations after antidepressant therapy.

Psychopharmacology (Berl). 2016 May; 233(9):1679–88.

34. Yovel G, Sirota P, Mazeh D, et al. Higher natural killer cell activity in schizophrenic patients: the impact of serum factors, medication, and smoking. *Brain Behavior and Immunity.* 2000 Sep;14(3): 153–69.

35. Schedlowski M, Jacobs R, Stratmann G, et al. Changes of natural killer cells during acute psychological stress. *J Clin Immunol.* 1993 Mar;13(2):119–26.

36. Segerstrom SC, Miller GE. Psychological stress and the human immune system: a meta-analytic study of 30 years of inquiry. *Psychol Bull.* 2004 Jul;130(4):601–30.

37. Duggal NA, Upton J, Phillips AC, Hampson P, Lord JM. NK cell immunesenescence is increased by psychological but not physical stress in older adults associated with raised cortisol and reduced perforin expression. *Age (Dordr).* 2015 Feb;37(1):9748.

38. Okun E, Griffioen KJ, Mattson MP. Toll-like receptor signaling in neural plasticity and disease. *Trends Neurosci.* 2011 May; 34(5):269–81.

39. Tanga FY, Nutile-McMenemy N, DeLeo JA. The CNS role of Toll-like receptor 4 in innate neuroimmunity and painful neuropathy. Proceedings of the National Academy of Sciences. *National Academy of Sciences.* 2005 Apr 19;102 (16):5856–61.

40. Hutchinson MR, Zhang Y, Brown K, et al. Non-stereoselective reversal of neuropathic pain by naloxone and naltrexone: involvement of toll-like receptor 4 (TLR4). *Eur J Neurosci.* 2008 Jul;28(1):20–9.

41. Hutchinson MR, Zhang Y, Shridhar M, et al. Evidence that opioids may have toll-like receptor 4 and MD-2 effects. *Brain Behavior and Immunity.* 2010 Jan;24 (1):83–95.

42. Qu J, Tao X-Y, Teng P, et al. Blocking ATP-sensitive potassium channel alleviates morphine tolerance by inhibiting HSP70-TLR4-NLRP3-mediated

neuroinflammation. *J Neuroinflammation. BioMed Central.* 2017 Nov 25; 14(1):228.

43. Hutchinson MR, Northcutt AL, Hiranita T, et al. Opioid Activation of Toll-Like Receptor 4 Contributes to Drug Reinforcement. *Journal of Neuroscience.* 2012 Aug 15;32(33):11187–200.

44. Pandey GN, Rizavi HS, Ren X, Bhaumik R, Dwivedi Y. Toll-like receptors in the depressed and suicide brain. *Journal of Psychiatric Research.* 2014 Jun 1;53 (C):62–8.

45. Hung Y-Y, Kang H-Y, Huang K-W, Huang T-L. Association between toll-like receptors expression and major depressive disorder. *Psychiatry Research.* 2014 Dec 15;220(1–2):283–6.

46. Latz E, Xiao TS, Stutz A. Activation and regulation of the inflammasomes. *Nat Rev Immunol.* 2013 Jun;13(6):397–411.

47. Alcocer-Gómez E, de Miguel M, Casas-Barquero N, et al. NLRP3 inflammasome is activated in mononuclear blood cells from patients with major depressive disorder. *Brain Behavior and Immunity.* 2014 Feb;36:111–7.

48. Zhang Y, Liu L, Liu YZ, et al. NLRP3 Inflammasome Mediates Chronic Mild Stress-Induced Depression in Mice via Neuroinflammation. *Int J Neuropsychopharm.* 2015 May 29;18 (8):pyv006–6.

49. Kim HK, Andreazza AC, Elmi N, Chen W, Young LT. Nod-like receptor pyrin containing 3 (NLRP3) in the post-mortem frontal cortex from patients with bipolar disorder: A potential mediator between mitochondria and immune-activation. *Journal of Psychiatric Research.* 2016 Jan 1;72(C):43–50.

50. Heneka MT, Kummer MP, Stutz A, et al. NLRP3 is activated in Alzheimer's disease and contributes to pathology in APP/PS1 mice. *Nature.* 2013 Jan 23;493 (7434):674–8.

51. Iwata M, Ota KT, Li X-Y, et al. Psychological Stress Activates the Inflammasome via Release of Adenosine Triphosphate and Stimulation of the Purinergic Type 2X7 Receptor. *Biological Psychiatry.* 2016 Jul 1;80(1):12–22.

52. Smith KJ, Au B, Ollis L, Schmitz N. The association between C-reactive protein, Interleukin-6 and depression among older adults in the community: A systematic review and meta-analysis. *Exp Gerontol.* 2018 Feb 1;102:109–32.

53. Valkanova V, Ebmeier KP, Allan CL. CRP, IL-6 and depression: a systematic review and meta-analysis of longitudinal studies. *J Affect Disord.* 2013 Sep 25;150(3):736–44.

54. Wium-Andersen MK, Ørsted DD, Nielsen SF, Nordestgaard BG. Elevated C-reactive protein levels, psychological distress, and depression in 73, 131 individuals. *JAMA Psychiatry.* 2013 Feb;70 (2):176–84.

55. Khandaker GM, Pearson RM, Zammit S, Lewis G, Jones PB. Association of serum interleukin 6 and C-reactive protein in childhood with depression and psychosis in young adult life: a population-based longitudinal study. *JAMA Psychiatry.* 2014 Oct;71(10):1121–8.

56. Uher R, Tansey KE, Dew T, et al. An inflammatory biomarker as a differential predictor of outcome of depression treatment with escitalopram and nortriptyline. *Am J Psychiatry.* 2014 Dec 1;171(12):1278–86.

57. Inoshita M, Numata S, Tajima A, et al. A significant causal association between C-reactive protein levels and schizophrenia. *Sci Rep.* 2016 May 19;6 (1):26105.

58. Fernandes BS, Steiner J, Bernstein H-G, et al. C-reactive protein is increased in schizophrenia but is not altered by antipsychotics: meta-analysis and implications. *Mol Psychiatry.* 2016 Apr;21 (4):554–64.

59. Fernandes BS, Steiner J, Molendijk ML, et al. C-reactive protein concentrations across the mood spectrum in bipolar disorder: a systematic review and meta-analysis. 2016 Dec;3(12):1147–56.

60. Khakzad MR, Javanbakht M, Shayegan MR, et al. The complementary role of high sensitivity C-reactive protein in

the diagnosis and severity assessment of autism. *Research in Autism Spectrum Disorders*. 2012 May 5;6(3):1032–7.

61. Orsini F, De Blasio D, Zangari R, Zanier ER, De Simoni M-G. Versatility of the complement system in neuroinflammation, neurodegeneration and brain homeostasis. *Front Cell Neurosci*. 2014;8:380.

62. Sekar A, Bialas AR, de Rivera H, et al. Schizophrenia risk from complex variation of complement component 4. *Nature*. 2016 Feb 11;530(7589):177–83.

63. Haijma SV, Van Haren N, Cahn W, et al. Brain volumes in schizophrenia: a meta-analysis in over 18 000 subjects. *Schizophr Bull*. 2013 Sep;39(5):1129–38.

64. Osimo EF, Beck K, Reis Marques T, Howes OD. Synaptic loss in schizophrenia: a meta-analysis and systematic review of synaptic protein and mRNA measures. *Mol Psychiatry*. 2019 Apr;24(4):549–61.

65. Dantzer R, O'Connor JC, Freund GG, Johnson RW, Kelley KW. From inflammation to sickness and depression: when the immune system subjugates the brain. *Nat Rev Neurosci*. 2008 Jan;9 (1):46–56.

66. Banks WA. Blood-brain barrier transport of cytokines: a mechanism for neuropathology. *Curr Pharm Des*. 2005;11 (8):973–84.

67. Krueger JM, Rector DM, Roy S, et al. Sleep as a fundamental property of neuronal assemblies. 2008 Nov 5;9(12): 910–9.

68. Rachal Pugh C, Fleshner M, Watkins LR, Maier SF, Rudy JW. The immune system and memory consolidation: a role for the cytokine IL-1beta. *Neurosci Biobehav Rev*. 2001 Jan;25(1):29–41.

69. Allan SM, Tyrrell PJ, Rothwell NJ. Interleukin-1 and neuronal injury. *Nat Rev Immunol*. 2005 Aug;5(8):629–40.

70. Conductier G, Blondeau N, Guyon A, Nahon J-L, Rovère C. The role of monocyte chemoattractant protein MCP1/CCL2 in neuroinflammatory diseases. *Journal of Neuroimmunology*. 2010 Jul 27;224 (1–2):93–100.

71. Eyre HA, Air T, Pradhan A, et al. A meta-analysis of chemokines in major depression. *Prog Neuropsychopharmacol Biol Psychiatry*. 2016 Jul 4;68:1–8.

72. Leighton SP, Nerurkar L, Krishnadas R, et al. Chemokines in depression in health and in inflammatory illness: a systematic review and meta-analysis. *Mol Psychiatry*. 2017 Nov 14;7(1):72–58.

73. Stuart MJ, Baune BT. Chemokines and chemokine receptors in mood disorders, schizophrenia, and cognitive impairment: a systematic review of biomarker studies. *Neurosci Biobehav Rev*. 2014 May;42:93–115.

74. Haapakoski R, Mathieu J, Ebmeier KP, Alenius H, Kivimäki M. Cumulative meta-analysis of interleukins 6 and 1β, tumour necrosis factor α and C-reactive protein in patients with major depressive disorder. *Brain Behavior and Immunity*. 2015 Oct;49:206–15.

75. Rodrigues-Amorim D, Rivera-Baltanás T, Spuch C, et al. Cytokines dysregulation in schizophrenia: A systematic review of psychoneuroimmune relationship. *Schizophrenia Research*. 2018 Jul;197:19–33.

76. Miller GE, Cole SW. Clustering of depression and inflammation in adolescents previously exposed to childhood adversity. *Biological Psychiatry*. 2012 Jul 1;72(1):34–40.

77. Baumeister D, Akhtar R, Ciufolini S, Pariante CM, Mondelli V. Childhood trauma and adulthood inflammation: a meta-analysis of peripheral C-reactive protein, interleukin-6 and tumour necrosis factor-α. *Mol Psychiatry. Nature Publishing Group*; 2016 May;21(5):642–9.

78. Musselman DL, Lawson DH, Gumnick JF, et al. Paroxetine for the prevention of depression induced by high-dose interferon alfa. *N Engl J Med*. 2001 Mar 29;344(13):961–6.

79. Corvin A, Morris DW. Genome-wide Association Studies: Findings at the Major Histocompatibility Complex Locus in Psychosis. *Biological Psychiatry*. 2014 Feb 15;75(4):276–83.

80. Schizophrenia Working Group of the Psychiatric Genomics Consortium. Biological insights from 108 schizophrenia-associated genetic loci. *Nature*. 2014 Jul 24;511(7510):421–7.

81. Kebir H, Kreymborg K, Ifergan I, et al. Human TH17 lymphocytes promote blood-brain barrier disruption and central nervous system inflammation. *Nat Med*. 2007 Oct;13(10):1173–5.

82. Reboldi A, Coisne C, Baumjohann D, et al. C-C chemokine receptor 6-regulated entry of TH-17 cells into the CNS through the choroid plexus is required for the initiation of EAE. *Nat Immunol*. 2009 May;10(5):514–23.

83. Stromnes IM, Cerretti LM, Liggitt D, Harris RA, Goverman JM. Differential regulation of central nervous system autoimmunity by T(H)1 and T(H)17 cells. *Nat Med*. 2008 Mar;14(3):337–42.

84. Avgustin B, Wraber B, Tavcar R. Increased Th1 and Th2 immune reactivity with relative Th2 dominance in patients with acute exacerbation of schizophrenia. *Croatian Medical Journal*. 2005 Apr;46(2):268–74.

85. Brambilla P, Bellani M, Isola M, et al. Increased M1/decreased M2 signature and signs of Th1/Th2 shift in chronic patients with bipolar disorder, but not in those with schizophrenia. *Transl Psychiatry*. 2014 Jul 1;4(7):e406–6.

86. Debnath M, Berk M. Th17 pathway-mediated immunopathogenesis of schizophrenia: mechanisms and implications. Schizophrenia Bulletin. Oxford University Press; 2014 Nov;40(6):1412–21.

87. Ding M, Song X, Zhao J, et al. Activation of Th17 cells in drug naïve, first episode schizophrenia. *Prog Neuropsychopharmacol Biol Psychiatry*. 2014 Jun 3;51:78–82.

88. Fernandez-Egea E, Vértes PE, Flint SM, et al. Peripheral Immune Cell Populations Associated with Cognitive Deficits and Negative Symptoms of Treatment-Resistant Schizophrenia. *PLoS ONE*. 2016;11(5):e0155631.

89. Røge R, Møller BK, Andersen CR, Correll CU, Nielsen J. Immunomodulatory effects of clozapine and their clinical implications: what have we learned so far? *Schizophrenia Research*. Elsevier B.V. 2012 Sep 1;140(1–3):204–13.

90. Chen M-L, Tsai T-C, Lin Y-Y, et al. Antipsychotic drugs suppress the AKT/NF-kB pathway and regulate the differentiation of T-cell subsets. *Immunology Letters*. Elsevier B.V. 2011 Oct 30;140(1–2):81–91.

91. Chen M-L, Tsai T-C, Wang L-K, et al. Clozapine inhibits Th1 cell differentiation and causes the suppression of IFN-γ production in peripheral blood mononuclear cells. *Immunopharmacol Immunotoxicol*. 2012 Aug;34(4):686–94.

92. O'Sullivan D, Green L, Stone S, et al. Treatment with the antipsychotic agent, risperidone, reduces disease severity in experimental autoimmune encephalomyelitis. *PLoS ONE*. 2014;9(8):e104430.

93. Shatz CJ. MHC class I: an unexpected role in neuronal plasticity. *Neuron*. 2009 Oct 15;64(1):40–5.

94. de Graaf MT, Smitt PAES, Luitwieler RL, et al. Central memory CD4+ T cells dominate the normal cerebrospinal fluid. *Cytometry B Clin Cytom*. 2011 Jan;80(1):43–50.

95. Nikkilä H, Müller K, Ahokas A, et al. Abnormal distributions of T-lymphocyte subsets in the cerebrospinal fluid of patients with acute schizophrenia. *Schizophrenia Research*. 1995 Feb;14(3):215–21.

96. Moalem G, Leibowitz-Amit R, Yoles E, et al. Autoimmune T cells protect neurons from secondary degeneration after central nervous system axotomy. *Nat Med*. 1999 Jan;5(1):49–55.

97. Kipnis J, Mizrahi T, Hauben E, et al. Neuroprotective autoimmunity: naturally occurring CD4+CD25+ regulatory T cells suppress the ability to withstand injury to the central nervous system. *Proc Natl Acad Sci USA*. National Acad Sciences. 2002 Nov 26;99(24):15620–5.

98. Kipnis J, Cardon M, Avidan H, et al. Dopamine, through the extracellular signal-regulated kinase pathway, downregulates CD4+CD25+ regulatory T-cell activity: implications for neurodegeneration. *J Neurosci. Society for Neuroscience.* 2004 Jul 7;24(27):6133–43.

99. Walsh JT, Zheng J, Smirnov I, Lorenz U, Tung K, Kipnis J. Regulatory T cells in central nervous system injury: a double-edged sword. *J Immunol.* 2014 Nov 15;193(10):5013–22.

100. Kipnis J, Gadani S, Derecki NC. Pro-cognitive properties of T cells. *Nat Rev Immunol.* 2012 Sep;12(9):663–9.

101. Dalmau J, Tüzün E, Wu H-Y, et al. Paraneoplastic anti-N-methyl-D-aspartate receptor encephalitis associated with ovarian teratoma. *Ann Neurol.* 2007 Jan;61(1):25–36.

102. Lennox BR, Palmer-Cooper EC, Pollak T, et al. Prevalence and clinical characteristics of serum neuronal cell surface antibodies in first-episode psychosis: a case-control study. *Lancet Psychiatry.* 2017 Jan;4(1):42–8.

103. Brimberg L, Mader S, Jeganathan V, et al. Caspr2-reactive antibody cloned from a mother of an ASD child mediates an ASD-like phenotype in mice. *Mol Psychiatry.* 2016 Dec;21(12):1663–71.

104. Brudek T, Winge K, Folke J, et al. Autoimmune antibody decline in Parkinson's disease and Multiple System Atrophy; a step towards immunotherapeutic strategies. *Mol Neurodegener.* 2017 Jun 7;12(1):44.

105. Iliff JJ, Wang M, Liao Y, et al. A paravascular pathway facilitates CSF flow through the brain parenchyma and the clearance of interstitial solutes, including amyloid β. Science Translational Medicine. *American Association for the Advancement of Science.* 2012 Aug 15;4(147):147ra111–1.

106. Louveau A, Smirnov I, Keyes TJ, et al. Structural and functional features of central nervous system lymphatic vessels. *Nature.* 2015 Jun 1;523(7560):337–41.

107. Aspelund A, Antila S, Proulx ST, et al. A dural lymphatic vascular system that drains brain interstitial fluid and macromolecules. *J Exp Med.* 2015 Jun 29;212(7):991–9.

108. Da Mesquita S, Fu Z, Kipnis J. The Meningeal Lymphatic System: A New Player in Neurophysiology. *Neuron.* 2018 Oct 24;100(2):375–88.

109. Louveau A, Da Mesquita S, Kipnis J. Lymphatics in neurological disorders: a neuro-lympho-vascular component of multiple sclerosis and Alzheimer's disease? *Neuron.* Elsevier Inc. 2016 Sep 7;91(5):957–73.

110. Harrison NA, Brydon L, Walker C, et al. Inflammation causes mood changes through alterations in subgenual cingulate activity and mesolimbic connectivity. *Biological Psychiatry.* 2009 Sep 1;66(5):407–14.

111. Harrison NA, Doeller CF, Voon V, Burgess N, Critchley HD. Peripheral Inflammation Acutely Impairs Human Spatial Memory via Actions on Medial Temporal Lobe Glucose Metabolism. *Biological Psychiatry.* 2014 Oct 1;76(7):585–93.

112. Tracey KJ. Reflex control of immunity. *Nat Rev Immunol.* 2009 Jun;9(6):418–28.

113. Bellinger DL, Millar BA, Perez S, et al. Sympathetic modulation of immunity: Relevance to disease. *Cell Immunol.* 2008;252(1–2):27–56.

114. Sloan EK, Capitanio JP, Tarara RP, et al. Social Stress Enhances Sympathetic Innervation of Primate Lymph Nodes: Mechanisms and Implications for Viral Pathogenesis. *Journal of Neuroscience.* 2007 Aug 15;27(33):8857–65.

115. Pacheco R, Riquelme E, Kalergis AM. Emerging evidence for the role of neurotransmitters in the modulation of T cell responses to cognate ligands. *Cent Nerv Syst Agents Med Chem.* 2010 Mar;10(1):65–83.

116. Ilani T, Ben-Shachar D, Strous RD, et al. A peripheral marker for schizophrenia: Increased levels of D3 dopamine receptor mRNA in blood lymphocytes. *Proc Natl*

Acad Sci USA. National Acad Sciences. 2001 Jan 16;98(2):625–8.

117. Brito-Melo GEA, Nicolato R, de Oliveira ACP, et al. Increase in dopaminergic, but not serotoninergic, receptors in T-cells as a marker for schizophrenia severity. *Journal of Psychiatric Research.* 2012 Jun 1;46 (6):738–42.

118. Nagai Y, Ueno S, Saeki Y, et al. Decrease of the D3 dopamine receptor mRNA expression in lymphocytes from patients with Parkinson's disease. *Neurology.* 1996 Mar 1;46(3):791–5.

119. Thomson CA, McColl A, Cavanagh J, Graham GJ. Peripheral inflammation is associated with remote global gene expression changes in the brain. *J Neuroinflammation.* 2014 Apr 8;11(1):73.

120. Miller AH, Raison CL. The role of inflammation in depression: from evolutionary imperative to modern treatment target. *Nature.* 2016 Jan;16 (1):22–34.

121. Harrison NA. Brain Structures Implicated in Inflammation-Associated Depression. *Curr Top Behav Neurosci.* 2017;31:221–48.

122. Capuron L, Ravaud A, Neveu PJ, et al. Association between decreased serum tryptophan concentrations and depressive symptoms in cancer patients undergoing cytokine therapy. *Mol Psychiatry.* 2002 Jun 18;7(5):468–73.

123. Capuron L, Gumnick JF, Musselman DL, et al. Neurobehavioral effects of interferon-alpha in cancer patients: phenomenology and paroxetine responsiveness of symptom dimensions. *Neuropsychopharmacology.* 2002 May;26 (5):643–52.

124. Krause D, Myint A-M, Schuett C, et al. High Kynurenine (a Tryptophan Metabolite) Predicts Remission in Patients with Major Depression to Add-on Treatment with Celecoxib. *Front Psychiatry.* 2017;8:16.

125. Abbasi S-H, Hosseini F, Modabbernia A, Ashrafi M, Akhondzadeh S. Effect of celecoxib add-on treatment on symptoms and serum IL-6 concentrations in patients with major depressive disorder: randomized double-blind placebo-controlled study. *J Affect Disord.* 2012 Dec 10;141 (2–3):308–14.

126. O'Connor JC, Lawson MA, André C, et al. Induction of IDO by bacille Calmette-Guérin is responsible for development of murine depressive-like behaviour. *J Immunol.* 2009 Mar 1;182(5): 3202–12.

From Psychoneuroimmunology to Immunopsychiatry: An Historical Perspective

Keith W. Kelley

2.1 Introduction

It was the best of times, it was the worst of times,
it was the age of wisdom, it was the age of foolishness,
it was the epoch of belief, it was the epoch of incredulity,
it was the season of Light, it was the season of Darkness,
it was the spring of hope, it was the winter of despair . . .
Charles Dickens, A Tale of Two Cities, *1859*

More than a century after Dickens published his best known historical novel, it was the worst of times for the fledging field of psychoneuroimmunology (PNI). But now it is the best of times for this field that emphasizes an integrative physiological approach to biomedical research. This renaissance in PNI has laid a solid brick-and-mortar foundation for the emerging field of immunopsychiatry. Indeed, before one can understand the importance of the emerging field of immunopsychiatry, one must first grasp the historical developments of PNI. The best and worst of times for immunopsychiatry has yet to be written. *Laissez les bon temps rouler*!

2.2 Immunology Research in the 1970s

Immunology was a relatively new discipline in the 1970s, particularly if the early work on vaccines is excluded. Examples include the classic nineteenth-century discoveries by Edward Jenner of the smallpox vaccine, and Louis Pasteur's work on the rabies vaccine and the germ theory of disease. Between 1901 and 1960, five immunologists were awarded the Nobel Prize (von Behring, Metchnikoff, Bordet, Landsteiner and Medawar/Burnet). Edelman and Porter unravelled the chemical structure of antibodies, for which they were awarded a Nobel Prize in 1972. But it was not known until the 1960s and 1970s that one set of lymphocytes was derived from the thymus gland and is a predominant player in cellular immunity (T cells). The other type of lymphocyte was discovered to come from the bone marrow and is needed for synthesizing antibodies (B cells). Monoclonal antibodies did not appear until 1975 following their production by Kohler and Milstein. Human interferon-α was not purified until 1978, and after sequencing, cloning and expression in bacteria, was the first recombinant cytokine approved by the Food and Drug Administration (FDA) for human use in 1986. It was not until the late 1970s that two leukocyte-derived proteins were discovered: IL-1 (i.e., endogenous pyrogen; lymphocyte activating factor) and IL-2 (i.e., T-cell growth factor) and were recognized as the first two cytokines. There were no

ELISA kits, no validated monoclonal antibodies, no RT-PCR, no regulatory T cells, no Toll-like receptors, no danger-associated molecular patterns, no cytokine receptor signalling pathways, no M-1 or M-2 macrophages, no RNAseq, no check-point inhibitors and no bioinformatics. Necrosis was the only form of cell death known to scientists; the programmed cell death processes of apoptosis, pyroptosis and necroptosis had not been discovered. In the clinic, flow cytometers and magnetic resonance imaging equipment were not to be found, both technologies becoming commercially available only in the 1980s.

The retrovirus that causes AIDS was discovered in 1983, which led to a very public debate between the Frenchman Luc Montagnier and the American scientist Robert Gallo about who originally discovered the human immunodeficiency virus (HIV). The AIDS epidemic was rapidly spreading at that time, with nearly 450,000 Americans dying of this disease and more than 300,000 others living with it. Ultimately, Montagnier shared the 2008 Nobel Prize in Physiology or Medicine with his former student, Françoise Barré-Sinoussi, for their discovery of HIV.

It is noteworthy that development of the AIDS epidemic occurred concurrently with the evolution of the field of PNI. Indeed, it was the field of PNI that reported some of the earliest observations that profound behavioural changes occur in some patients as AIDS progresses (1,2), including severe cognitive and behavioural changes. This was of course before effective treatments for HIV had been discovered. Moreover, at this point in time, HIV was considered to infect only CD4$^+$ T lymphocytes. Despite this dogma that HIV infected only peripheral T cells, the behavioural changes caused by HIV led to a focus on the brain, and it was PNI scientists who addressed this issue. Indeed, the National Institutes of Health (NIH) provided substantial research funding for PNI research via establishing AIDS committees, requests for AIDS grant applications and specialized study sections. We now know that there are macrophage-trophic strains of HIV and that HIV-infected CD4$^+$ T cells can enter the brain within four months of infection and can replicate in a compartmentalized fashion in the central nervous system (3).

The AIDS epidemic reinforced the perspective that immunology is a field of study associated with only infectious, autoimmune and oncologic diseases. While disease and vaccines remain a cornerstone (4), modern immunology research today encompasses much more than attempts to prevent or cure these kinds of diseases. Inflammation is no longer taught in medical schools as only a local regional process consisting of the five classic signs of heat (*calor*), pain (*dolor*), redness (*rubor*), swelling (*tumor*) and loss of function (*functio laesa*). In its place, the concept of chronic, systemic inflammation is now recognized as a major player in costly diseases ranging from cardiovascular to metabolic to mental health disorders. The idea that organs of the immune system are interconnected with all other physiologic systems and functions to maintain health of the entire body, including the brain, was not appreciated. Indeed, this idea was often scoffed at. But an early pioneer in the field, George Solomon, hung a sign in his laboratory in the 1960s at the Veterans Administration Hospital in Palo Alto, California that read, 'Psychoimmunology' (personal communication with Susan Solomon). As this emerging field grew, various names were used to describe it, like neuroimmunomodulation, behavioural immunology and psychosocial neuroimmunology. But it was not until 1980 that Robert Ader coined the term PNI (5). This name stuck and continues to be used today. This interdisciplinary field of PNI forms the historical and scientific basis of immunopsychiatry, a word that was coined a few years later. The first

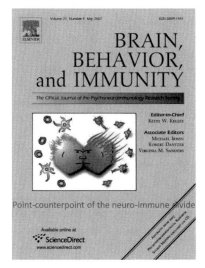

Volume 21, Number 4, May 2007   ISSN 0889-1591

BRAIN,
BEHAVIOR,
and IMMUNITY

The Official Journal of the Psychoneuroimmunology Research Society

Editor-in-Chief
KEITH W. KELLEY

Associate Editors
MICHAEL IRWIN
ROBERT DANTZER
VIRGINIA M. SANDERS

Point-counterpoint of the neuro-immune divide

Available online at
ScienceDirect
www.sciencedirect.com

Perspective is Everything

Dan "the immunologist" Aycroyd: "Neuroimmunology is neither neurobiology nor immunology. At best, this discipline has often been referred to as the third rail of immunology for those with insufficient drive to focus on the serious primary issues of immunology such as thymic selection and self/nonself recognition."

Jane "the neuroimmunologist" Kurton: "Dan, let me try to address your comments calmly and rationally. Let us consider your issue about serotonin. Who gets to call a molecule an interleukin, a chemokine or even an anaphylactotoxin is a manner of who placed their flag on that site first! Serotonin clearly is a major product of activated platelets and a classical mediator of inflammation."

Carson and Lo. 2007. *Brain, Behavior, and Immunity* 21:367

Figure 2.1 A view of interdisciplinary research involving neuroscience and immunology. This original figure from (9) earned the cover of the May 2007 issue of *Brain, Behavior, and Immunity*. The illustration vividly portrays the chasm that existed between neuroscientists and immunologists at the end of the twentieth and beginning of the twenty-first centuries (reprinted with permission from Elsevier Ltd).

scientist to use the term immunopsychiatry was Branislav D. Jankovic from the Institute of Immunology in Zagreb. This was in a 1985 article (6) in which he specifically referred to the neuromodulating activity of anti-brain antibodies that were described nearly three decades earlier.

The proposal that an interdisciplinary approach to biomedical research was needed that combined immunology, neuroscience and psychology was not greeted with much enthusiasm (7). 'Disdain' might be a better way to describe it. Clinician scientist Wallace Sampson was quoted as saying 'Most of what PNI involves is the measurement of artifacts' (8). As a more graphic example, Monica Carson and David Lo are both very well-respected scientists in the immunology (Lo) and neuroscience (Carson) communities. They published an amusing article in the form of an original *Saturday Night Live* point/counterpoint skit between Dan 'Aykroyd' and Jane 'Curtin' (9). One quote from this article, as presented in Figure 2.1, provides a flavour of the contempt that once existed between neuroscientists and immunologists. With the benefit of hindsight, the reason for this discord was that so little was known about the immune system in the early 1970s. Cytokines, and many other discoveries that were yet to be made, were unknown. But now, PNI has a firm scientific basis. It has given birth to immunopsychiatry, thus joining at the hip the immune system and brain in modern biomedical research.

2.3 The Immunology Laboratory of the 1970s

Imagine a modern, well-equipped immunology research laboratory at a major university or pharmaceutical company in the United States during the 1970s. There was a safety cabinet, a phase-contrast inverted and upright microscope, cell-harvesting equipment, gamma counter, beta counter, anion-exchange and gel-filtration sephadex columns, an ultracentrifuge and animal housing for the rabbits and sheep that were used for producing polyclonal antibodies. Missing were a microplate reader, flow cytometer, high-speed tabletop centrifuge, magnetic beads for cell separation, PCR thermocyclers, ultraviolet cameras for photographing RT-PCR gels, processers to develop films of Western blots and software to quantitate the bands. Pan T cells were identified not by flow cytometry but by their ability to bind erythrocytes to create fragile T-cell rosettes that were counted manually under a light microscope. RNA was isolated in an ultracentrifuge through high-density caesium chloride that often required spin times greater than 12 hours. Steady-state expression of RNA was measured by the insensitive technique of Northern blotting and RNase protection assays. There was a mimeograph machine and a very slow-speed copying machine in the central office. If you wanted to read a scientific paper, you did not click *PubMed* online or search for it on Google. Instead, you walked to the library, dug it out of the shelves and read it in the carrels or copied it so it could be read later. If you were a poor graduate student, you lugged as many of the bound journals as you could carry back to the departmental office in order to copy the relevant papers that were often free of charge. Reviews of NIH grant applications were mailed to applicants as a carbon copy on a pink sheet of paper (i.e., pink sheets). There were no tower or laptop computers with Microsoft Office suite software for word processing in Word, saving data in Excel or creating slides in PowerPoint. All scientific papers and grant applications were prepared on a typewriter. Several hard copies of these documents were sent by US mail to editorial offices of journals or to granting agencies. There was no online submission of any type, which only began in earnest after 2000. Email did not become widely available until the mid-1980s, and the computing power of today's smartphones was far beyond the horizon.

2.4 Specialization, a Key Theme During the Past 50 Years

Biomedical research is not immune to fads. Hot-ticket items often appear in the form of specialization, at least until these new-fad technologies are incorporated into mainstream biomedical research. For most of the 1980s and 1990s, well-trained molecular biologists were in demand for the best jobs in both academia and industry. These scientists were experts in creating plasmids that contained DNA sequences for a given protein and then expressing those vectors in prokaryotic and eukaryotic cells. No matter that these scientists had little to no training in neuroscience, behaviour, immunology or physiology. Systemic and conditional knock-out and knock-in animals were subsequently developed. Optogenetic tools became available and the more recent development of CRISPR (Clustered Regularly Interspaced Short Palindromic Repeats) technology to edit specific genes now holds substantial promise. It is certain that all of these new technologies advanced biomedical research. However, they came at the cost of training new Ph.D. graduates as technical experts rather than as integrative physiologists.

The trend towards increasing specialization continues today in the medical profession with the creation and expansion of numerous board specialities. In the United States, the American Board of Medical Specialties, formed in 1933, is one of three agencies that certify medical specialists. Physicians are eligible to become diplomates in 24 types of specialities. Most of these medical boards have subspecialties, like the 21 subspecialties in internal medicine and the 13 in psychiatry. The vast majority of American physicians carry diplomatic status in at least one boarded speciality, which then provides privileges at local hospitals. The academic biomedical research community has fallen in line with this approach of training specialists. Professors train their graduate students as neuroscientists, immunologists, geneticists, molecular biologists or statisticians. Integrative physiological research, as must be done in brain, behaviour and immunology projects, has not been in vogue for the past 50 years.

The practice of biomedical specialization is changing for at least three major reasons. First, growth and acceptance of the idea that the brain and immune system communicate with one another to affect nearly all aspects of human health. As such, for many biomedical research endeavours, it is more prudent and cost-effective to evaluate integrative physiological systems with a team of experts instead of studying the immune and central nervous systems in isolation. Second, the Institute of Medicine has recommended that a panel of measures on social and behavioural risk factors be included in every person's electronic medical record (10), which requires interdisciplinary training of physicians and biomedical research scientists(11). Third is recognition that more is needed in hospitals than the standard cadre of specialists. As but one example, the American Board of Physician Specialties recently created the American Board of Hospital Medicine (ABHM). The responsibilities of these boarded physicians are to provide general medical care for patients while they are in the hospital (12). Physicians boarded with the ABHM work with other medical specialists and their staff to coordinate hospital patient care. They respond to both patients and their caregivers by answering questions and responding to their concerns in an attempt to optimize the hospital experience of both the patients and family.

2.5 Early Research on Immune-Brain Communication

Now that the stage is set, PNI research during the past 50 years can be better understood in its proper context. That is not to imply that no research was conducted on mind-body interactions prior to the 1970s. Indeed, there is a rich history beginning Before Common Era (BCE). Certainly, early Egyptian, Chinese, Indian and Greek medicine incorporated many aspects of mind-body relationships (Figure 2.2, 13). But it took centuries before medical sciences discovered the existence of pathogenic microbes and how they caused disease. One notable example was the death of an American president, James Garfield, shortly after he was elected president in 1881. Unable to find an assassin's bullet in his body, several physicians inserted their unsterilized fingers into the wound to search for it. Not surprisingly, Garfield died of sepsis four months after being shot.

Growing knowledge of the immune system and its role in protecting against infections emerged in the next century. For PNI, a number of themes emerged even prior to the 1970s, such as research on stress, placebo, biofeedback and meditation. In 1964, the innovative psychiatrist George F. Solomon proposed that emotional stress was somehow related to immunological dysfunction (14). He published a number of original studies that tested this hypothesis, and most of his early work as well as the effect of a variety of stressors on animals was summarized in a review in 1980 (15). By 1981, the first book that was entirely devoted to the field of PNI was published (16). It contained chapters by leading scientists at the time, one of which summarized the early major contributions by Russian scientists (17). For example, one chapter described the early experiments by Korneva that showed destruction of the posterior hypothalamus in rabbits suppressed their immune response. Other Russian scientists demonstrated that an intravenous injection of antigen caused changes in electrical activity of the posterior hypothalamus. Professor Korneva's chapter and a subsequent paper (18) discussed and cited

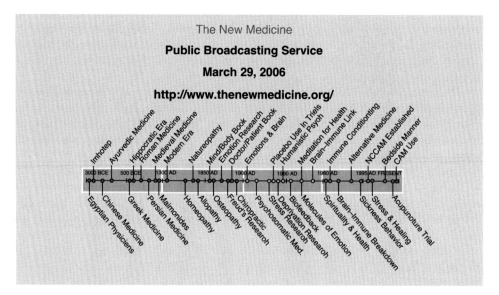

Figure 2.2 A general summary of the major trends in the development of integrative medicine that form a basis for the emerging field of immunopsychiatry (http://thenewmedicine.org/timeline.html; published with permission from TPT National Productions).

many of the early and original observations published in Russian scientific journals on the role of the hypothalamus in regulating the immune system. By 1993, the field was gaining some traction with the public, as noted by the well-respected journalist and commentator, Bill Moyers (19). He created a television series that featured pioneers in PNI such as Bob Ader, David Felten and Margaret Kemeny. Today, this interdisciplinary field of PNI is recognized as giving birth to the emerging field of immunopsychiatry (20).

Slowly, the idea that psychological events might affect the immune system began to be accepted (8). However, at the end of the twentieth century, PNI research clearly remained outside mainstream science. It was considered by most experts to be a pejorative term. The word immunopsychiatry had not yet even been coined. This uninformed state of the art provided a formidable obstacle for scientists trying to obtain grant funding for PNI research from major funding agencies like the NIH, National Science Foundation, European Research Foundation, Medical Research Council or Wellcome Trust. The idea that the brain could do things that would affect the immune system did not sit well with most immunologists. And certainly the possibility that something from the immune system could cause changes in neuronal circuits in the brain was nearly heresy.

2.6 Scientific Meetings that Led to Creation of Two Scholarly Societies

Not only were more original data and review papers on PNI beginning to be published in the 1970s and 1980s, scientific meetings were organized to more rapidly promote the dissemination of new results on neuroimmune interactions. One of the first was held in 1982 in Leningrad, Russia (now St Petersburg) at the Institute of Experimental Medicine. It was organized by Professor E. A. Korneva (21) and the title was 'Meeting of all union problems commission on physiology of immune homeostasis'. It was here that that the International Society of Neuroimmunomodulation (ISNIM) was conceived and plans were made for the first meeting of this society. That successful gathering was held in 1986 in Dubrovnik, Yugoslavia (now Croatia). In 1994, the first issue of the ISNIM-sponsored journal, *Neuroimmunomodulation*, appeared with Karger as the publisher. The 2017 impact factor of *Neuroimmunomodulation* was 2.24. The First International Workshop on Neuroimmunomodulation in the United States was held in 1984 on the NIH campus in Bethesda, Maryland under the auspices of the NIH (22). A summary slide from that NIH conference and the memento from the Dubrovnik meeting (Figure 2.3) provide a visual image of the state of the art of neuroimmune interactions during the early 1980s. The slide from the NIH conference clearly portrays the novel idea of reciprocal interactions between the brain and immune system. Both hormones and nerves emanating from the central nervous system were projected to affect the three main types of leukocytes that were

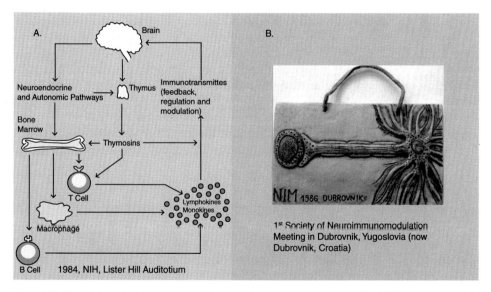

Figure 2.3 State of the art of research in neuroimmune interactions in the early 1980s. (A) The First International Workshop on Neuroimmunomodulation was held in 1984 in the NIH campus in Bethesda, Maryland, United States under the auspices of the NIH (22). This figure conceptualizes some of the earliest thinking in the field of PNI. It was one of the first to include a brain in the same figure with cells of the immune system. Note that a lot more was known about how the brain might affect the immune system rather than the major theme today that the immune system affects the brain. But clearly the figure portrays reciprocal communication between the immune system and brain, even though there was little to no understanding of how that occurred. In this scenario, it was mainly hormones like ACTH, glucocorticoids and catecholamines that affect lymphoid cells. Thymosins were included because they are thymic hormone-like peptides that affect leukocytes and other physiological systems. The concept of this figure was handicapped because only two cytokines were well accepted at that time, IL-1 (the monokine) and IL-2 (the lymphokine). However, this figure got the story straight by hypothesizing that products from both lymphoid and myeloid cells act on the brain to affect activation of neuroendocrine and autonomic systems. (B) The plaster memento given to registrants at the first ISNIM meeting in 1986 in Dubrovnik, Yugoslavia. The figure depicts a neuronal cell body with its axon terminal in contact with a lymphoid cell. Immunologists considered this to be heretical. But a recent paper using simple fluorescence clearly visualized macrophages in direct contact with sympathetic neurons in white adipose tissue (23). These neuron-associated macrophages, named sympathetic neuron-associated macrophages (SAM), import and catabolize norepinephrine, thereby impairing its lipolytic property in adipose tissue and contributing to obesity.

well accepted at that time: T cells, B cells and macrophages. The T-cell population synthesized and secreted the only known lymphokine, T-cell growth factor, now known as IL-2. Macrophages synthesized the only known monokine at that time, IL-1. Both these cytokines were hypothesized to somehow affect the brain.

In the United States, the NIH conference of 1984 spurred a subsequent meeting between leading immunologists and psychologists that was held in Tanque Verde Ranch near Tucson, Arizona (24). Imagine immunologists sitting across the table from psychologists! Following the meeting, Professor Cohen concluded, '. . . that we are on dangerous ground in the attempt to fuse the two fields of inquiry which are themselves still "soft". This gathering led to a series of subsequent meetings dubbed 'Research Perspectives in PNI'. The first was held in Boulder, Colorado, the next in Rochester, New York, and then Columbus, Ohio. The final one was held in Boulder, Colorado in 1993, and it was there that the Psychoneuroimmunology Research Society (PNIRS) was formally created (25). I became the first dues-paying member of this new scientific society on 23 April, 1993 by paying $50 to Secretary-Treasurer Bruce Rabin (Figure 2.4). Today, annual dues for the PNIRS are $230.

The first formal meeting of PNIRS was held in November of 1994 in Key Biscayne, Florida (26). The next one was in 1996 in Santa Monica, California, and a PNIRS meeting has been held every year since (for a list of meeting sites and many of the meeting programmes, see 27). Every third year, beginning in 1998, annual PNIRS meetings have been held in Western Europe. Beginning in 2012, the PNIRS reached out to China in the form of organizing symposia at major scientific meetings throughout the mainland and Taiwan (28). After a few years, this global approach to PNI research was so successful that the official name of this endeavour was changed from PNIRS**China** to PNIRS**Asia-Pacific**. These PNIRS**Asia-Pacific** symposia have been held in many cities on the mainland of China, Taiwan, Australia, Japan and South Korea. Activities from this initiative are now posted and

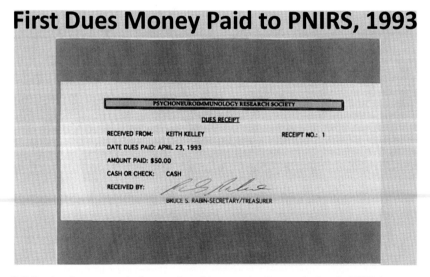

Figure 2.4 Receipt of payment as the first member of the new scientific organization, the PNIRS. An amount of $50 was paid by Keith W. Kelley for the first-year annual dues with the receipt issued by the new Secretary-Treasurer, Bruce S. Rabin. (26, reprinted with permission from Elsevier Ltd).

have been recently summarized (29) and new meetings updated regularly at the PNIRS home page (https://pnirs.org/pnirsasia-pacific). Although no formal PNIRS meeting has yet been held in the Asia-Pacific region, outreach of the PNIRS**Asia-Pacific** committee makes it likely that will happen in the coming years. Indeed, the entire study of reciprocal relationships between the immune system and the brain has gone global during the past five years, with prestigious meetings devoted to the topic being held in Barcelona, Paris, Berlin and Brisbane. The latest, entitled, 'Neuro-immune axis: reciprocal regulation in development, health, and disease', was organized in 2019 as a *Cell* symposium in Long Beach, California and included scientific editors from both *Cell* and *Neuron* (30). The objective of this meeting was to 'explore the interface between the nervous and immune systems during development, homeostasis, and disease. The meeting will examine the mediators, mechanisms, and implications of neuroimmune crosstalk in the central and peripheral nervous systems. It will also cover emerging areas such as the neuronal regulation of peripheral immune function and the influence of the microbiota on the brain'. Clearly, understanding how the immune and nervous systems interact to affect our health has finally become a mainstream topic. The growing field of immunopsychiatry is now poised to continue to advance this field of science.

A major factor that promoted the entire field of PNI was creation of a new journal that first appeared in 1987, *Brain, Behavior, and Immunity* (31). Beginning on 1 January, 2000, *Brain, Behavior, and Immunity*, which was founded as an Academic Press journal, became the official journal of the PNIRS (26). Elsevier purchased Academic Press shortly thereafter, and to this date *Brain, Behavior, and Immunity* has remained in the large stable of Elsevier of academic journals. Since that time, both growth and prestige PNI research has skyrocketed, at least as assessed by both the number of annual submissions (<100 in 2000 to ~900 in 2017) and the impact factor (~2 in 2000 to >6 in 2017) of *Brain, Behavior, and Immunity* (28). This rise in impact factor has led to it ranking in the top 10% to 15% of all global journals published in both immunology and neurosciences. As such, *Brain, Behavior, and Immunity* has been coined 'the best immunology journal in the neurosciences' for nearly the past 20 years because it has remained the highest ranked journal in both the categories of neurosciences and Immunology, as assessed by the Web of Science. Beginning in 2019, Elsevier facilitated *Brain, Behavior, and Immunity* to become ranked in psychiatry as well, and it is already in the top 10% of all scientific journals published in psychiatry (15th out of 146 psychiatry journals).

It turns out that the 1986 conceptualization from the neuroimmunomodulation meeting in Dubrovnik was correct (Figure 2.3). A novel subset of macrophages was recently discovered to reside in very close contact with sympathetic nerves in white adipose tissue. These cells exist in both humans and mice and have been designated sympathetic neuron-associated macrophages (SAMs) (23). These myeloid cells import and degrade norepinephrine from the neurons, thereby preventing lipolysis that is needed to reduce the amount of adipose tissue. Inhibition of SAMs increases brown adipose tissue and thermogenesis, leading to a reduction in obesity. As such, neurons not only are in direct contact with myeloid cells, but this connection has important functional outcomes in terms of the American obesity epidemic. This finding is important for the growing field of immunopsychiatry because obesity is known to be associated with a number of mood and personality disorders (32). And certainly many more cytokines other than IL-1 and IL-2, such as interferon-α, have been shown to affect the brain, leading to abnormal behaviours.

2.7 Historical Basis of Immunopsychiatry: The Immune System as a Sixth Sense

The fundamental notion of immunopsychiatry is that mental health is driven, at least in part, by the immune system (20). I credit the conceptual basis for this paradigm-shifting idea to Edwin J. Blalock, who in 1984 was in the Department of Microbiology at the University of Texas Medical Branch in Galveston. Professor Blalock proposed that the immune system is really a sensory system that serves as our sixth sense (33). He introduced and supported the radical idea that the immune system is in constant dialogue with the brain. Even though Professor Blalock's paper was published in the official scientific journal of the American Association of Immunologists, the idea that the immune system could serve a sensory system to inform the brain about events occurring in the periphery was not well accepted by immunologists. Yet, the beauty of this idea was simple. All of us have been sick at one time or another. As but one example, the influenza virus causes numerous discomforting symptoms, including fever, headache, lack of appetite, drowsiness, disrupted cognitive function, fatigue and achiness. For at least the first five of these seven symptoms, the brain is required. As is well known, the classic five sensory systems are seeing, hearing, touching, tasting and smelling, But none of these senses has the ability to detect a pathogen. Blalock was a visionary who offered a conceptual explanation for how a lung infection with influenza can lead to the brain inducing symptoms of sickness that we have all experienced. His conception of the immune system as a sensory system has now been accepted and recently updated to include proprioception as a sixth sense and input from the immune system as the seventh sense (34). It was this early, provocative view of reciprocal immune to brain communication that forms an important historical conceptual basis for development of this new field of immunopsychiatry. That said, with the foundation of immunopsychiatry being PNI, the emerging field of immunopsychiatry is not without significant conceptual issues. As pointed out by Konsman (35), '. . . immunopsychiatry can be considered as a field of translational research in which hypotheses generated by basic science are tested in a clinical context'. In order to successfully advance clinical medicine, Konsman advises that much clearer criteria are needed to define concepts and constructs than those being utilized today in immunopsychiatry.

2.8 PNI Focus Moves the Needle from Efferent to Afferent Communication

Efferent signals from brain to immune system. The field of PNI began with a top-down approach. That is, the main interest was efferent signals sent from the brain to the rest of the body. The major emphasis of PNI research during the 1970s and 1980s was devoted to understanding how stress-induced glucocorticoids and catecholamines affect immunocompetence (36,37). Seen through the prism of a rear-view mirror, it is noteworthy that there were only limited lymphocyte populations to study, amounting to T helper and T suppressor cells (the latter now known as regulatory T cells, or Tregs), B cells and natural killer (NK) cells. Flow cytometry was only a developing technology in the 1980s, so labelling multiple epitopes on cells to define specific lymphoid and myeloid populations was not possible. Worse, functional assays of immune competence both in vivo (e.g., vaccine response, hypersensitivity reactions) and in vitro (mitogen proliferation and natural killer cell assays) were quite limited. These limitations, coupled with the challenges of conducting clinical studies with human psychiatric disorders like schizophrenia, led Stein et al. (36) to characterize immunopsychiatric studies as 'findings in search of meaning'. Other hormones, such as growth hormone, insulin-like growth factor-I, prolactin and thyroid-stimulating hormone were in the news because they all had significant effects on the immune system (38). Although these types of studies are no longer the most prominent in the PNI literature, important results of this type continue to be reported. For example, Farhart et al. (39) recently discovered a phenomenal increase in lung and blood bacteria following infection with *Streptococcus pneumoniae* in mice deficient in growth hormone. This reduction in host resistance to the thymus-independent antigen was associated with a reduced IgM response.

Another important and classic example of the early focus on how stress affects the immune system was published by Janice Kiecolt-Glaser and colleagues (40). Instead of focusing exclusively on patients, she tested the hypothesis that caregivers of patients might be affected. She used dependent variables consisting of both mental health and immune system readouts. Kiecolt-Glaser found that family caregivers of patients with Alzheimer's disease experienced more distress and loneliness than control subjects. Furthermore, caregivers had fewer T helper cells, a lower helper-suppressor T-cell ratio and reduced resistance to the latent Epstein–Barr virus. In the context of with what is known today, her findings seem obvious. But it was the psychologist Professor Kiecolt-Glaser who recognized this issue early on and brought it to the attention of the medical community. She continues today with her productive research programme aimed at understanding health issues of caregivers (41).

Tai chi is a mild physical exercise that combines stretching with mindfulness and provides bidirectional communication between the brain and immune system. A remarkable study was published by Michael Irwin et al. (42) that showed how tai chi affects the immune system. He asked whether 15 weeks of tai chi movements would improve the immune response to herpes zoster, the virus that causes shingles, in elderly humans. The results were clear, with tai chi increasing varicella zoster virus-specific cell-mediated immunity, particularly in older adults with the poorest health functioning. These experiments provide just one more example of how engaging the mind and body can elicit a positive effect on the immune system. As a note, tai chi not only improves a vaccine response in the geriatric subjects, it also improves sleep quality in the elderly (43) and reduces symptoms of depression in breast cancer survivors (44).

Afferent signals from immune system to brain. In 1987, *Science* magazine published two papers showing that a cytokine produced by the immune system communicates with the brain. These two papers ultimately caused a paradigm shift by moving PNI research away from efferent signals from the brain to the periphery and toward afferent signals sent by the immune system to the brain. Hugo Besedovsky and colleagues were the first to define this afferent immune signal that was sent to the brain. In a series of groundbreaking papers, many of which appeared in Science magazine he conclusively showed that an intraperitoneal injection of recombinant IL-1 causes an increase in plasma adrenocorticotropic hormone (ACTH) and corticosterone (45). It was well known that the periventricular nucleus of the hypothalamus is a region of the brain that links the nervous system to the endocrine system via the pituitary gland, ultimately leading to an increase in plasma glucocorticoids. Pre-injection of an antiserum to corticotropin-releasing factor (CRF) prior to systemic IL-1 totally prevented the increase in plasma corticotropin-releasing hormone. In that same issue of *Science*, Robert Sapolsky reported equally convincing findings by showing that an intravenous injection of IL-1 caused a dose-dependent increase in secretion of hypothalamic CRF and plasma corticosterone (46). Immunoneutralization of CRF prevented the IL-1-induced increase in corticosterone. Authors of both papers concluded that there must be an immunoregulatory feedback circuit between the immune system and brain. These two back-to-back publications ultimately changed the face and subsequent course of PNI research because they clearly demonstrated that an afferent signal known to be produced by macrophages can activate parvocellular neurosecretory cells of the periventricular nucleus.

The following year, another paper appeared in the *Journal of Immunology* that advanced the emerging concept of reciprocal communication systems between the immune system and brain (47). IL-1 was given several names prior to its cloning. In addition to being an endogenous pyrogen, it also was known as thymocyte stimulating factor. Before ELISA assays became available, this property of IL-1 was used in a bioassay to measure its activity because it helped to increase thymocyte proliferation in vitro. But, when IL-1 was injected systemically in vivo, Morrissey et al. found that it caused the thymus to nearly totally regress. This surprising finding was explained based on the results of both Besedovsky and Sapolsky discussed above. IL-1-induced thymic involution was caused by inducing the cascade of IL-1-→CRF-→ACTH-→corticosterone-→reduction in size of the thymus gland. This example shows how an afferent signal arising from the immune system can be detected by the brain, which in turn mounts an efferent response that down-regulates the size of a primary lymphoid organ. This is a classic example of reciprocal communication between the immune and central nervous systems.

Where is the "P" in PNI? Early clinical studies with cytokines reinforced the possibility that systemic cytokines could have major effects on the central nervous system. Interferon-α was the first cytokine to be cloned, expressed and made available for clinical studies in the 1980s. This was followed by identification, cloning and availability of other cytokines like IL-1 and IL-2. Both interferon-α and IL-2 were hypothesized to be useful for treatment of a variety of cancers. But the earliest phase I clinical trials established that systemic administration of these cytokines caused a variety of adverse effects, including lethargy, fever, malaise and disorientation (48). These CNS-mediated symptoms were argued to be due to toxicity caused by injection of high doses of cytokines into very sick patients. Clearly these early data established that peripheral cytokines can have major effects on the brain, but the results were viewed as pure pharmacological rather than physiological effects.

Those preclinical studies have now led to a better understanding of the side-effects caused by some of the newest antibody-based treatments for a variety of cancers as well as those for organ transplants. This immunotherapy includes treatments with chimeric antigen receptor (CAR) T cells and bispecific antibodies. Symptoms following these treatments are strikingly similar to sickness behaviours and can be mild to life-threatening. They include myalgia, inappetence, fever, secondary headaches, fever, somnolence and chronic fatigue. The origin of these symptoms is now considered to be caused by a variety of cytokines that are induced by the cancer treatments. This phenomenon is known as the cytokine release syndrome (49). Research in this area is growing because these adverse consequences to cancer therapy often limit the amount and duration of treatment.

The *Journal of Immunology* published a supplement on neuroimmunomodulation in 1985 (50). This supplement contained 28 articles written by leading scientists. Of particular relevance to this book on immunopsychiatry, only a single article was devoted to human and animal behaviour, focusing on clinical depression and the immune system (51). Behaviour was clearly outside mainstream PNI science. Even at the 2004 annual meeting of PNIRS in Titisee, Germany, research on behaviour was not mainstream. So much so, in fact, that Professor Michael Irwin organized an informative discussion session entitled, 'The 'P' in PNIRS – A discussion over beer' (52). Since that time, behaviour and inflammation have been key topics in PNI. As but one example that has emerged since that time, emotional stress is also now well accepted to increase blood levels of cytokines in humans, many of which can affect human behaviours. For example, a recent meta-analysis focused on inflammatory activity in response to acute laboratory stress (53). Acute stress caused significant increases in IL-1β, IL-6, IL-10 and tumour necrosis factor (TNF).

The vagus as an important neural afferent signal from the immune system to the brain. In the early 1990s, the first evidence for a direct afferent neural route from the immune system to the brain was published. The group of Dwight Nance demonstrated that the immediate early gene, *c-fos*, is induced in the hypothalamus and brain stem following injection of lipopolysaccharide (LPS; 54). The following year, this same group showed that the LPS-induced induction of neuronal *c-fos* was blocked by a subdiaphragmatic vagotomy (55). That same year, Bluthé et al. (56) showed that LPS-induced sickness behaviour could also be abrogated by a vagal neurotomy inferior to the diaphragm. Vagotomy also impaired acute inflammation-induced hyperalgesia (57), increase in corticosterone (58) and induction of IL-1 in the brain (59). In all of these cases, the inflammatory stimulus was injected intraperitoneally. However, when the same stimulus was given intravenously, subdiaphragmatic vagotomy was not effective (60). This result confirmed the earlier work of Wan et al. (55) with a behaviour rather than *c-fos* as the dependent variable. These data were novel and exciting because they established a neuronal pathway by which an inflammatory stimulus arising in the abdominal cavity could communicate with the brain. The potential importance of the vagus as a pathway linking the periphery to the brain has now been extended to the gut. Although tested mostly in non-human primates, this 'wandering nerve' has recently been established to be an important communication pathway that permits gut microbiota to influence a variety of brain functions (61).

Sickness to depression: the discovery. It was these types of behavioural research experiments with cytokines that ultimately reinforced the potential importance of immune cell-derived messengers as afferent signals to the brain. Perhaps one of the most significant early reviews that form an evolutionary basis for immunopsychiatry was published by B. L. Hart (62). He concluded, 'the behavior of sick animals and people is not a maladaptive response or the effect of debilitation, but rather an organized, evolved behavior strategy to facilitate the role of fever in combating viral and bacterial infections'. By using the newly defined IL-1 receptor antagonist injected by both the intracerebroventricular and peritoneal routes, Kent et al. (63) subsequently established that the fever-inducing properties of IL-1 could be separated from its ability to induce sickness behaviours. Measurement of a variety of sickness behaviours was then proposed as a new target that could be used to develop therapeutics (64). Reports of sickness behaviour have increased substantially since that time. But it was Raz Yirmiya who first recognized similarities between sickness behaviour and depression in rodents (65) and subsequently in humans (66). He published the first experimental evidence demonstrating a role for the immune system in depressive-like behaviour. He assessed anhedonia using preference of rodents for saccharin rather than water and several measurements of male sexual behaviour following systemic injection with increasing amounts of lipopolysaccharide. The results showed that rats treated with LPS drank less saccharin and engaged in fewer sexual activities, some of which could be prevented by chronic treatment with the antidepressant imipramine.

Immune afferent signals in humans. Preclinical experiments such as those described above quickly justified the importance of testing the bottom-up afferent hypothesis in humans. The initial report on the psychiatric effects of immunotherapy was conducted by Lucile Capuron in the late 1990s, as reported in a short Letter to the Editor in the *New England Journal of Medicine* (67). These workers reported a relationship between depressive symptoms in ten patients with malignant melanoma before and four weeks after treatment with interferon-α. Further reports testing this possibility were conducted by Andrew Miller's research group at Emory University. He took advantage of the FDA's approval of interferon-α for treatment of patients diagnosed with hepatitis C as well as malignant melanoma. These workers used a double-blind, placebo-controlled study design with 40 patients diagnosed with malignant melanoma. Major depression developed in nearly half the patients who received chronic, high-dose, interferon-α therapy (68). Importantly, the selective serotonin reuptake inhibitor paroxetine significantly reduced the incidence of major depression among patients receiving interferon-α.

Coupled with several early clinical reports showing a relationship between cytokines and various indices of depression in cancer patients, inflammatory theories of depression began to appear at the turn of the twenty-first century. At that time, the elevation in glucocorticoids caused by chronic stress had long been considered to be an important cause of major depression. However, Raison and Miller (69) argued that while it was well known that depression causes heightened production of glucocorticoids, they argued that it was diminished glucocorticoid signalling that was responsible for psychiatric disorders caused by stress. They presented a compelling argument that the impairment in glucocorticoid signalling caused by inflammatory conditions may be more important than the hypothalamic-pituitary axis for major depression. Indeed, it is now known that inflammatory cytokines are responsible for reduced responses to glucocorticoids (70). These early ideas of glucocorticoid resistance were recently substantiated in unmedicated patients with major depressive disorder (71). Interestingly, glucocorticoid resistance was identified only in monocytes but not T cells, thus adding a new layer of complexity to immunopsychiatry. These original ideas formed the scientific basis for testing the potential role of anti-inflammatory agents as treatments in major depression.

The entire field of hormone resistance induced by stress and pro-inflammatory cytokines is currently not well explored. Biomedical scientists often measure the concentrations of cytokines in various disorders, but not the responsiveness of hormone-responsive cells. In medical conditions like type 2 diabetes, rheumatoid arthritis, chronic heart disease and obesity, inflammatory cytokines are also elevated. Several reports have appeared showing that pro-inflammatory cytokines like TNF cause resistance to both insulin (72) and its closely related relative, insulin-like growth factor-I (38). Chronic stress in rodents induces glucocorticoid resistance in monocytes and increases the recruitment of these proinflammatory monocytes into the brain (73). Very low picogram concentrations of TNF cause resistance to IGF-I signalling in neurons, muscle myoblasts and cancer epithelial cells (7). An exciting recent clinical extension of these findings is that the protein tyrosine phosphatase Shp2 has been identified to impair signalling of the anti-inflammatory cytokine IL-10 in both colonic macrophages and monocytes of patients with inflammatory bowel disease (74). Given the emerging link between the gut microbiome, immune system and brain, the concept of pro-inflammatory cytokines impairing normal physiologic responses continues to emerge and to enhance our understanding of a variety of pathologies. Just as ELISAs have been developed to routinely measure pictogram quantities of cytokines in a variety of clinical settings, validated assays are now needed to measure cellular responsiveness and the signalling pathways associated with specific receptor activation.

2.9 Major Advances in PNI During the Past 50 Years

Scientists engaged in the integrative field of PNI research have been important contributors to new knowledge because they have discovered interrelationships between the brain and immune systems. Because of their work and persistence, some of the concepts that were taught to medical and graduate students 50 years ago are no longer accepted. A short list of the major ones is summarized in Figure 2.5 and discussed below.

Acute versus chronic stress. The concept of homeostasis developed by Walter Cannon (75) and Hans Selye's ideas about stress (76) dominated much of the thinking of scientists engaged in PNI research until 2000. Cannon's definition of homeostasis is a process by which steady states in the body are maintained. Selye coined the phrase 'General Adaptation Syndrome', which consists of the three phases of alarm, resistance and exhaustion. But, as pointed out by Bruce McEwen, physiological processes in the body are not homeostatic but rather in a constant state of motion because they are always fluctuating (77,78). By borrowing from the early work on the limitations of the concept of homeostasis to account for the daily fluctuations in blood pressure according to the individual's activities (79), McEwen developed a new concept of stress termed allostatic load. The essential idea of allostasis is that physiologic systems are always adapting to environmental demands in real

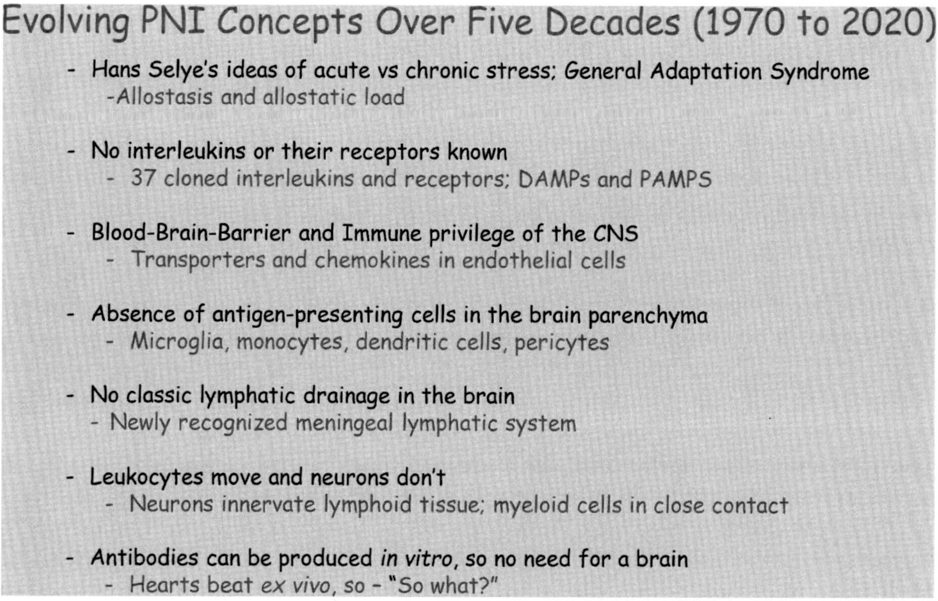

Evolving PNI Concepts Over Five Decades (1970 to 2020)

- Hans Selye's ideas of acute vs chronic stress; General Adaptation Syndrome
  - Allostasis and allostatic load

- No interleukins or their receptors known
  - 37 cloned interleukins and receptors; DAMPs and PAMPS

- Blood-Brain-Barrier and Immune privilege of the CNS
  - Transporters and chemokines in endothelial cells

- Absence of antigen-presenting cells in the brain parenchyma
  - Microglia, monocytes, dendritic cells, pericytes

- No classic lymphatic drainage in the brain
  - Newly recognized meningeal lymphatic system

- Leukocytes move and neurons don't
  - Neurons innervate lymphoid tissue; myeloid cells in close contact

- Antibodies can be produced *in vitro*, so no need for a brain
  - Hearts beat *ex vivo*, so – "So what?"

Figure 2.5 Old and new concepts in PNI that changed from 1970 to 2020. A short discussion of each is presented in the text.

time and in anticipation of events to come. Chronic stress increases the cost for these physiologic changes. These ideas were particularly relevant to mental health disorders like depression and anxiety and their risk factors such as cardiovascular disease, diabetes, social economic status and early life experiences.

Early discoveries in immunology encouraged PNI scientists to test the hypothesis that stress can increase susceptibility to infection by affecting the immune system. It has been known since the days of Louis Pasteur that cold stress increases disease susceptibility to pathogens like *Bacillus anthracis* (80) and *Staphylococcus aureus* (81). Of course, this is not because stress causes disease, but rather that stress interacts with pathogenic microorganisms to exacerbate disease symptoms (7). This message about the importance of interactions was clearly sent by the group of Sheldon Cohen in 1991 (82). These scientists exposed human subjects to a variety of respiratory viruses at doses that increased both respiratory infections and clinical cold symptoms. By using three different measures of psychological stress, they reported that stress increased in a dose-response fashion the severity of acute respiratory illness. This was caused by increased rates of infection rather than increased frequency of symptoms. These data answered the age-old question as to whether stress can cause the common cold, which is a clear 'no' because respiratory infections cannot occur in the absence of a pathogen. But the Cohen data showing that increasing psychological stress augments the severity of infection provides a clear example of a microbe-by-environment interaction.

The same concept in the form of a genetic-by-environment interaction was highlighted a few years later (83). These workers reported data on 847 subjects with short and long polymorphisms in the promoter region of the serotonin transporter. They found that subjects who were homozygous for the short allele of the promoter displayed more symptoms of depression in response to life stress than those subjects who were homozygous for the long allele. This concept of interaction, in all of its forms in all kinds of psychiatric conditions, cannot be underestimated in PNI research.

Interleukins, DAMPS and PAMPS. It is amazing that early pioneers in PNI research could have even begun to correctly interpret their data in the absence of knowledge about the existence of any cytokine. The discovery of 37 interleukins, their receptors and intracellular signalling pathways is perhaps the greatest contributor to the advances that have been made in PNI during the past 50 years. The laboratory of France Haour was the first to show strong binding of radio-labelled IL-1 in coronal sections of the brains of mice (84). The strongest binding occurred in the dentate gyrus, choroid plexus, granule neurons of the hippocampus, meninges and pituitary. The first neuroanatomical description of the localization of interleukin-1 receptor mRNA using *in situ* hybridization was done in the laboratory of Errol de Souza (85). We now know that other cytokine receptors are expressed on neurons (e.g., TNF on dorsal horn afferents in the spinal cord; 86), And, the reciprocal case is also true in that cells of the immune system can express receptors for neurotransmitters (e.g., acetylcholine on macrophages; 87). Indeed, the scientific basis for the emergence and growth of immunopsychiatry rests with these discoveries of cytokine receptors on neurons as well as neurotransmitter receptors on cells of the immune system.

Following closely behind the identification of cytokines and their receptors in terms of importance to the field of immunopsychiatry was the watershed discovery of pattern recognition receptors. These molecules are critically important for proper functioning of the innate immune system. Bruce Beutler at the University of Texas Southwestern Medical

Center and Jules Hoffmann in the CNRS at the University of Strasbourg shared the 2011 Nobel Prize in Physiology or Medicine (88) for their discovery of Toll-like receptors. Pattern recognition receptors are formed of two classes, known as pathogen-associated molecular patterns (PAMPs) and danger-associated molecular patterns (DAMPs) (89,90), both of which are coupled with the more recent discovery of inflammasomes (91). Compounds like extracellular ATP, adenosine, polysaccharides, high-mobility group box 1 (HMGB1) and DNA are all part of the vocabulary of immunologists and neuroscientists who are now engaged in physiological research ranging from vaccine development to neuropathic pain to mood disorders to links between the gut microbiome and health. As but one example, a recent report demonstrated that microbiota in processed foods, particularly minced meat, stimulate Toll-like receptors -1 and -2 to cause hepatic inflammation and to ultimately affect cardiovascular health (92). The importance of the discovery of pattern recognition receptors in understanding and advancing the fields of PNI and immunopsychiatry cannot be understated.

Blood-Brain-Barrier and immune privilege of the central nervous system. In 1960, Peter Medawar as the 'Father of Transplantation' shared the Nobel Prize with Frank Macfarlane Burnet for groundbreaking discoveries on acquired immunological tolerance. Since that time, professors of neuroscience have long preached to their students the truism and importance of the blood-brain-barrier (BBB) that is largely responsible, along with the lack of lymphatic drainage, for conferring immune privilege to the central nervous system. But of course many substances gain entrance to the brain parenchyma by a variety of passive and active transport systems. Brain endothelial cells, pericytes and astrocytes in the neuro-vascular unit all contribute to passive transmembrane diffusion and transport mechanisms involving solute carriers, adsorptive transcytosis and receptor-mediated transcytosis (93). But recent discoveries are changing the view of the BBB as an impermeable barrier that separates the blood and the brain. While it has been accepted for years that substances like glucose and even cytokines can be actively transported across the BBB, the role of chemo-kines and cytokines on activity of endothelial cells is only now coming into focus (94). For example, the monocyte attracting chemokine C-C motif chemokine ligand (CCL)-2 impairs expression of tight junctions (95). Pericytes synthesize nitric oxide and a variety of inter-leukins and cytokines following exposure to LPS (96). Another example is the change in behaviour that occurs following the rise in interferon-α caused by a viral infection (97). It turns out that it is not the interferon-α receptor on brain neuronal cells that drives virus-induced sickness behaviour. Instead, it is expression of chain 1 of this receptor on brain endothelial and epithelial cells that drives the synthesis and movement of CXCL10 into the parenchyma. This chemokine then binds to CXCR3 on CNS neurons and induces sickness behaviour and changes in cognition. New findings such as these and many others are forcing a re-evaluation of the original concept of the BBB as an impassable barrier that separates the brain from blood, which is evolving to the concept that the BBB also serves very important functions as a blood-brain-interface (BBI) (94).

Absence of antigen-presenting cells in the brain parenchyma. The BBB is not the only reason that the original concept of immune privilege was engrained in neuroscience and medical textbooks. Immunologists subsequently discovered three other characteristics of the brain that were considered to be important contributors to the dogma of immune privilege of the brain: (a) absence of antigen-presenting cells, (b) limited expression of both class I and class II major histocompatibility proteins, which are required for graft rejection, and (c) lack of lymphoid drainage in the central nervous system. Technological advances have now established that the evidence for all three of these conditions is flawed. First, significant advances have been made in flow cytometry by coupling heavy metal-stable isotopes to antibodies with defined specificities followed by analysis by mass spectrometry (cytometry time of flight; CyTOF). Using this approach, the laboratory of Asya Rolls demonstrated that all the major phenotypes of immune cells – CD4 T cells, CD8 T cells, B cells, NK cells, monocytes, dendritic cells and other myeloid cells – are present in the central nervous system (98). It is noteworthy that around 80% of these cells are in the meninges and choroid plexus and not in the parenchyma. Consistent with these findings, recent reviews established that nearly all of the currently known myeloid cell subsets are found in the central nervous system (99,100). The beneficial and detrimental effects of parenchymal microglia and perivascular microphages are currently a hot topic of investigation. That is because these cells process and present antigenic peptides in the context of type II major histocompatibility antigens, phagocytose developing and dying cells in the brain, synthesize and secrete a variety of neuroactive substances, including reactive oxygen species, prostaglandins, nitric oxide, cytokines, chemokines and matrix proteases (101). Second, it is true that there is limited expression of class I and II major histocompatibility antigens in the central nervous system. However, what was missing from the early studies was the discovery that several cytokines, particularly interferon-γ, strongly increase expression of these proteins on antigen-presenting cells in the CNS (102). Given that many cytokines are synthesized in the brain in response to stimuli outside the brain, it is apparent that expression and function of major histocompatibility proteins can be upregulated in the brain parenchyma during inflammation. Third, new findings reject the long-held view that there is no lymphatic drainage system in the brain (see next section). The entire original concept of the BBB must be modified based on the past 50 years of research in PNI.

No classic lymphatic drainage in the brain. Throughout the history of neuroscience, there has been a search for the pathway(s) by which cerebrospinal fluid exits the brain and finds its way into the periphery. The studies of Cserr, Harling-Berg and Knopf (103) used tracers to discover that cerebrospinal fluid can follow the arachnoid sheaths of the olfactory nerve, which then passes through the cribriform plate to the nasal mucosa and on to the systemic lymphatics. The more recent discovery by Maiken Nedergaard and colleagues of a glymphatic system provided another pathway for clearing macromolecules and waste products like β-amyloid from the brain (104). Now, two reports not only document but visualize a lymphatic drainage system in the meninges of the brain. Both papers used a variety of antibodies that recognize proteins expressed in peripheral lymphatic endothelial cells (105,106); and both reported the existence of lymphatic vessels along the dural sinuses that exit through the foramina at the base of the skull. These meningeal lymphatic vessels transport both cerebrospinal fluid and lymphocytes (107). Recent findings show that the size of these lymphatic vessels can be increased or decreased by various members of the vascular endothelial growth factor family (108). These discoveries offer a new approach for understanding the functional importance of these vessels in immunopsychiatry and other clinically significant central nervous system disorders.

Leukocytes move and neurons do not. The early findings of Suzanne and David Felten (109) clearly established that tyrosine-positive nerve terminals can be visualized in the spleen. These sympathetic noradrenergic nerve fibres were detected throughout the white pulp and were in close contact with both lymphoid and myeloid cells. Although leukocytes migrate through the spleen whereas the neurons are more stationary, both T and B lymphocytes and resident macrophages and dendritic cells are exposed to the neurotransmitter norepinephrine that is released from sympathetic terminals. That is a big part of the reason why early research in PNI was focused on efferent rather than afferent communication systems. Even though these seminal findings established an anatomical basis for neuroimmunomodulation, the results begged the question: Is there a role for catecholamines in immune regulation? Clearly, that answer is 'yes', as established by the elegant publications by Virginia Sanders over many years of research on T cells (110) and by Shamgar Ben-Eliyahu (111) and Manfred Schedlowski et al. (112) on natural killer cells in rats and humans. This important line of research continues, with the newest data suggesting that the release of norepinephrine from sympathetic nerve terminals rather than circulating epinephrine is likely responsible for the stress-enhanced metastasis of tumour cells (113). The newest results from a large research group in China showed that the stress-induced rise in epinephrine acts through lactate dehydrogenase A (LDHA) to promote development of breast cancer stem cells in mice (114). This paper also established that this pathway appears to be conserved in human breast cancer patients. Importantly, a large drug screen identified Vitamin C as an agent capable of inhibiting this LDHA-mediated glycolysis-dependent pathway and its association with development of the stem-like properties of breast cancer cells (114).

Dwight Nance was the first to establish that the thymus has very limited, if any, parasympathetic innervation (115). Indeed, it appears that the major organs of the immune system, including the thymus, bone marrow, spleen and lymph nodes, are all hardwired with sympathetic but not parasympathetic nerves. That is in contrast to most organs of the body. At the turn of the new century, Kevin Tracey's laboratory reported that the parasympathetic neurotransmitter acetylcholine suppresses TNF synthesis by LPS-stimulated macrophages (116). Newer findings showed that the T helper subset $CD^4+CD44^{hi}CD62L^{lo}$ expresses choline acetyltransferase, an enzyme required for synthesis of acetylcholine (117,118). Electrical stimulation of the vagus nerve suppresses TNF production in mice injected with LPS, an effect that is mediated by the nicotinic acetylcholine receptor alpha7 subunit (117). The nicotinic acetylcholine receptor alpha7 subunit is found on macrophages (87). Much of the TNF produced during sepsis is derived from the spleen, and sectioning of splenic nerves prevented the ability of vagal stimulation to inhibit the production of TNF (119).

As noted above, there is very little parasympathetic innervation of the spleen (120,121,122,123). As such, it now appears that activation of the vagus causes the splenic nerve to release norepinephrine that in turn stimulates splenic T cells to produce acetylcholine (122). It is noteworthy that 80% of vagal fibres are afferent rather than efferent. Recent data show that selective stimulation of afferent vagal fibres almost fully inhibits the ability of LPS to increase plasma TNF (124). Bilateral sectioning of splanchnic sympathetic nerves blocked this effect. These results show clearly that sympathetic terminals of splanchnic nerves are involved in the cholinergic anti-inflammatory pathway, although all the details are not yet fully understood.

Antibodies can be produced in vitro, so no need for the brain. Classic physiological principles make this argument untenable (125). An example using physiology of the heart makes this point. Known for over a century, the Frank–Starling law of the heart can be simplified to mean that the more blood the heart receives, the more blood the heart pumps. Of course, this law assumes that all other factors remain constant, so the Frank–Starling law is based upon the intrinsic function of the myocardium and can pump for years outside the body in an ex vivo system. But it is also well known that the heart is regulated by the nervous and endocrine systems. Acetylcholine slows heart rate, norepinephrine increases heart rate and epinephrine from the adrenal medulla increases not only heart rate but the force of contractions. Without the regulation provided by these exogenous factors, it would be difficult to simply walk across the room, much less run away from a ferocious animal in the middle of a jungle. It is therefore clear that cells of the immune system can produce antibodies and perform other functions both in vitro and in vivo under constant, steady-state conditions. But when the immune system is challenged, such as during an infection, growth of tumour cells, a stressful environment, obesity, wounding or degenerating neurons, a number of exogenous molecules are recruited for allostasis. As such, physiological principles dictate as false the original argument that there is no need for a brain to regulate the immune system.

Coda. The remarkable history of PNI forms the foundation of the emerging field of immunopsychiatry. Most of the progress has occurred during the past 50 years. Thanks to important advances in a number of technologies, biomedical scientists from a variety of disciplines have made discoveries that refute a number of 'gold standard concepts' in both neuroscience and immunology. New techniques and approaches for studying glial biology both in vivo and in vitro are particularly exciting (126). More importantly, these updated concepts have changed the course of health care. Exercise in all forms, mindfulness-based meditation and manipulation of the gut-immune-brain axis are moving these discoveries into changes in lifestyle that are improving the health of all of us (28).

References

1. Solomon GF. Psychoneuroimmunologic approaches to research on AIDS. *Ann NY Acad Sci.* 1987;496:628–36.

2. Kiecolt-Glaser JK, Glaser R. Psychological influences on immunity: implications for AIDS. *Amer Psychol.* 1988;43:892–8.

3. Sturdevant CB, Joseph SB, Schnell G, et al. Compartmentalized replication of R5 T Cell-Tropic HIV-1 in the central nervous system early in the course of infection. *PLOS Pathogens.* 2015. doi.org/10.1371/journal .ppat.1004720

4. Rapuoli R, Santoni A, Mantovani, A. Vaccines: an achievement of civilization, a human right, our health insurance for the future. *J Exp Med.* 2018;216:7–9.

5. Ader R. Psychosomatic and psychoimmunologic research. *Psychosomatic Research.* 1980;42; 307–21.

6. Janković BD. From immunoneurology to immunopsychiatry: neuromodulating activity of anti-brain antibodies. *Int Rev Neurobiol.* 1985;26:249–314.

7. Kelley KW. Norman Cousins lecture. From hormones to immunity: the physiology of immunology. *Brain Behav Immun.* 2004;18:95–113.

8. Benowitz S. Psychoneuroimmunology finds acceptance as science adds evidence. *The Scientist.* 1996. www.the-scientist.com /research/psychoneuroimmunology-finds- acceptance-as-science-adds-evidence -57912

9. Carson MJ, Lo DD. Perspective is everything: an irreverent discussion of CNS-immune system interactions as viewed from different scientific traditions. *Brain Behav Immun.* 2007;21: 367–73.

10. Institute of Medicine. *Capturing Social and Behavioral Domains and Measures in Electronic Health Records. Phase 2.* Washington, DC, National Academies Press; 2014.

11. Pantell MS, Prather AA, Downing,JM, et al. Association of social and behavioral risk factors with earlier onset of adult hypertension and diabetes. *JAMA Network Open.* 2019;2:e193933. doi:10.17226/18951

12. Anonymous. The expanding role of hospital medicine and the co-management of patients. *In Focus*, FOJP Service Corporation. 2013;21:1–20. https://hicgroup.com/sites/default/files/InFocus_Spring13_0.pdf

13. National Public Radio. Timeline. 2006. http://thenewmedicine.org/timeline.html

14. Solomon GF, Moss RH. Emotions, immunity, and disease; a speculative theoretical integration. *Arch Gen Psychiatry*. 1964;11:657–74.

15. Kelley KW. Stress and immune function: a bibliographic review. *Ann Rech Vet*. 1980; 11:445–78.

16. Ader R. *Psychoneuroimmunology*. Academic Press, New York; 1981;1–688.

17. Spector NH, Korneva EA. Neurophysiology, immunophysiology and neuroimmunomodulation. In Ader R, ed. *Psychoneuroimmunology*. Academic Press, New York; 1981:449–69.

18. Korneva EA. Beginnings and main directions of psychoneuroimmunology. *International Journal of Psychophysiology*. 1989;7:1–18.

19. Moyers B. Healing & the mind. 1993. https://billmoyers.com/series/healing-and-the-mind/

20. Pariante CM. Psychoneuroimmunology or immunopsychiatry. *The Lancet Psychiatry*. 2015;2:197–8.

21. Korneva EA. On the history of immunophysiology: first steps and main trends. In Berczi I, ed. *New Insights to Neuroimmune Biology*. Elsevier, Amsterdam; 2010:33–50.

22. Kerza-Kwiatecki AP. Conference report. First international workshop on neuroimmunomodulation (NIM). *J Neuroimmunol*. 1985;10:97–9.

23. Pirzgalska RM, Seixas E, Seidman JS, et al. Sympathetic neuron–associated macrophages contribute to obesity by importing and metabolizing norepinephrine. *Nature Medicine*. 2017;23:1309–18.

24. Cohen JJ. Methodological issues in behavioural immunology. *Immunology Today*. 1987;8:33–4.

25. Laudenslager ML. Research perspectives in psychoneuroimmunology IV, 1993. *Psychoneuroendocrinology*. 1994;19:751–63.

26. Kelley KW. Presidential Address: it's time for psychoneuroimmunology. *Brain Behav Immun*. 2001;15:1–6.

27. Anonymous. Past meeting sites. 2019a. https://pnirs.org/meetings/pastmeetings.cfm

28. Kelley KW. To boldly go where no one has gone before. *Brain Behav Immun*. 2017;66:1–8.

29. Kelley KW, Peng, YP, Liu Q, et al. PsychoNeuroImmunology goes east: Development of the PNIRS China affiliate and its expansion into PNIRS Asia-Pacific. Brain Behav Immun 88:75–87. doi.org/10.1016/j.bbi.2020.04.026.

30. Anonymous. Neural-immune axis. Reciprocal regulation in development, health and disease. 2019c. www.cell-symposia.com/neuroimmunology-2019

31. Ader R, Cohen N, Felten DL. Editorial: brain, behavior, and immunity. *Brain Behav Immun*. 1987;1:1–6.

32. Petry NM, Barry D, Pietrzak RH, et al. Overweight and obesity are associated with psychiatric disorders: results from the national epidemiologic survey on alcohol and related conditions. *Psychosom Med*. 2008;70:288–97.

33. Blalock JE. The immune system as a sensory organ. *J Immunol*. 1984;132:1067–70.

34. Kipnis J. Immune system. The 'seventh sense'. *J Exp Med*. 2018;215:397–8.

35. Konsman JP. Inflammation and depression: a nervous plea for psychiatry to not become immune to interpretation. *Pharmaceuticals*. 2019;12:29. https://doi.org/10.3390/ph12010029

36. Stein M, Miller AH, Trestman RL. Depression, the immune system, and health and illness. *Arch Gen Psychiatry*. 1991;48:171–7.

37. Stein M. Future directions for brain, behavior, and the immune system. *Bull NY Acad Med*. 1992;68:390–410.

38. Kelley KW, Weigent DA, Kooijman R. Protein hormones and immunity. *Brain Behav Immun.* 2007;21:384–92.

39. Farhat K, Bodart G, Charlet-Renard C, et al. Growth hormone (GH) deficient mice with GHRH gene ablation are severely deficient in vaccine and immune responses against *Streptococcus pneumoniae. Front Immunol.* 2018;9:1–15(article 2175).

40. Kiecolt-Glaser JK, Glaser R, Shuttleworth, EC, et al. Chronic stress and immunity in family caregivers of Alzheimer's disease victims. *Psychosom Med.* 1987;49:523–35.

41. Wilson SJ, Padin AC, Birmingham DJ, et al. When distress becomes somatic: dementia family caregivers' distress and genetic vulnerability to pain and sleep Problems. *Gerontologist.* 2018. doi:10.1093/geront/gny150

42. Irwin MR, Olmstead R, Oxman MN. Augmenting immune responses to varicella zoster virus in older adults: a randomized, controlled trial of Tai Chi. *J Am Geriatr Soc.* 2007;55:511–17.

43. Irwin MR, Olmstead R, Carrillo C, et al. Tai chi chih compared with cognitive behavioral therapy for the treatment of insomnia in survivors of breast cancer: a randomized, partially blinded, noninferiority trial. *J Clin Oncol.* 2017;35:2656–65.

44. Lavretsky H, Altstein LL, Olmstead RE, et al. Complementary use of Tai chi chih augments escitalopram treatment of geriatric depression: a randomized controlled trial. *Am J Geriatr Psychiatry.* 2011;19:839–50.

45. Berkenbosch F, van Oers J, del Rey A, et al. Corticotropin-releasing factor-producing neurons in the rat activated by interleukin-1. *Science.* 1987;238:524–6.

46. Sapolsky R, Rivier C, Yamamoto G, et al. Interleukin-1 stimulates the secretion of hypothalamic corticotropin-releasing factor. *Science.* 1987;238:522–4.

47. Morrissey PJ, Charrier K, Alpert A, et al. In vivo administration of IL-1 induces thymic hypoplasia and increased levels of serum corticosterone. *J Immunol.* 1988;141:1456–63.

48. Dantzer R, Kelley KW. Stress and immunity: An integrated view of relationships between the brain and the immune system. *Life Sciences.* 1989;44:1995–2008.

49. Shimabukuro-Vornhagen A, Godel P, Subklewe M, et al. Cytokine release syndrome. *J ImmunoTherapy of Cancer.* 2018;656. doi: 10.1186/s40425-018-0343-9

50. Goetzl EJ. Forward. *J Immunol.* 1985; 135:738. doi: 10.1186/s40425-018-0343-9

51. Stein M, Keller SE, Schleifer SJ. Stress and immunomodulation: the role of depression and neuroendocrine function. *J Immunol.* 1985;135:827–33.

52. Irwin MR. The "P" in PNIRS – A discussion over beer. 2004. https://pnirs .org/resources/docs/Program%20Booklet %202004.pdf

53. Marsland A, Walsh C Lockwood K, et al. The effects of acute of psychological stress on circulating and stimulated inflammatory markers: A systematic review and meta-analysis. *Brain Behav Immun,* 2017;64:208–19.

54. Wan W, Janz L, Vriend CY, et al. Differential induction of *c-Fos* immunoreactivity in hypothalamus and brain stem nuclei following central and peripheral administration of endotoxin. *Brain Res Bull.* 1993;32:581–7.

55. Wan W, Wetmore L, Sorensen C, et al. Neural and biochemical mediators of endotoxin and stress-induced *c-fos* expression in the rat brain. *Brain Res Bull.* 1994;34:7–14.

56. Bluthé RM, Walter V, Parnet P, et al. Lipopolysaccharide induces sickness behaviour in rats by a vagal mediated mechanism. *C R Acad Sci III.* 1994;317:499–503.

57. Watkins LR, Wiertelak EP, Goehler LE, et al. Neurocircuitry of illness-induced hyperalgesia. *Brain Res.* 1994;639:283–99.

58. Fleshner M, Goehler LE, Hermann J, et al. Interleukin-1 beta induced corticosterone elevation and hypothalamic NE depletion is vagally mediated. *Brain Res Bull.* 1995;37:605–10.

59. Layé S, Bluthé RM, Kent S, et al. Subdiaphragmatic vagotomy blocks induction of IL-1 beta mRNA in mice brain in response to peripheral LPS. *Am J Physiol.* 1995;268:R1327–31.

60. Bluthé RM, Michaud B, Kelley KW, et al. Vagotomy blocks behavioural effects of interleukin-1 injected via the intraperitoneal route but not via other systemic routes. *Neuroreport.* 1996;7:2823–7.

61. Fülling C, Dinan TG, Cryan JF. Gut microbe to brain signaling: What happens in vagus . . . *Neuron.* 2019;101:998–1002.

62. Hart BL. Biological basis of the behavior of sick animals. *Neurosci Biobehav Rev.* 1988;12:123–137.

63. Kent S, Bluthé RM, Dantzer R, et al. Different receptor mechanisms mediate the pyrogenic and behavioral effects of interleukin 1. *Proc Natl Acad Sci USA.* 1992a;89:9117–20.

64. Kent S, Bluthé RM, Kelley KW, et al. Sickness behavior as a new target for drug development *TIPS.* 1992b;13:24–28.

65. Yirmiya R. Endotoxin produces a depressive-like episode in rats. *Brain Research.* 1996;711:163–74.

66. Reichenberg A, Yirmiya R, Schuld A, et al. Cytokine-mediated emotional and cognitive disturbances in humans. *Archives of General Psychiatry.* 2001;58:445–52.

67. Capuron L, Ravaud A. Prediction of the depressive effects of interferon alfa therapy by the patient's initial affective state. *N Engl J Med.* 1999;340:1370.

68. Musselman DL, Lawson DH, Gumnick JF, et al. Paroxetine for the prevention of depression induced by high-dose interferon alfa. *N Engl J Med.* 2001;344:961–6.

69. Raison CL, Miller AH. When not enough is too much: the role of insufficient glucocorticoid signaling in the pathophysiology of stress-related disorders. *Am J Psychiatry.* 2003;160:1554–65.

70. Pace TW, Hu F, Miller AH. Cytokine-effects on glucocorticoid receptor function: relevance to glucocorticoid resistance and the pathophysiology and treatment of major depression*Brain Behav Immun.* 2007;21:9–19.

71. Hasselmann H, Gamradt S, Taenzer A, et al. Pro-inflammatory monocyte phenotype and cell-specific steroid signalling alterations in unmedicated patients with major depressive disorder. *Front Immunol.* 2018;9:1–9(article 2693).

72. Hotamisligil GS, Shargill NS, Spiegelman BM. Adipose expression of tumor necrosis factor-alpha: direct role in obesity-linked insulin resistance. *Science.* 1993;259:87–91.

73. Niraula A, Wang Y, Godbout JP, et al. Corticosterone production during repeated social defeat causes monocyte mobilization from the bone marrow, glucocorticoid resistance, and neurovascular adhesion molecule expression. *J. Neuroscience.* 2018;38:2338–40.

74. Xiao P, Zhang H, Zhang Y, et al. Phosphatase Shp2 exacerbates intestinal inflammation by disrupting macrophage responsiveness to interleukin-10. *J Exp Med.* 2019:216(2):337–49. doi:10.1084/jem20181198

75. Cannon W. The wisdom of the body. *Physiol Rev.* 1929;9:399–431.

76. Selye H. Stress and the General Adaptation Syndrome. *Br Med J.* 1950;1:1383–92.

77. McEwen BS, Stellar E. Stress and the individual: mechanisms leading to disease. *Arch Intern Med.* 1993;153:2093–101.

78. McEwen BS. Allostasis and allostatic load: implications for neuropsychopharmacology. *Neuropsychpharmacology.* 1999;22:108–24.

79. Sterling P, Eyer J. Allostasis: A new paradigm to explain arousal pathology. In Fisher S and Reason J, eds. *Handbook of Life Stress, Cognition and Health.* John Wiley and Sons, New York; 1988;629–49.

80. Kelley KW, Curtis SE, Dantzer R. Disease-environment interactions: Another contribution of Louis Pasteur. 2009. www .brainimmune.com/disease-environment-interactions-another-contribution-of-louis -pasteur-1878/

81. Previte JJ, Berry LJ. The effect of environmental temperature on the host–parasite relationship in mice. *J Infect Dis.* 1962;119:201–9.

82. Cohen S, Tyrrell DA, Smit. AP. Psychological stress and susceptibility to the common cold. *N Engl J Med.* 1991;325:606–12.

83. Caspi A, Sugden K, Moffitt TE, et al. Influence of life stress on depression: moderation by a polymorphism in the 5-HTT gene. *Science.* 2003;301:386–9.

84. Ban E, Milon G, Prudhomme N, et al. Receptors for interleukin-1 (alpha and beta) in mouse brain: mapping and neuronal localization in hippocampus. *Neuroscience.* 1991;43:21–30.

85. Cunningham ET, Wada Jr, E, Carter DB, et al. Localization of interleukin-1 receptor messenger RNA in murine hippocampus. *Endocrinology.* 1991;28:2666–8.

86. Holmes GM, Hebert SL SL, Rogers RC, et al. Immunocytochemical localization of TNF type 1 and type 2 receptors in the rat spinal cord. *Brain Res.* 2004;1025:210–19.

87. Wang H, Yu M, Ochani M, et al. Nicotinic acetylcholine receptor α7 subunit is an essential regulator of inflammation. *Nature.* 2003;421:384–8.

88. O'Neill LAJ, Golenbock D, Bowie AG. The history of Toll-like receptors – redefining innate immunity. *Nature Reviews Immunology.* 2013;13:453–60.

89. Matzinger P. Tolerance, danger, and the extended family. *Annual Review of Immunology.* 1994;12:991–1045.

90. Seong SY, Matzinger P. Hydrophobicity: an ancient damage-associated molecular pattern that initiates innate immune responses. *Nature Reviews Immunology.* 2004;4:469–78.

91. Fleshner M, Frank M, Maier SF. Danger signals and inflammasomes: stress-evoked sterile inflammation in mood disorders. *Neuropsychopharmacology.* 2017;42:36–45.

92. Faraj TA, Stover C, Erridge C. Dietary toll-like receptor stimulants promote hepatic inflammation and impair reverse cholesterol transport in mice via macrophage-dependent interleukin-1 production. *Front Immunol.* 2019;10:1404. doi.org/10.3389/fimmu.2019.01404

93. Erickson MA, Banks WA. Neuroimmune axes of the blood–brain barriers and blood–brain interfaces: bases for physiological regulation, disease states, and pharmacological interventions. *Pharmacol Rev.* 2018;70:278–314.

94. Banks WA. From blood-brain barrier to blood-brain interface: new opportunities for CNS drug delivery. *Nat Rev Drug Discov.* 2016;15:275–92.

95. Stamatovic SM, Shakui P, Keep RF, et al. Monocyte chemoattractant protein-1 regulation of blood-brain barrier permeability. *J Cereb Blood Flow Metab.* 2005;25:593–606.

96. Kovac A, Erickson MA, Banks WA. Brain microvascular pericytes are immunoactive in culture: cytokine, chemokine, nitric oxide and LRP-1 expression in response to lipopolysaccharide. *J Neuroinflammation.* 2011;8:139. doi: 10.1186/1742-2094-8-139

97. Blank T, Detje CN, Spieß A. et al. Brain endothelial- and epithelial-specific interferon receptor chain 1 drives virus-induced sickness behavior and cognitive impairment. *Immunity.* 2016;44:901–12.

98. Korin R, Ben-Shaanan TL, Schiller M, et al. High-dimensional, single-cell characterization of the brain's immune compartment. *Nat Neurosci.* 2017;20:1300–9.

99. Mrdjen D, Pavlovic A, Hartmann FJ. et al. High-dimensional single-cell mapping of central nervous system immune cells reveals distinct myeloid subsets in health, aging, and disease. *Immunity.* 2018;48:380–95.

100. Herz J, Filiano AJ, Smith A, et al. Myeloid cells in the central nervous system. *Immunity.* 2017;6:943–56.

101. Galloway DA, Phillips AEM, Owen DRJ, Moore CS. Phagocytosis in the brain: homeostasis and disease. *Frontiers in Immunology.* 2019;10:1–15.

102. John GR, Lee SC, Brosnan CF. Cytokines: powerful regulators of glial cell activation. *Neuroscientist.* 2003;9:10–22.

103. Cserr HF, Harling-Berg CJ Knopf PM. Drainage of brain extracellular fluid into blood and deep cervical lymph and its immunological significance. *Brain Pathol.* 1992;2:269–76.

104. Iliff JJ, Wang M, Liao Y. et al. A paravascular pathway facilitates CSF flow through the brain parenchyma and the clearance of interstitial solutes, including amyloid β. *Sci Transl Med.* 2012;4:147ra111.1–11.

105. Louveau A, Smirnov I, Keyes TJ. et al. Structural and functional features of central nervous system lymphatic vessels. *Nature.* 2015;523:337–41.

106. Aspelund A, Antila S, Proulx ST. et al. A dural lymphatic vascular system that drains brain interstitial fluid and macromolecules. *J Exp Med.* 2015;212:991–9.

107. Louveau A, Herz J, Alme MN, et al. CNS lymphatic drainage and neuroinflammation are regulated by meningeal lymphatic vasculature. *Nat Neurosci.* 2018;21:1380–91.

108. Antila S, Karaman S, Nurmi H, et al. Development and plasticity of meningeal lymphatic vessels. *J Exp Med.* 2017;214:3645–67.

109. Felten DL, Ackerman KD, Wiegand SJ, et al. Noradrenergic sympathetic innervation of the spleen: I. Nerve fibers associate with lymphocytes and macrophages in specific compartments of the splenic white pulp. *J Neurosci Res.* 1987;18:28–36.

110. Sanders VM. The beta2-adrenergic receptor on T and B lymphocytes: do we understand it yet? *Brain Behav Immun.* 2012;26:195–200.

111. Shakhar G, Ben-Eliyahu S. In vivo beta-adrenergic stimulation suppresses natural killer activity and compromises resistance to tumor metastasis in rats. *J Immunol.* 1998;60:3251–8.

112. Schedlowski M, Jacobs R Stratmann G, et al. Changes of natural killer cells during acute psychological stress. *J Clin Immunol.* 1993;13:119–26.

113. Walker AK, Martelli D, Ziegler AL, et al. Circulating epinephrine is not required for chronic stress to enhance metastasis. *Psychoneuroendocrinology.* 2019;99:191–5.

114. Cui B, Luo Y, Tian P, et al. Stress-induced epinephrine enhances lactate dehydrogenase A and promotes cancer stem-like cells. *J Clin Invest.* 2019;129:1030–46. doi.org/10.1172/JCI121685

115. Nance DM, Hopkins DA, Bieger D. Re-investigation of the innervation of the thymus gland in mice and rats. *Brain Behav Immun.* 1987;1:134–47.

116. Borovikova LV, Ivanova S, Zhang M, et al. Vagus nerve stimulation attenuates the systemic inflammatory response to endotoxin. *Nature.* 2000;405:458–62.

117. Rosas-Ballina M, Olofsson PS, Ochani M, et al. Acetylcholine-synthesizing T cells relay neural signals in a vagus nerve circuit. *Science.* 2011;334:98–101.

118. Olofsson PS, Steinberg BE, Sobb, R, et al. Blood pressure regulation by CD4+ lymphocytes expressing choline acetyltransferase. *Nat Biotechnol.* 2016;34:1066–71.

119. Huston JM, Ochani M, Rosas-Ballina M, et al. Splenectomy inactivates the cholinergic anti-inflammatory pathway during lethal endotoxemia and polymicrobial sepsis. *J Exp Med.* 2006;203:1623–8.

120. Nance DM, Sanders VM. Autonomic innervation and regulation of the immune system. *Brain Behav Immun.* 2007;21:736–45.

121. Bratton BO, Martelli D, McKinley MJ, et al. Neural regulation of inflammation: no neural connection from the vagus to splenic sympathetic neurons. *Exp Physiol.* 2012;97:1180–5.

122. Marteelli D, McKinley MJ, McAllen RM. The cholinergic anti-inflammatory pathway: A critical review. *Antonomic Neuroscience: Basic and Clinical.* 2014;182:65–9.

123. Gautron L, Rutkowski JM, Burton MD, et al. Neuronal and nonneuronal cholinergic structures in the mouse gastrointestinal tract and spleen. *J Comp Neurol*. 2013;521:3741–67.

124. Komegae EN, Farmer DGS, Brooks VL, et al. Vagal afferent activation suppresses systemic inflammation via the splanchnic anti-inflammatory pathway. *Brain Behav Immun*. 2018;73:441–9.

125. Kelley KW. Immunological consequences of changing environmental stimuli. In Moberg GP, ed. *Animal Stress*. Bethesda, MD: American Physiological Society; 1985:193–233.

126. Guttenplan KA, Liddelow SA. Astrocytes and microglia: models and tools. *J Exp Med*. 2019;216(1):71–83. http://doi.org/10.1084/jem.20180200

Stress, Immune System and the Brain

Julie-Myrtille Bourgognon, Alison McColl, Maria
Suessmilch, Rajeev Krishnadas and Jonathan Cavanagh

3.1 Introduction

Stress encompasses the psychological perception of pressure from the environment, and the body's physiological response to it. The sources of stress have evolved over time, from predation and natural disasters, to things like interpersonal conflicts and economic insecurities. While in the past, stressors evoked a very acute physical 'fight or flight' response, these events are rare in today's terms. In contrast, the stressors we experience in the modern world are arguably more trivial – they are not often immediately life threatening – however they are more persistent, manifesting as a chronic, low level source of anxiety in our daily lives. The natural stress response involves multiple systems and is designed to provide short-term beneficial effects to the individual to help see them through a threatening situation. It is thought this response is mediated largely through glucocorticoid (GC) production and will rapidly normalize following the stressful event. In the event of chronic exposure to stress, some of these short-term physiological changes fail to return to 'normality', and as a result, the nature of our homeostasis is altered. This chapter will focus on the changes to the immune system and brain mediated through exposure to stress, with particular emphasis on the detrimental effects of chronic stress.

3.2 Controlling the Stress Response

The hypothalamic-pituitary-adrenal (HPA) axis and the autonomic nervous system (ANS) mediate the hormonal and neural response to stress respectively, and are key to understanding how stress influences other body systems (1). While these two systems, presented diagrammatically in Figure 3.1, are separate enough to control independent stress-response cascades, their overlapping neural circuitry and physiological function allows homeostasis to be reached following exposure to stress (1).

Acute stress evokes well-orchestrated physiological changes that together encompass the 'fight or flight' response. This response is driven by the sympathetic nervous system (SNS) and is facilitated by descending nerve fibres that innervate organs and activate physiological changes throughout the body (2). For example, a sharp rise in blood pressure and the reallocation of blood and glucose to the muscles prepares the body for movement (1). The upregulation of neurotransmitters and hormones, to which almost all immune cells express receptors, directs the mobilization and activation of leukocytes from the bone marrow and secondary lymphoid pools into the blood and lymphatic vessels (3). This extravasation of leukocytes and the concurrent increase in blood levels of pro-inflammatory cytokines prepares the host for potential infection or wounding in a non-specific manner. The combined actions of the HPA axis and ANS result in a potent and immediate response

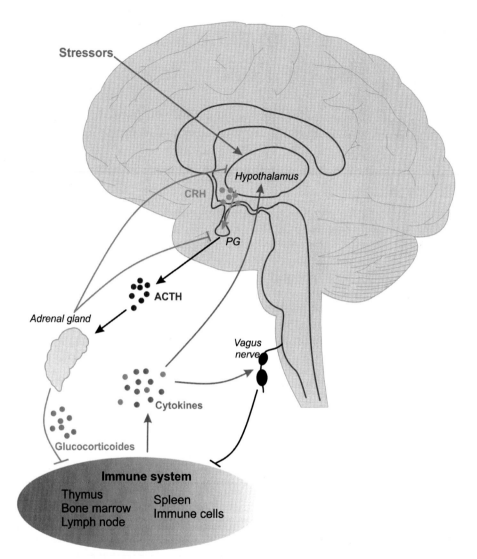

Figure 3.1 Schematic representation of the communication network between the HPA axis, the ANS and the immune system in response to stress (modified from Sternberg, Nature Reviews Immunology, 2006 (4)). Exposure to stressors like pro-inflammatory cytokines leads to the production of corticotropin-releasing hormone (CRH) from the hypothalamus into the vicinity of the pituitary gland (PG). This triggers the release of adrenocorticotropic hormone (ACTH), which promotes the production of glucocorticoids. Glucocorticoids regulate inflammation via their anti-inflammatory properties and also downregulate the HPA axis in order to maintain homeostasis. Another negative-feedback control of systemic inflammation is provided by the vagus nerve fibres following their activation by pro-inflammatory molecules. (A black and white version of this figure will appear in some formats. For the colour version, please refer to the plate section.)

that aims to neutralize threat and return the body to homeostasis (3,4). The acute stress response is self-limiting and quickly resolves, mediated through several efficient negative feedback loops. Thus, this fundamental system confers a survival advantage to the host without being harmful in itself.

3.3 Stress and the Immune System

Over the last 30 years or so, a significant amount of research has been directed towards understanding the effect of stress on various facets of the immune system and the immune response. As mentioned, stress can influence the production of inflammatory mediators and the activation and mobilization of immune cells (4). In the context of chronic stress, the continued or repeated activation of this process will dampen the host's ability to resolve the response leading to prolonged changes in the immune system. Such changes have been reported in a number of different species, from Atlantic salmon to rodents and humans, and can affect multiple components of the immune system. This series of events is thought to increase the risk of several age-related inflammatory conditions such as cardiovascular disease and Alzheimer's disease (5,6).

Chapter 1 in this book has already provided an overview of the multiple communication pathways that exist between the immune system and the brain. These include the afferent and efferent signalling arms of the inflammatory reflex, the recently described glymphatic system and the active transport systems within the blood-brain-barrier (BBB). Thus, the immune system and the central nervous system (CNS) are more intimately linked than historically thought and changes in peripheral immune components following exposure to stress can be relayed to the brain through several defined mechanisms. These pathways may be key to the onset of neuropsychiatric conditions in response to stress-mediated immune changes and are highlighted in Figure 3.2. Indeed, there is some evidence to suggest that chronic stress induces a vulnerability to psychiatric disorders by altering neural circuitry (7,8).

3.4 Preclinical Models of Stress

With a growing interest in the pathophysiology of the stress response and in the potentially negative consequences following exposure to stress, a number of preclinical rodent models have been established to interrogate, among other things, the immunological response to stressful stimuli. Since long-term immune changes are most commonly reported following chronic stress, we will focus on some of the most representative animal models presented in the literature. As always, it is important to consider the nature of the stimulus in the various models used to study stress. A variety of stimuli produce patterns of inflammation in the brain. Pathogens and pathogen-mimics, such as lipopolysaccharide (LPS) and poly-IC (PIC), are *acute* systemic immune challenges and while similar immune-mediated inflammatory pathways will be engaged by stress models, the nature of these responses are distinctive in terms of magnitude and length. Nonetheless, activation of these pathways provides an opportunity to explore the consequences of neuroinflammation on neural cells.

3.4.1 Repeated Social Defeat (RSD)

The RSD model is arguably the most common rodent model of social stress. This model involves the introduction of a large, aggressive male mouse into the home cage of a resident mouse of a different strain. The natural hierarchy formation behaviour displayed by rodents means these confrontations will result in the resident mouse being subjected to bouts of social defeat by the aggressor mouse (9). While each interaction will last only five–ten minutes, this exposure is repeated for several consecutive days. The RSD model has been used extensively to study the neuroimmune effects of chronic stress (10) and is accompanied

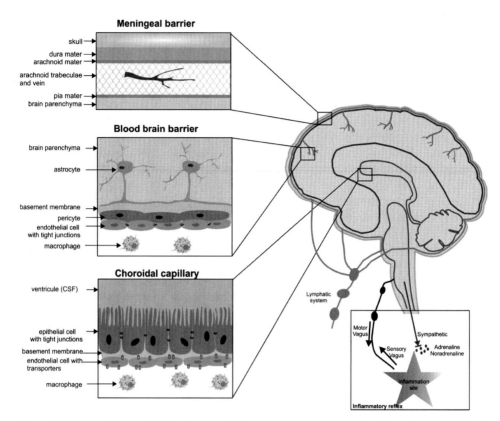

Figure 3.2 **Routes of communication between the immune system and CNS.** The different facets of the blood-brain interface can become leaky or break down following inflammation or physical trauma. In the meningeal barrier, the pia mater allows cerebrospinal fluid (CSF) that circulates in the subarachnoid space to enter the brain interstitial fluid. The BBB is formed by small blood capillaries that infiltrate into the deeper structures of the brain. Any leakage from the blood into the brain is prevented by the presence of pericytes and astrocytes wrapped around the endothelial cells bearing tight junctions. The choroid plexus is formed by epithelial cells with tight junctions in order to prevent the passage of molecules from the CSF into the brain. However, the choroidal endothelial cells contain transporters that allow selective active transport of substances into and out of the CSF. The lymphatic drainage system is another tool for the organism to filter inflammatory signals as well as maintain water and solute balance, homeostasis and metabolism. Finally, the inflammatory reflex is a neural circuit that regulates the immune response to injury and infection The vagus nerve sends the inflammatory information via the nucleus tractus solitarius to the forebrain where the information is integrated, and a response is sent back via the efferent vagus branch of the inflammatory reflex to peripheral organs in order to suppress pro-inflammatory cytokine release. Sympathetic output directs adrenaline and noradrenaline to the inflammation site to attenuate the response. (A black and white version of this figure will appear in some formats. For the colour version, please refer to the plate section.)

by the activation of stress-reactive neurocircuitry, prolonged anxiety-like behaviour, microglial activation and increased cytokine signalling (11). Therefore, this model serves as a fundamental source of the preclinical data we will mention in the next section.

3.4.2 Chronic Unpredictable/Mild/Variable Stress (CUS/CMS/CVS)

The CUS/CMS/CVS model is, as the name suggests, a series of mild yet unpredictable stressors that are inflicted in short intervals (hours) over a period of weeks (12). Studies will use a rotation of, for example, damp bedding, cage shaking, restraint, foot shock, cold swimming, white noise and cage tilting. This model was initially used in the 1980s to investigate the effects of several antidepressants, demonstrating that downstream behavioural changes and anhedonia could be prevented with concurrent chronic antidepressant therapy (13,14). The behavioural and physiological changes following this model bear a distinct similarity to the symptoms of depression, with one review stating that the only symptoms of depression not mirrored by this model are those that are only accessible via verbal enquiry (15). Thus, due to its validity and translational potential, the CUS model is largely associated with stress-induced depression.

3.4.3 Chronic Restraint/Immobilization Stress (CRS/CIS)

As the name suggests, this model involves restraining rodents, most often in a cylindrical tube, for one–two hours per day for several days or weeks. This model is more often used in its acute form, where rodents are exposed to restraint on a single occasion, due to some reports of habituation following multiple exposures, however there is a developing literature surrounding its repeated use. This is a particularly relevant model in the context of stress-mediated changes in brain structure and function, which will be discussed later in Section 3.5.

3.4.4 Early Life Stress (ELS)

Maternal separation is one of the most commonly used forms of ELS in rodents. Separation normally lasts for a period of several hours and is repeated for several consecutive days (typically during the first two postnatal weeks) (16). ELS has also been applied in the form of the limited bedding and nesting model (17), or as a 'two-hit' model using maternal separation followed by either limited bedding or early weaning (18). There is some controversy as to whether ELS mimics neglect, abuse or both, but variations of this model are generally thought to represent childhood maltreatment/adversity.

While these stress models are commonly used to study the mechanisms and consequences of the stress response, it is important to highlight that these models are not without their limitations. There is a significant amount of literature reporting the importance of experimental variables such as rodent strain, sex, age, source of animals and ambient conditions for the outcome of these experiments. This is not to mention the extensive variation that exists with regards to the models themselves; for example, the exposure time to the stressor, the length of the model and the nature of the stressor, even within a defined model. Despite an attempt by some to ratify this by publishing standardized protocols, the sensitivity of the stress response to all these factors means the preclinical stress biology literature is highly heterogeneous. With this in mind, it is difficult to generalize 'the stress response' and particular attention should be paid to the methodologies when surveying the literature.

3.4.5 Stress Effects on Peripheral Immune Cells

The nature of the stressor and the duration of exposure can impact on the proliferation, release and function of leukocytes to promote a more specialized immune response. The activation and mobilization of immune cells from the bone marrow (BM) is particularly important in this regard as it is the site of proliferation and maturation of mesenchymal stromal cells (MSCs), specialized stem cells that are able to differentiate into a range of cell types as required. RSD increases monocyte and granulocyte progenitor cells in the BM, although the overall BM cell numbers initially decrease, largely due to a loss of mature cells (19,20). Monocytes begin to accumulate in the circulation after two or three cycles of RSD and continue to increase with subsequent exposures (19,21). This same pattern is not seen in lymphocyte populations, with RSD in fact reducing T and B cell numbers in BM and circulation, suggesting a shift towards the production of innate immune cells (19). This myelopoietic response is noted alongside increased norepinephrine (NE) in BM stroma, and is mediated via the chemokine CXCL12, an important molecule in both neurodevelopment and immune homeostasis. Indeed, blocking NE signalling (using either genetic deletion or pharmacological inhibition) restores CXCL12 expression and reduces circulating mono-cytes and neutrophils (22–24). Thus, RSD activates sympathetic NE signalling that reduces CXCL12 and promotes myeloid cell production and mobilization. These RSD-induced circulating monocytes are less mature and more inflammatory than 'homeostatic' mono-cytes, displaying potent phagocytic capacity, increased reactive oxygen species (ROS) production and increased pro-inflammatory cytokine production (19–21). Thus, RSD stress-induced monocytes are mobilized and exhibit a pro-inflammatory phenotype (25,26).

RSD causes an initial increase in GCs when the aggressor mouse is first introduced into the home cage. This returns to baseline a few hours after cessation of the stress cycle and does not have a lasting effect on homeostatic levels (24). However, the RSD-induced myeloid cells are resistant to the inhibitory effects of GCs. The normal negative feedback loop of GCs leads to the increased transcription of anti-inflammatory molecules (27), however, after RSD, this mechanism is impaired and GC-insensitive monocytes begin to accumulate. The repeated and chronic nature of the stress is important as the GC resistance is only noted after six RSD cycles and will persist for at least ten days after stress termination (28). These GC-resistant circulating monocytes are thought to be particularly important in the neuroinflammatory stress response as they have been shown to traffic to the brain in an adoptive transfer model and will home to perivascular spaces of regions associated with fear/anxiety, for example the hypothalamus, amygdala and hippocampus (21,23). This monocyte infiltration occurs despite the BBB remaining intact (assessed using Evans Blue). These cells are evident in the brain after three RSD cycles and peak after six cycles and correlate with IL-1b upregulation and anxiety-like behaviour. These observations persist for at least eight days after the last cycle of RSD but are no longer apparent after 24 days (29). The absence of chemokine receptors CCR2 or CX3CR1 (using CCR2KO and CX3CR1KO mice respectively) prevented monocyte recruitment to the brain after RSD, but these inflammatory monocytes were still released into the circulation, suggesting monocyte recruitment to the brain is an active process mediated via chemokine signalling (21).

Indeed, RSD induced the expression of adhesion molecules that could facilitate immune cell entry into the brain (30). For example, increased expression of E-selectin was observed in stress-reactive brain regions where monocyte trafficking occurs. In addition, intracellular adhesion molecule (ICAM) and vascular cell adhesion molecule (VCAM) expression was increased on BBB endothelial cells after six cycles of RSD and correlated temporally with monocyte recruitment into the brain. These adhesion molecules are important mediators of the migration of leukocytes from the blood into the tissues and changes in expression are thought to be in response to pro-inflammatory cytokines and chemokines (31). Microglia and macrophages are also potential sources of matrix metalloproteinases (MMPs), a family of degrading enzymes that help break down the extracellular matrix and endothelial cell tight junctions of the BBB. These enzymes are thought to be important for facilitating leukocyte migration from the perivascular space into the brain parenchyma and are increased in response to inflammation and stress (32,33). Indeed, genome-wide transcriptional profiling indicates splenic monocytes upregulate several MMPs in response to RSD implicating this as a potential mechanism of entry, however further studies are needed to determine if monocyte infiltration into the brain is truly MMP-mediated.

While a lot of effort has been made to characterize this monocyte-associated stress response, it is important to note that it cannot be generalized to all other rodent models of chronic stress. It is also important to note that some of the response to RSD could be due to exposure to biting from the aggressor, which results in local inflammation and increased pain. This would act as an initial immune insult and could offer an additional priming effect, however daily treatment with the anxiolytic drug Clonazepam, prevents myelopoiesis without affecting the magnitude of biting, indicating that biting alone could not account for the whole RSD response (34). CUS has been associated with increases in haematopoietic stem cells (HSCs, progenitor cells that are able to differentiate into any kind of blood cell) in the BM, prior to an increase of circulating inflammatory monocytes and neutrophils (22). This response is thought to be mediated through an NE-induced reduction in CXCL12, in keeping with the findings from the RSD studies, however the migration of these leukocytes into the brain was not examined.

There is also evidence to suggest that chronic stress can have a modulatory effect on the adaptive immune system, although much of the literature has been explored in the context of cancer. Frick et al. reported accelerated tumour progression and decreased survival when CRS was used alongside a T cell lymphoma model (35). This was thought to be the result of impaired cytotoxic T cell responses against tumour cells alongside a general suppression of T cell activity. Similarly, Budiu et al. reported that stress was associated with increased tumour angiogenesis, increased metastasis, attenuated T cell responses and decreased survival in a mouse model of breast cancer (36). Interestingly, their results were differentially regulated depending on the nature of the stressor, comparing both restraint and social isolation models. These findings have been supported by other rodent studies that indicate immune impairment is mediated through the suppression of tumour-specific cytotoxic T cells and the secretion of IFN γ (37).

3.4.6 Stress Effects on CNS-Resident Microglia

In addition to the mobilization and activation of peripheral immune cells, stress can mediate direct effects on brain-resident immune cells. Microglia represent 10–15% of all brain cells and are tissue-resident macrophages that originate from the yolk sac and colonize the brain early in embryogenesis, before BBB formation (38). Frank et al. have described microglia as immunosensors of the stress response as they express neuroendocrine receptors, neurotransmitter receptors and immune receptors, making them sensitive to all components of the physiological stress response (39). Morphological changes in microglia in response to stress have been well documented, however it can prove challenging when trying to unify the findings. Some report hyper-ramification and longer, thicker processes (40), while others describe de-ramification and a retraction of processes (23), albeit using different models of stress. Nonetheless, there is a strong consensus to suggest that microglia are sensitive to stress of varying natures and are quick to respond in one way or another (41).

Stress-induced NE and GCs can activate microglia, particularly in regions of the brain that have been associated with the stress response (hypothalamus, pituitary, hippocampus, amygdala). Blocking either β-adrenergic or GC receptors can prevent this (23). Reader et al. report that, with regards to RSD, microglia are characterized by an altered neuroinflammatory profile; increased cytokines (IL-1b, IL-6, TNF-α), increased CCL2 and reduced anti-inflammatory regulation of neuron-derived CX3CL1 and CX3CR1 (11). Microglia also change morphology and become amoeboid, akin to activation. These microglia are 'primed' and produce an exaggerated inflammatory response upon subsequent immune challenge. This is noted alongside reduced social interaction and open field exploration, suggesting an increase in anxiety-like behaviour (29). A recent review by Churchward et al. described a 'niche' role for microglia that supports the homeostatic maintenance and function of the nervous system into adulthood, moving away from the idea that microglia are somewhat senescent until activated (42). They highlight that, in addition to the direct effects of microglial activation following exposure to stress or inflammation, the interruption of these crucial 'niche' functions could lead to deficits in plasticity, neurocircuitry and neurogenesis if not promptly reinstated. The use of minocycline (a drug used to inhibit microglial activation) provides some evidence to support this theory as it attenuates pro-inflammatory cytokine increase and protects against stress-associated deficits in cognitive memory tasks and depressive-like and anxiety-like behaviours, indicating that the activation of microglia mediates behavioural and cognitive alterations (41). It is important to note, however, that minocycline can also affect other immune cell types making it difficult to infer a causal role for microglia specifically (43). Nonetheless, chronic stress exposure can affect microglia morphology and sensitivity and disrupt crucial homeostatic functions, while, in parallel, peripheral immune cells can be mobilized to the brain. The cumulative effect of this cellular stress response is outlined in Figure 3.3.

3.4.7 The Immune Priming Effects of Stress

There is significant evidence to suggest that exposure to stress could prime the immune system and moderate neuroinflammation following a subsequent insult. However, the literature is mixed as to the downstream effects of this, with some suggesting prior exposure to stress imparts a pro-inflammatory priming effect, whereas others suggest an anti-inflammatory, protective effect.

Wohleb et al. propose that RSD stress confers a lasting stress-sensitivity phenotype (29). On day 24 post RSD cycles, when almost all stress phenotypes had normalized, mice were exposed to a 'sub-threshold' stress (a single 2-hour exposure to the aggressor that alone would not induce monocyte trafficking, microglia activation or anxiety-like behaviour). Stress-sensitized mice re-established anxiety-like behaviour and exaggerated social avoidance, along with reinstated monocyte trafficking to the brain, activation of microglia and elevated pro-inflammatory cytokine signalling. Interestingly, in this context, monocyte trafficking did not appear to be dependent on egress from the BM, rather primed monocytes are thought to have been released from a splenic reservoir of newly differentiated monocytes (29). Indeed splenectomy prior to 'sub-threshold' stress exposure attenuated the response (29,44). Like monocyte egress from the BM, release of splenic monocytes is thought to be driven by NE signalling and can be prevented using a peripheral sympathetic inhibitor, such as guanethidine (44). Administration of this, or β-adrenergic receptor antagonists, prior to stress re-exposure prevented monocyte trafficking, anxiety-like behaviour and microglial cytokine expression, irrespective of the intervention being able to cross the BBB. In addition, Cohen et al. have hypothesized that chronic stress-induced GC resistance may

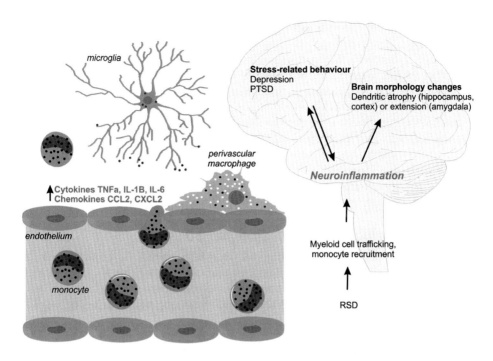

Figure 3.3 Stress-induced microglia activation and macrophage recruitment to the brain following RSD have long-term effects on brain morphology and behaviour. Repeated social defeat triggers inflammatory monocytes to cross the BBB and differentiate into perivascular and parenchymal macrophages. These cells and activated microglia contribute to the neuroinflammatory signalling and the enhanced production of cytokines and chemokines, which are involved in specific regional morphology changes and stress-related behaviour. (A black and white version of this figure will appear in some formats. For the colour version, please refer to the plate section.)

dampen the anti-inflammatory effects of GCs and induce prolonged production of pro-inflammatory mediators – an effect already alluded to regarding the GC-resistant monocyte pathway in the RSD/CUS models (45).

Kelly et al. performed a comparison study examining the response to LPS and PIC following either one-week of continuous corticosterone (CORT) exposure, or 90 days of intermittent CORT exposure (every other week). They report that a single week-long exposure to CORT significantly increased the expression of a number of inflammatory cytokines in the brain following LPS and PIC administration compared with controls, and that this priming effect was evident even with a 30-day lag period prior to inoculation (46). Furthermore, repeated CORT exposure over a 90-day period induced a response in the brain that was ten-fold higher than the exaggerated response observed following single CORT exposure. These findings suggest that prolonged exposure to stress increases susceptibility to immune insults by an order of magnitude, highlighting the potential danger of persistent stressors.

Brachman et al. attempted to investigate whether lymphocytes retain memory of psychosocial stress by adoptively transferring lymphocytes from RSD or control mice into Rag2KO mice, which lack mature lymphocytes (7). In contrast to Kelly et al., they reported that mice receiving cells from stressed donors displayed lower levels of blood pro-inflammatory cytokines, microglia akin to a neuroprotective anti-inflammatory phenotype, increased hippocampal neuron proliferation and higher levels of plasma CORT, when compared with those receiving cells from healthy donors. The authors propose that this memory-driven, anti-inflammatory state is a potential mechanism of resilience, which we discuss later in Section 3.9. It is, however, possible that stress memory is retained by cells other than lymphocytes, and it is important to consider the overall developmental and immune consequences of lacking mature lymphocytes.

Overall, the experiments described in this section detail a potential pathway wherein repeated stress generates a bone marrow response that facilitates the mobilization of pro-inflammatory leukocytes into the circulation. Subsequently, changes in chemokines, adhesion molecules and MMPs may allow these cells to infiltrate into the brain and alter CNS homeostasis by acting on brain-resident immune cells. While we have mentioned the altered state and activation status of specific cell types, stress can also induce changes in brain structure and connectivity, which will be discussed in the following section.

3.5 Stress-Induced Changes in Brain Structure

There is already a significant amount of work describing the experience-induced plasticity of the brain with regards to its structure and connections (47). Several regions of the brain such as the prefrontal cortex (PFC), the hippocampus and amygdala adapt to stress by changing their morphology and reshaping the cellular network and chemistry.

3.5.1 Cortex Morphology

The PFC is the most evolved brain region and plays a key role in decision-making and executive control, behavioural adaptation and working memory (48–50). Chronic restraint stress has been associated with dendritic atrophy of the medial PFC (mPFC), as apical spine density and length are reduced (by 16% and 20% respectively) (51–53). However, this effect is not uniform across the PFC as dendritic extension has been described in the lateral orbitofrontal cortex (OFC), a subregion of the PFC involved in emotion and social recognition (54). Chronic restraint stress led to a 43% increase arborization in the OFC, whereas apical and branching were reduced in mPFC (55). As we have already mentioned, stress can influence microglia morphology and function (56). In turn, these modifications can modulate the morphology of the mPFC. Following CUS, layer 1 of the mPFC of rodents is remodelled by brain-resident microglia and displays a reduction in dendritic spine density, particularly in male mice (57). This effect is mediated by the neuronal colony-stimulating factor 1 receptor (CSF1 R) expression and correlates with the expression of anxiety- and depressive-like behaviours.

3.5.2 Amygdala Morphology

The amygdala detects threats and processes emotions (58). Chronic stress exposure leads to dendritic extension in the amygdala with cells of the basolateral amygdala (BLA) undergoing a marked increase in apical dendritic arborization and spine density (59). Chronic immobilization stress elicits permanent dendritic hypertrophy in BLA principal neurons (60). An fMRI study on the effect of unpredictable early stress in mice described strengthened connectivity between the amygdala and the PFC and hippocampus (61).

3.5.3 Hippocampus Morphology

The hippocampus is involved in short- and long-term memory processing and consolidation as well as spatial memory. An MRI study demonstrated that rats that experienced CRS showed a reduction in hippocampus volume (62). Anatomical reconstruction of neuron-specific Nissl-stained tissue allows for precise localization of this volume loss and shows that it is detected particularly in the dentate gyrus, and CA1 and CA3 regions (63). However, the degree of volume reduction varies according to the type of stress, as CUS results in moderate CA3 atrophy compared to CRS (59). Furthermore, stress-induced shrinkage of dendrites of hippocampal CA3 and dentate gyrus neurons, loss of spines in CA1 neurons (64,65) and a significant atrophy of the CA1 pyramidal cell dendrites were described in adulthood following chronic neonatal bedding stress (66). Like much of the stress response, the timing and type of stressor will differentially affect brain structures. Mice exposed to CIS demonstrated dendritic retraction of CA3 short-shaft pyramidal neurons as well as a retraction of dendrites of dorsal CA1 pyramidal neurons (67). Similarly, the dentate gyrus undergoes a reduction of neuronal cells following chronic stress (68), among which are cells undergoing proliferation (69). The shortening and loss of dendritic spines has been linked to a more active microglial phagocytosis of cellular elements in mice subjected to CUS (70). This key role of microglia depends on CX3CL1 activity and is necessary for the development of depressive-like symptoms (70).

3.6 Neuroplasticity as a Mediator for Psychiatric Pathology

The morphological changes triggered by stress that we have described above are accompanied by a remodelling of neuronal connections in order to adjust the brain cell response to the new, stress-related environment. These modifications are mostly studied using electrophysiology and involve an array of molecules such as neurotransmitters, neurotrophic factors and hormones. For instance, neuronal cell recordings performed in rat hippocampal slices showed that acute stress causes an imbalance of synaptic plasticity, favouring long-term depression (LTD) over long-term potentiation (LTP), leading to synaptic hypofunction, destabilization and neuronal loss (71,72). Adrenal steroids play an important role in modulating hippocampal structure under stress as these molecules interact with an array of chemicals that modulate the brain stress response such as gamma-aminobutyric acid (GABA), glutamate and extracellular molecules such as neural cell adhesion molecules.

Brain-derived neurotrophic factor (BDNF) is involved in the maturation of GABAergic circuits and studies have shown that BDNF levels are dynamically modulated during chronic stress. CIS elevates BDNF levels in the BLA, an increase that lasts for at least 21 days after the termination of stress (73). This temporal response is consistent with earlier findings on CIS-induced dendritic hypertrophy in the BLA (60), which was also reported 21 days later. However, this effect is not homogenous in all brain regions. Indeed, in the hippocampal CA3 region, CIS triggers a decrease in BDNF levels that reverses to basal levels within this 21-day period, suggesting that BDNF is differentially regulated depending on the region of the brain (73).

Inflammatory molecules can cause glutamate-related neurotoxicity as they impact on almost all aspects of glutamate neurotransmission, including multiple cellular effects that influence both release and reuptake mechanisms (74). Cytokines like TNF may amplify and alter the magnitude and propagation of intracellular Ca^{2+} oscillations to transfer immune signals and to mediate changes in neural activity (75). Further, in the context of inflammation, glial cells and trafficking macrophages increase surface expression of cysteine/glutamate exchanger (Xc) transporters that extrude glutamate into the extrasynaptic space in exchange for cysteine. These Xc transporters release large volumes of glutamate in close proximity to extrasynaptic binding sites that, when stimulated chronically, trigger apoptosis. Thus, inflammatory cytokines may be an important mechanism for glutamate toxicity in the context of stress-induced inflammation.

3.7 Clinical Studies of Stress and the Immune System

This chapter has focused on the preclinical studies examining the stress-induced immune response in rodents thus far; however, there is also a significant amount of clinical evidence to support stress-related immune changes in humans. We will discuss some of the broad findings that best echo the preclinical work presented earlier in Sections 3.4–3.6.

A large meta-analysis highlighted that the severity and chronicity of stressors can impact on the outcome of several immunological parameters (76). This is in keeping with preclinical work, where results are varied, and the nature of stress can affect experimental findings. The meta-analysis reported that chronic stress could affect nearly every aspect of the functional immune system, including adaptive T cell and antibody responses (76). Some studies have reported reduced GC receptor-mediated transcription and a heightened inflammatory profile of circulating monocytes, suggesting a pro-inflammatory phenotype that is insensitive to GC-medicated immunosuppression. Miller et al. reported this pattern following genome-wide expression analysis of peripheral blood monocytes from familial caregivers of brain cancer patients and matched, non-carer, controls (77). This was reported alongside a two-fold increase in circulating C-reactive protein (CRP) in the caregivers. In addition, an in vitro study examining blood leukocytes isolated from patients with post-traumatic stress disorder (PTSD) identified higher levels of spontaneously produced IL-1, IL-6 and TNF-α when compared with healthy controls. Furthermore, this study highlighted that immune priming may occur, as subsequent exposure to LPS, a potent immune stimulus, resulted in exaggerated IL-6 production.

Neuroimaging techniques such as MRI have been the investigative tool of choice in exploring the relationship between the immune-mediated stress response and brain structure and connectivity. In keeping with preclinical findings, specific regions implicated include the amygdala, hippocampus, mPFC, anterior cingulate cortex and insula (78). For example, stress-mediated increases in neural activity in the amygdala are associated with increases in IL-6 and individuals showing stronger coupling between the amygdala and the dorsomedial PFC also showed a heightened inflammatory response to stress (79). Childhood stress studies have also demonstrated changes in amygdala volume, but are conflicting as to whether the volume increases (80) or decreases (81). If we consider PTSD an example of a stress-induced human condition, meta-analytical data reveal alterations in volume, function, and functional connectivity of the hippocampus, thought to be mediated through the upregulation of pro-inflammatory cytokines (82).

Finally, maternal stress is thought to be a significant risk factor for negative outcomes in offspring and stress during pregnancy is highly associated with the onset of neuropsychiatric disorders, including schizophrenia and depression (83). In addition, some studies have reported that stress during pregnancy is associated with reduced head circumference at birth and a reduction in brain volume (84), although other studies have been unable to replicate this (85). It has been proposed that the negative effects of maternal stress on offspring are mediated through changes in the immune system, specifically dysregulation of glucocorticoid: immune coordination.

While clinical studies often struggle to demonstrate causative links, many of the findings from preclinical work, including changes in immune status and brain connectivity, have also been shown in humans following exposure to stress. Further work is required to clarify the mechanisms of this response in humans; however, these findings further support the idea of stress interacting with the immune system and the CNS.

3.8 Stress in the Context of the Bayesian Brain

We have thus far presented an overview of the literature that associates stress with immune system and brain changes, however biological data is often limited due to its correlative nature. To attempt to overcome this, and to allow us to understand the causal relationship with behaviour, it is possible to apply a mathematical model as a framework. In this section of the chapter, we will examine stress in the context of the Bayesian brain and predictive processing.

Current predictive processing theories hypothesize that the brain is not just a stimulus-response organ, but also an inference engine that actively generates statistical models (predictions) of the world it lives in (86–89). In this context, the brain uses its sensory inputs to actively sample information from its world in order to gather evidence for the model it has generated. Here, the brain maximizes the evidence (model) of its world – both its external and internal milieu. Therefore, the sensory input is compared against the brain's own model of the world, and if the sensory input matches (provides good enough evidence for) the brain's model of the world, status quo is maintained. However, if the sensory input does not match the existing (prior) model, a *prediction error* is generated. Within a hierarchical neuronal framework, as in the brain, predictions generated within the higher levels (within the deep pyramidal cells) are compared to the lower level sensory evidence and, given a mismatch; prediction error signals are generated (within the superficial pyramidal cells). The brain maintains itself within a limited set of states. In fact, Friston et al. suggest that because the brain (being a self-organising living agent that resists a tendency to disorder) maintains itself within a limited set of states, it actively minimizes a mathematical quantity called 'free energy' (surprisal/surprise). This 'free energy' is the long-term average of all the prediction errors we alluded to above, given a model of the world (87,88,90). On experiencing a sensory input, the brain minimizes prediction error using one of the following three strategies: 1) the internal model is updated, in order to match them to the sensory samples from the world (perception); 2) the brain actively changes its sampling space, until the sensory input matches its internal model (action); or 3) the sensory input, and hence the prediction error, is ignored (biased attention), by adjusting the gain (precision) through neuromodulatory mechanisms (88,91). While experimental evidence for predictive processing theories is sparse, this framework provides a strong theoretical background against which neuroimmune signalling and stress can be tested.

3.8.1 Stress as Uncertainty (Persistent Expected Surprise)

In keeping with the above framework, Peters et al. suggest that in the long run, the brain minimises 'expected free energy' thereby minimising 'expected surprise' – also known as entropy or *uncertainty* (92). In line with Mason (1959), they quantify any condition as stressful if it is novel, unpredictable and uncontrollable, for example any situation that increases uncertainty (93). In other words, we feel uncertain when we anticipate and cannot avoid an increase in the 'expected surprise'. An increase in uncertainty is associated with 1) activation of locus coeruleus (LC) and NE release, which, through neuromodulation, leads to enhanced cortical information transmission, resulting in precision allocation to sensory input/ prediction error; 2) activation of the SNS, allocating more energy to the brain; and 3) activation of the HPA axis, that suspends cortical plasticity (learning) (94). Persistent uncertainty and the activation of the above systems leads to failure of allostasis (an adaptive process for maintaining homoeostasis) and increased allostatic load (the wear and tear on the body and brain as a result of persistent stress) (94). Within the predictive processing context, Peters et al. redefine stress as 'the individual's state of uncertainty about what needs to be done to safeguard physical and mental wellbeing' (92). They suggest that altering the functional and structural neuronal architecture often makes it possible to avoid or master states of uncertainty. They define three forms of stress. 'Good stress' refers to episodes of uncertainty that leads to a successful updating of the internal model of the world (hence, uncertainty resolution). 'Tolerable stress', where an updating of the internal model of the world is not successful, however, habituation leads to a partial resolution of the uncertainty. And finally, 'toxic stress', which refers to persistent unresolved uncertainty due to a failure of model updating and habituation. In this case, the damaging effects of stress consequently prevail, leading to poor physical and mental outcomes. Redefining stress as above gives us the opportunity to incorporate stress, or uncertainty, within the neuronal predictive processing framework (PPF), thereby enabling us to quantify it more formally.

3.8.2 Immune Response and Stress within the Bayesian Brain

Seth and others have used the PPF to try to explain how the brain generates models (within the visceromotor cortex (VMC)) about bodily states (internal milieu), and how interoceptive sensory input provides the evidence for the model the brain has generated (89,91,95). Here, interoception refers to any sensory input that reaches the brain through vagal afferents (96,97). These sensations have a predominantly visceral origin, and they are integrated within the brain stem hub and within the thalamic nuclei, before they are relayed to the viscerosensory cortex (VSC) (96–98). Within the PPF, an inflammatory response that is signalled to the brain is considered an 'interoceptive surprise/uncertainty', which is essentially a mismatch between viscerosensory input and the brain's generative model of the body's inflammatory state. While several theoretical models have been proposed, here we describe briefly the EPIC model proposed by Barret and Simmons to demonstrate how, within a PPF, an inflammatory response in the periphery can activate interoceptive pathways and initiate an allostatic/ behavioural response. Within the context of the EPIC model, the agranular anterior insula and ACC are thought to act as the viscero-motor centres that estimate the 'balance' between the available immune/inflammatory resources, such as cytokines, and the predicted require ments (the model) based on past experience. Based on this estimation, the VMC sends out 'prediction' signals to the VSC (posterior insula) and 'motor' signals to the LC, SNS and HPA axis in order to maintain allostasis/homeostasis. The VSC computes the difference between prior VMC predictions and thalamic interoceptive input based on Bayesian active inference. This 'prediction error' signal is transmitted back to the VMC to allow modification of its 'prediction' or the 'motor' signals, as shown in Figure 3.4. In health,

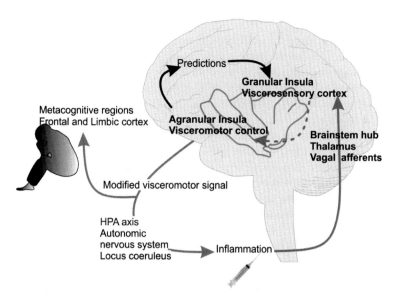

Figure 3.4 **Bayesian-brain connections.** Blue arrow represents visceromotor predictions (model) of the inflammatory state of the body. The red arrow represents the inflammatory stimulus that is conveyed to the brain through interoceptive/humoral pathways. The mismatch between predictions and incoming sensory signals give rise to prediction error signals (dotted red arrow), conveyed back to the VMC. This leads to activation of LC, SNS and HPA axis – that lead to allostatic/homoeostatic control. Failure of this system would lead to metacognitive appraisal of the homoeostatic/allostatic dyscontrol, manifesting as fatigue/ depressive symptoms. (A black and white version of this figure will appear in some formats. For the colour version, please refer to the plate section.)

the 'prediction' matches the 'sensory' signals, and there is no additional bottom up information transfer. Furthermore, the agranular VMC is somewhat insensitive to small fluctuations in available inflammatory resources, resulting in relatively stable 'predictions' and the temporal stability of homeostasis in health. The viscerosensory/ prediction mismatch would ideally trigger a homeostatic response that corrects the dyshomeostasis. Here, there is perhaps a very strong link between the nervous system, the endocrine system and the immune system, perhaps through Tracey et al.'s 'inflammatory reflex' (99,100). Stephan et al. suggest that any failure to correct this (leading to an increase in inflammatory markers and hence surprise/uncertainty), leads to a metacognitive recognition of the failure and persistent uncertainty, which materialize through subjective feelings of fatigue and depression (101). In other words, a persistent inflammatory response induces higher order beliefs about lack of control and low self-efficacy beliefs. In this context, fatigue is the metacognitive detection of an ongoing fruitless effort to regulate homeostasis.

While the interoceptive Bayesian models are primarily postulated from neuronal pathways signalling via the interoceptive viscerosensory system, there are other pathways through which circulating inflammatory markers can signal the brain. Of particular theoretical relevance is that humoral sensing circumventricular organs like the subfornical organ, which have fenestrated capillaries that allow exposure to large molecules like inflammatory cytokines, form part of the key viscerosensory paths in the brain (98,102). Studies that link neuroimmune signalling using the Bayesian model should consider these alternative pathways.

3.9 Resilience

One mechanism of defence the body uses in response to stress, particularly psychological stress, is resilience. Resilience is the ability to adapt to stressful events using a strategic multistep process of recovery and is exhibited by most people to varying degrees. It ultimately defines an individual's ability to 'bounce back'. This is also an important component of one's adaptive threshold to stimulus. For example, when a stressor is experienced time and time again, the stress response is designed to adapt to the increased exposure and limit the extent of the stress response with each recurring episode. However, this is not preserved from one person to another and habituation is inconsistent.

Neuroendocrine hormones have been associated with stress and differentially modulate the activity of discrete brain regions. CORT delivery increases corticotropin-releasing factor (CRF) mRNA concentrations in the central nucleus of the amygdala (103) and facilitates the encoding of emotion-related memory (104). Adrenal steroids such as cortisol have biphasic effects on hippocampal excitability and cognitive function and memory (105) that may contribute to adaptive alterations in behaviours induced by cortisol during the acute response to stress. Another adrenal steroid released under stress is dehydroepiandrosterone (DHEA). This is thought to be neuroprotective and displays anti-GC (106,107) and anti-glutamatergic activity in several tissues in the context of stress. In the brain it acts as a NMDAR positive allosteric modulator and a $GABA_AR$ negative allosteric modulator (108). In hippocampal neurons, DHEA decreases GC levels (109) and exerts an antidepressant action by restoring cortisol-induced suppression of LTP in dentate gyrus neurons (110). Moreover, other studies have reported an elevated cortisol-DHEA ratio in patients diagnosed with major depression (111) and DHEA has been successfully used to counteract depression symptoms in humans (112).

Resilience is also characterized by morphological modifications to brain regions that are sensitive to stress. Krzystyniak et al. subjected mice to RSD and noticed that the resilient individuals, who had received a prophylactic-ketamine treatment, displayed an increase in spine density in the CA1 and CA3 regions of the hippocampus as well as in the PFC, whereas the spine density was significantly lower in anhedonic mice (113). The authors also described an effect of ketamine treatment on the spine length-to-head width ratio, which reflects more mature synaptic connections and stable network. Using a similar paradigm, Wang et al. described how the prophylactic treatment with two phytochemicals, dihydrocaffeic acid and malvidin-3'-O-glucoside, promoted resilience and reversed RSD-induced synaptic structural and functional alterations in the nucleus accumbens via the modulation of IL-6 and the GTPase Rac1 (114). The authors show that RSD stress significantly increased the number of postsynaptic density protein 95 (PSD-95) immunoreactive puncta compared to the vehicle-treated unstressed mice.

Together, these findings suggest that resilient behaviour represents a distinct, active neurobiological process (not simply the absence of vulnerability), however the unique nature of stress reactivity can make it difficult to predict vulnerability to or resilience against stress on an individual basis.

3.10 Summary

There is considerable evidence demonstrating the intricate relationship between stress, the immune system and the brain. While this relationship is essential for maintaining homeostasis after exposure to acute stress, it is becoming increasingly apparent that chronic stress can lead to irreversible changes in immune and neuroendocrine systems that have downstream negative effects on the brain. As such, exposure to chronic stress is thought to predispose to both age-related inflammatory diseases and neuropsychiatric conditions including depression and anxiety. While the literature regarding this field is increasingly comprehensive, it is becoming more and more apparent that the downstream effects of chronic stress are sensitive to the subtleties of the environment in which they have been assessed and care should be taken when attempting to generalize any mechanistic findings. Nonetheless, the field warrants further study in order to maximize our understanding of the complex relationship between stress, the immune system and the brain and to identify potential therapeutic targets.

References

1. Ulrich-Lai YM, Herman JP. Neural regulation of endocrine and autonomic stress responses. *Nature Reviews Neuroscience*. 2009;10:397.

2. Morey JN, Boggero IA, Scott AB, Segerstrom SC. Current directions in stress and human immune function. *Current Opinion in Psychology*. 2015;5:13–7.

3. Dhabhar FS, Malarkey WB, Neri E, McEwen BS. Stress-induced redistribution of immune cells – From barracks to boulevards to battlefields: a tale of three hormones – Curt Richter Award Winner. *Psychoneuroendocrinology*. 2012;37 (9):1345–68.

4. Sternberg EM. Neural regulation of innate immunity: a coordinated nonspecific host response to pathogens. *Nature Reviews Immunology*. 2006;6:318.

5. McEwen BS. Physiology and neurobiology of stress and adaptation: central role of the brain. *Physiological Reviews*. 2007;87 (3):873–904.

6. Bisht K, Sharma K, Tremblay M-È. Chronic stress as a risk factor for Alzheimer's disease: roles of microglia-mediated synaptic remodeling, inflammation, and oxidative stress. *Neurobiology of Stress*. 2018;9: 9–21.

7. Brachman RA, Lehmann ML, Maric D, Herkenham M. Lymphocytes from chronically stressed mice confer antidepressant-like effects to naive mice. *The Journal of Neuroscience*. 2015;35(4):1530.

8. American Psychological Association. From stress to inflammation and major depressive disorder: a social signal transduction theory of depression (press release). 2014.

9. Kudryavtseva NN, Bakshtanovskaya IV, Koryakina LA. Social model of depression in mice of C57BL/6J strain. *Pharmacology Biochemistry and Behavior*. 1991;38 (2):315–20.

10. Weber MD, Godbout JP, Sheridan JF. Repeated social defeat, neuroinflammation, and behavior: monocytes carry the signal. *Neuropsychopharmacology*. 2017;42 (1):46–61.

11. Reader BF, Jarrett BL, McKim DB, et al. Peripheral and central effects of repeated social defeat stress: monocyte trafficking, microglial activation, and anxiety. *Neuroscience*. 2015;289:429–42.

12. Willner P. The chronic mild stress (CMS) model of depression: history, evaluation and usage. *Neurobiology of Stress*. 2016;6:78–93.

13. Willner P, Towell A, Sampson D, Sophokleous S, Muscat R. Reduction of sucrose preference by chronic unpredictable mild stress, and its restoration by a tricyclic antidepressant. *Psychopharmacology*. 1987;93(3):358–64.

14. Muscat R, Willner P. Suppression of sucrose drinking by chronic mild unpredictable stress: a methodological analysis. *Neuroscience & Biobehavioral Reviews*. 1992;16(4):507–17.

15. Willner P. Validity, reliability and utility of the chronic mild stress model of depression: a 10-year review and evaluation. *Psychopharmacology*. 1997;134 (4):319–29.

16. Murthy S, Gould E. Early life stress in rodents: animal models of illness or resilience? *Frontiers in Behavioral Neuroscience*. 2018;12:157.

17. Walker C-D, Bath KG, Joels M, et al. Chronic early life stress induced by limited bedding and nesting (LBN) material in rodents: critical considerations of methodology, outcomes and translational potential. *Stress*. 2017;20(5):421–48.

18. George ED, Bordner KA, Elwafi HM, Simen AA. Maternal separation with early weaning: a novel mouse model of early life neglect. *BMC Neuroscience*. 2010;11 (1):123.

19. Engler H, Bailey MT, Engler A, Sheridan JF. Effects of repeated social stress on leukocyte distribution in bone marrow, peripheral blood and spleen. *Journal of Neuroimmunology*. 2004;148(1):106–15.

20. Powell ND, Sloan EK, Bailey MT, et al. Social stress up-regulates inflammatory gene expression in the leukocyte transcriptome via β-adrenergic induction of myelopoiesis. Proceedings of the National Academy of Sciences. 2013;110 (41):16574.

21. Wohleb ES, Powell ND, Godbout JP, Sheridan JF. Stress-induced recruitment of bone marrow-derived monocytes to the brain promotes anxiety-like behavior. *The Journal of Neuroscience*. 2013;33(34):13820.

22. Heidt T, Sager HB, Courties G, et al. Chronic variable stress activates hematopoietic stem cells. *Nature Medicine*. 2014;20:754.

23. Wohleb ES, Hanke ML, Corona AW, et al. β-adrenergic receptor antagonism prevents anxiety-like behavior and microglial reactivity induced by repeated social defeat. *The Journal of Neuroscience*. 2011;31 (17):6277.

24. Hanke ML, Powell ND, Stiner LM, Bailey MT, Sheridan JF. Beta adrenergic blockade decreases the immunomodulatory effects of social disruption stress. *Brain, Behavior, and Immunity*. 2012;26(7):1150–9.

25. Bailey MT, Engler H, Powell ND, Padgett DA, Sheridan JF. Repeated social defeat increases the bactericidal activity of splenic macrophages through a Toll-like receptor-dependent pathway. *American Journal of Physiology-Regulatory,*

Integrative and Comparative Physiology. 2007;293(3):R1180–R90.

26. Powell ND, Bailey MT, Mays JW, et al. Repeated social defeat activates dendritic cells and enhances Toll-like receptor dependent cytokine secretion. *Brain, Behavior, and Immunity*. 2009;23(2):225–31.

27. Gjerstad JK, Lightman SL, Spiga F. Role of glucocorticoid negative feedback in the regulation of HPA axis pulsatility. *Stress (Amsterdam, Netherlands)*. 2018;21 (5):403–16.

28. Avitsur R, Stark JL, Dhabhar FS, Padgett DA, Sheridan JF. Social disruption-induced glucocorticoid resistance: kinetics and site specificity. *Journal of Neuroimmunology*. 2002;124(1):54–61.

29. Wohleb ES, McKim DB, Shea DT, et al. Re-establishment of anxiety in stress-sensitized mice is caused by monocyte trafficking from the spleen to the brain. *Biological Psychiatry*. 2014;75(12):970–81.

30. Sawicki CM, McKim DB, Wohleb ES, et al. Social defeat promotes a reactive endothelium in a brain region-dependent manner with increased expression of key adhesion molecules, selectins and chemokines associated with the recruitment of myeloid cells to the brain. *Neuroscience*. 2015;302:151–64.

31. O'Carroll SJ, Kho DT, Wiltshire R, et al. Pro-inflammatory TNFα and IL-1β differentially regulate the inflammatory phenotype of brain microvascular endothelial cells. *Journal of Neuroinflammation*. 2015;12:131.

32. Lakhan SE, Kirchgessner A, Tepper D, Leonard A. Matrix metalloproteinases and blood-brain barrier disruption in acute ischemic stroke. *Frontiers in Neurology*. 2013;4:32.

33. Könnecke H, Bechmann I. The role of microglia and matrix metalloproteinases involvement in neuroinflammation and gliomas. *Clin Dev Immunol*. 2013;2013:914104.

34. Ramirez K, Niraula A, Sheridan JF. GABAergic modulation with classical benzodiazepines prevent stress-induced neuro-immune dysregulation and

behavioral alterations. *Brain, Behavior, and Immunity.* 2016;51:154–68.

35. Frick, LR, Arcos ML, Rapanelli M, et al. Chronic restraint stress impairs T-cell immunity and promotes tumor progression in mice. *Stress.* 2009;12(2):134–43.

36. Budiu RA, Vlad AM, Nazario L, et al. Restraint and social isolation stressors differentially regulate adaptive immunity and tumor angiogenesis in a breast cancer mouse model. *Cancer Clin Oncol.* 2017;6 (1):12–24.

37. Sommershof A, Scheuermann L, Koerner J, Groettrup M. Chronic stress suppresses anti-tumor TCD8+ responses and tumor regression following cancer immunotherapy in a mouse model of melanoma. *Brain, Behavior, and Immunity.* 2017;65:140–9.

38. Li Q, Barres BA. Microglia and macrophages in brain homeostasis and disease. *Nature Reviews Immunology.* 2017;18:225.

39. Frank M, Fonken L, Watkins L, Maier S. Microglia: Neuroimmune-sensors of stress. *Seminars in Cell & Developmental Biology.* 2019;94:176–85.

40. Hinwood M, Tynan RJ, Charnley JL, et al. Chronic stress induced remodeling of the prefrontal cortex: structural re-organization of microglia and the inhibitory effect of minocycline. *Cerebral Cortex.* 2012;23(8):1784–97.

41. Walker FR, Morandini J, Day TA, Hinwood M. Evidence that microglia mediate the neurobiological effects of chronic psychological stress on the medial prefrontal cortex. *Cerebral Cortex.* 2012;22(6):1442–54.

42. Churchward MA, Michaud ER, Todd KG. Supporting microglial niches for therapeutic benefit in psychiatric disorders. *Progress in Neuro-Psychopharmacology and Biological Psychiatry.* 2019;94:109648.

43. Garrido-Mesa N, Zarzuelo A, Gálvez J. Minocycline: far beyond an antibiotic. *British Journal of Pharmacology.* 2013;169 (2):337–52.

44. McKim DB, Patterson JM, Wohleb ES, et al. Sympathetic release of splenic monocytes promotes recurring anxiety following repeated social defeat. *Biological Psychiatry.* 2016;79(10):803–13.

45. Cohen S, Janicki-Deverts D, Doyle WJ, et al. Chronic stress, glucocorticoid receptor resistance, inflammation, and disease risk. Proceedings of the National Academy of Sciences of the United States of America. 2012;109(16):5995–9.

46. Kelly KA, Michalovicz LT, Miller JV, et al. Prior exposure to corticosterone markedly enhances and prolongs the neuroinflammatory response to systemic challenge with LPS. *PLoS ONE.* 2018;13(1): e0190546.

47. Markham JA, Greenough WT. Experience-driven brain plasticity: beyond the synapse. *Neuron Glia Biology.* 2004;1(4):351–63.

48. Lara AH, Wallis JD. The role of prefrontal cortex in working memory: a mini review. *Frontiers in Systems Neuroscience.* 2015;9:173.

49. Domenech P, Koechlin E. Executive control and decision-making in the prefrontal cortex. *Current Opinion in Behavioral Sciences.* 2015;1:101–6.

50. Hosokawa T, Nakamura S, Matsui Y, et al. The effect of inactivation of prefrontal cortex on immediate behavioral adaptation in group reversal task by offline repetitive transcranial magnetic stimulation (rTMS) in monkeys. *Brain Stimulation: Basic, Translational, and Clinical Research in Neuromodulation.* 2015;8(2):321.

51. Radley JJ, Rocher AB, Miller M, et al. Repeated stress induces dendritic spine loss in the rat medial prefrontal cortex. *Cerebral Cortex.* 2006;16(3):313–20.

52. Radley JJ, Sisti HM, Hao J, et al. Chronic behavioral stress induces apical dendritic reorganization in pyramidal neurons of the medial prefrontal cortex. *Neuroscience.* 2004;125(1):1–6.

53. Cook SC, Wellman CL. Chronic stress alters dendritic morphology in rat medial prefrontal cortex. *Journal of Neurobiology.* 2004;60(2):236–48.

54. Rempel-Clower NL. Role of orbitofrontal cortex connections in emotion. *Annals of*

the New York Academy of Sciences. 2007;1121(1):72–86.

55. Liston C, Miller MM, Goldwater DS, et al. Stress-induced alterations in prefrontal cortical dendritic morphology predict selective impairments in perceptual attentional set-shifting. *The Journal of Neuroscience.* 2006;26(30):7870–4.

56. Frederick Rohan W, Michael N, Kimberley J. Acute and chronic stress-induced disturbances of microglial plasticity, phenotype and function. *Current Drug Targets.* 2013;14(11):1262–76.

57. Wohleb ES, Terwilliger R, Duman CH, Duman RS. Stress-induced neuronal colony stimulating Factor 1 provokes microglia-mediated neuronal remodeling and depressive-like behavior. *Biological Psychiatry.* 2018;83(1):38–49.

58. Phelps EA, LeDoux JE. Contributions of the amygdala to emotion processing: from animal models to human behavior. *Neuron.* 2005;48(2):175–87.

59. Vyas A, Mitra R, Shankaranarayana Rao BS, Chattarji S. Chronic stress induces contrasting patterns of dendritic remodeling in hippocampal and amygdaloid neurons. *The Journal of Neuroscience.* 2002;22(15):6810–8.

60. Vyas A, Pillai AG, Chattarji S. Recovery after chronic stress fails to reverse amygdaloid neuronal hypertrophy and enhanced anxiety-like behavior. *Neuroscience.* 2004;128(4): 667–73.

61. Johnson FK, Delpech J-C, Thompson GJ, et al. Amygdala hyper-connectivity in a mouse model of unpredictable early life stress. *Translational Psychiatry.* 2018;8(1):49.

62. Lee T, Jarome T, Li S-J, Kim JJ, Helmstetter FJ. Chronic stress selectively reduces hippocampal volume in rats: a longitudinal magnetic resonance imaging study. *Neuroreport.* 2009;20(17):1554–8.

63. Schoenfeld TJ, McCausland HC, Morris HD, Padmanaban V, Cameron HA. Stress and Loss of Adult Neurogenesis Differentially Reduce Hippocampal Volume. *Biological Psychiatry.* 2017;82 (12):914–23.

64. McEwen BS. Stress and hippocampal plasticity. *Annual Review of Neuroscience.* 1999;22(1):105–22.

65. Magarin̄os AM, McEwen BS. Stress-induced atrophy of apical dendrites of hippocampal CA3c neurons: Involvement of glucocorticoid secretion and excitatory amino acid receptors. *Neuroscience.* 1995;69(1):89–98.

66. Brunson KL, Kramár E, Lin B, et al. Mechanisms of late-onset cognitive decline after early-life stress. *The Journal of Neuroscience.* 2005;25(41):9328–38.

67. Christian KM, Miracle AD, Wellman CL, Nakazawa K. Chronic stress-induced hippocampal dendritic retraction requires CA3 NMDA receptors. *Neuroscience.* 2011;174:26–36.

68. Pham K, Nacher J, Hof PR, McEwen BS. Repeated restraint stress suppresses neurogenesis and induces biphasic PSA-NCAM expression in the adult rat dentate gyrus. *European Journal of Neuroscience.* 2003;17(4):879–86.

69. Gould E, McEwen BS, Tanapat P, Galea LAM, Fuchs E. Neurogenesis in the dentate gyrus of the adult tree shrew is regulated by psychosocial stress and NMDA receptor activation. *The Journal of Neuroscience.* 1997;17(7):2492–8.

70. Milior G, Lecours C, Samson L, et al. Fractalkine receptor deficiency impairs microglial and neuronal responsiveness to chronic stress. *Brain, Behavior, and Immunity.* 2016;55:114–25.

71. Duman RS, Aghajanian GK, Sanacora G, Krystal JH. Synaptic plasticity and depression: new insights from stress and rapid-acting antidepressants. *Nature Medicine.* 2016;22:238.

72. Xiong W, Wei H, Xiang X, et al. The effect of acute stress on LTP and LTD induction in the hippocampal CA1 region of anesthetized rats at three different ages. *Brain Research.* 2004;1005(1):187–92.

73. Lakshminarasimhan H, Chattarji S. Stress leads to contrasting effects on the levels of brain derived neurotrophic factor in the hippocampus and amygdala. *PLoS ONE.* 2012;7(1):e30481.

74. Halassa MM, Fellin T, Haydon PG. The tripartite synapse: roles for gliotransmission in health and disease. *Trends in Molecular Medicine.* 2007;13 (2):54–63.

75. Volterra A, Meldolesi J. Astrocytes, from brain glue to communication elements: the revolution continues. *Nature Reviews Neuroscience.* 2005;6:626.

76. Segerstrom SC, Miller GE. Psychological stress and the human immune system: a meta-analytic study of 30 years of inquiry. *Psychological Bulletin.* 2004;130(4): 601–30.

77. Miller GE, Chen E, Sze J, et al. A functional genomic fingerprint of chronic stress in humans: blunted glucocorticoid and increased NF-kappaB signaling. *Biological Psychiatry.* 2008;64(4):266–72.

78. Miller AH, Haroon E, Raison CL, Felger JC. Cytokine targets in the brain: impact on neurotransmitters and neurocircuits. *Depression and Anxiety.* 2013;30(4):297–306.

79. Muscatell KA, Dedovic K, Slavich GM, et al. Greater amygdala activity and dorsomedial prefrontal-amygdala coupling are associated with enhanced inflammatory responses to stress. *Brain, Behavior, and Immunity.* 2015;43:46–53.

80. Evans GW, Swain JE, King AP, et al. Childhood cumulative risk exposure and adult amygdala volume and function. *Journal of Neuroscience Research.* 2016;94 (6):535–43.

81. Hanson JL, Nacewicz BM, Sutterer MJ, et al. Behavioral problems after early life stress: contributions of the hippocampus and amygdala. *Biological Psychiatry.* 2015;77(4):314–23.

82. Kim Y-K, Amidfar M, Won E. A review on inflammatory cytokine-induced alterations of the brain as potential neural biomarkers in post-traumatic stress disorder. *Progress in Neuro-Psychopharmacology and Biological Psychiatry.* 2019;91: 103–12.

83. Hantsoo L, Kornfield S, Anguera MC, Epperson CN. Inflammation: a proposed intermediary between maternal stress and offspring neuropsychiatric risk. *Biological Psychiatry.* 2019;85(2):97–106.

84. Lou HC, Hansen D, Nordentoft M, et al. Prenatal stressors of human life affect fetal brain development. *Developmental Medicine & Child Neurology.* 1994; 36(9):826–32.

85. Obel C, Hedegaard M, Brink Henriksen T, Jørgen N. Stressful life events in pregnancy and head circumference at birth. *Developmental Medicine & Child Neurology.* 2003;45(12):802–6.

86. Clark A. Whatever next? Predictive brains, situated agents, and the future of cognitive science. *Behav Brain Sci.* 2013;36 (3):181–204.

87. Friston K, Kilner J, Harrison L. A free energy principle for the brain. *J Physiol Paris.* 2006;100(1–3):70–87.

88. Hohwy J. *The Predictive Mind.* First edition. Oxford University Press, Oxford; 2013.

89. Seth AK, Friston KJ. Active interoceptive inference and the emotional brain. *Philos Trans R Soc Lond B Biol Sci.* 2016;371:(1708).

90. Friston K. The free-energy principle: a rough guide to the brain? *Trends Cogn Sci.* 2009;13(7):293–301.

91. Seth AK. Interoceptive inference, emotion, and the embodied self. *Trends Cogn Sci.* 2013;17(11):565–73.

92. Peters A, McEwen BS, Friston K. Uncertainty and stress: why it causes diseases and how it is mastered by the brain. *Prog Neurobiol.* 2017;156: 164–88.

93. Mason J. Hormones and metabolism: psychological influences on the pituitary-adrenal cortical. In Pincus C, ed. *Recent Progress In Hormone Research: Proceedings of the Laurentian Hormone Conference 1958.* Academic Press, New York and London; 1959.

94. McEwen BS. Stress, adaptation, and disease. Allostasis and allostatic load. *Ann N Y Acad Sci.* 1998;840:33–44.

95. Barrett LF, Simmons WK. Interoceptive predictions in the brain. *Nat Rev Neurosci.* 2015;16(7):419–29.

96. Craig AD. How do you feel? Interoception: the sense of the physiological condition of the body. *Nat Rev Neurosci.* 2002;3 (8):655–66.

97. Craig AD. Interoception: the sense of the physiological condition of the body. *Curr Opin Neurobiol.* 2003;13(4):500–5.

98. Critchley HD, Harrison NA. Visceral influences on brain and behavior. *Neuron.* 2013;77(4):624–38.

99. Tracey KJ. The inflammatory reflex. *Nature.* 2002;420(6917):853–9.

100. Tracey KJ. Reflex control of immunity. *Nat Rev Immunol.* 2009;9(6):418–28.

101. Stephan KE, Manjaly ZM, Mathys CD, et al. Allostatic self-efficacy: a metacognitive theory of dyshomeostasis-induced fatigue and depression. *Front Hum Neurosci.* 2016;10:550.

102. Lind RW. Bi-directional, chemically specified neural connections between the subfornical organ and the midbrain raphe system. *Brain Research.* 1986;384 (2):250–61.

103. Shepard JD, Barron KW, Myers DA. Corticosterone delivery to the amygdala increases corticotropin-releasing factor mRNA in the central amygdaloid nucleus and anxiety-like behavior. *Brain Research.* 2000;861(2):288–95.

104. Roozendaal B. Glucocorticoids and the regulation of memory consolidation. *Psychoneuroendocrinology.* 2000;25 (3):213–38.

105. Diamond DM, Fleshner M, Ingersoll N, Rose G. Psychological stress impairs spatial working memory: Relevance to electrophysiological studies of hippocampal function. *Behavioral Neuroscience.* 1996;110(4): 661–72.

106. McNelis JC, Manolopoulos KN, Gathercole LL, et al. Dehydroepiandrosterone exerts antiglucocorticoid action on human preadipocyte proliferation, differentiation, and glucose uptake. *American Journal of Physiology Endocrinology and Metabolism.* 2013;305 (9):E1134-E44.

107. Kalimi M, Shafagoj Y, Loria R, Padgett D, Regelson W. Anti-glucocorticoid effects of dehydroepiandrosterone (DHEA). *Molecular and Cellular Biology.* 1994; 131(2): 99–104.

108. Prough RA, Clark BJ, Klinge CM. Novel mechanisms for DHEA action. *Journal of Molecular Endocrinology.* 2016;56(3): R139–55.

109. Cardounel A, Regelson W, Kalimi M. Dehydroepiandrosterone protects hippocampal neurons against neurotoxin-induced cell death: mechanism of action (44437). Proceedings of the Society for Experimental Biology and Medicine. 1999;222(2):145–9.

110. Kaminska M, Harris J, Gijsbers K, Dubrovsky B. Dehydroepiandrosterone sulfate (DHEAS) counteracts decremental effects of corticosterone on dentate gyrus LTP. Implications for depression.*Brain Research Bulletin.* 2000;52(3):229–34.

111. Young AH, Gallagher P, Porter RJ. Elevation of the cortisol-dehydroepiandrosterone ratio in drug-free depressed patients. *American Journal of Psychiatry.* 2002;159(7):1237–9.

112. Wolkowitz OM, Reus VI, Keebler A, et al. Double-blind treatment of major depression with dehydroepiandrosterone. *American Journal of Psychiatry.* 1999; 156(4):646–9.

113. Krzystyniak A, Baczynska E, Magnowska M, et al. Prophylactic ketamine treatment promotes resilience to chronic stress and accelerates recovery: correlation with changes in synaptic plasticity in the CA3 subregion of the hippocampus. *International Journal of Molecular Sciences.* 2019; 20(7):1726.

114. Wang J, Hodes GE, Zhang H, et al. Epigenetic modulation of inflammation and synaptic plasticity promotes resilience against stress in mice. *Nature Communications.* 2018;9(1):477.

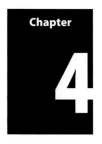

Chapter

4

The Role of Prenatal and Childhood Infection and Inflammation in Schizophrenia

Carly Apar, Fiona Conway, Genevieve Falabella and Alan S. Brown

4.1 Introduction

Schizophrenia is a neurodevelopmental disorder with both genetic and environmental determinants (1). Among potential environmental factors, intriguing new findings point to immune and infectious exposures. The plausibility for the relation of these exposures in the aetiology of schizophrenia is supported by the fact that this exposure alters prenatal and neonatal neurological development (1). In an effort to better understand these potential causes of schizophrenia, this chapter will review the literature on prenatal immune and infectious factors in relation to schizophrenia as well as discuss implications of these studies for the future of prevention and treatment. We review research findings accumulated over the past two decades, which have pointed to prenatal infection as a risk factor for schizophrenia, discuss potential causal mechanisms, and discuss the implications of this work for prevention and a better understanding of the pathogenesis of this disorder. We also review the current literature regarding childhood infection and schizophrenia.

4.2 Studies of Prenatal Infection and Schizophrenia

4.2.1 Ecological Studies

The earliest studies of maternal infection and schizophrenia utilized a research design known as an ecological study. This type of design makes use of naturally occurring epidemics in populations in order to make large scale comparisons and to understand the relationship between risk factors and disease. Several of these studies provided evidence of associations between influenza epidemics occurring at the time of pregnancy and schizophrenia among offspring. Some initial positive findings indicated that among cases of schizophrenia who were *in utero* during influenza epidemics in Finland, Denmark, England and Wales, a higher incidence of schizophrenia was observed in offspring compared to offspring in the same populations during non-epidemic periods (2–5). However, numerous studies failed to replicate these findings (6–9). These inconsistent findings are potentially explained by the fact that ecological studies are not based on documentation of infections during pregnancy among individuals. Rather, all pregnancies during an epidemic are classified as "exposed" to a particular infection (10). This can lead to misclassification of exposure if pregnant mothers were classified as "exposed" to infection merely because they were pregnant during an epidemic. It is estimated that approximately 70% of mothers that were pregnant during the 1957 type A2 influenza epidemic were misclassified as having been exposed to the infection when in fact they were unexposed (1). Conversely, some proportion of women who were pregnant during a period outside the time frame of an epidemic may have been classified as "unexposed" to an infection when in fact they were exposed.

4.2.2　Birth Cohort Studies

Birth cohort studies offer methodologic advantages to ecological studies in the analysis of maternal infection and schizophrenia. One key advantage is that infection exposure status can be determined in individual pregnancies. Infection status can be determined by analysis of biospecimens such as maternal sera or other body fluids. The latter approach can provide data on infection status based on antibody levels to the microbial agent, which reduces the likelihood of diagnostic misclassification that was characteristic of ecological studies. Other birth cohort studies are based on electronic medical records of infection. While the latter type of studies have yielded intriguing findings, one limitation is diagnostic misclassification which may occur if individuals carrying an infection while pregnant do not seek out treatment, a not uncommon occurrence in the case of influenza, for example (11).

Studies such as the Child Health and Development Study (CHDS) and the Collaborative Perinatal Project (CPP) can capture exposure to an infection even among untreated or misdiagnosed individuals, by the use of biomarkers of infection from archived maternal serum drawn during pregnancy to determine infection status.

Offspring were then followed up by databases and structured interviews in order to investigate the relationship between prenatal infections and schizophrenia risk. The data available from these studies also allows for adjustment of numerous potential covariates. More recently, studies utilizing national cohorts, such as the Finnish Prenatal Studies (FIPS), have provided further advantages to the above-mentioned birth cohort studies. The FIPS includes all births in Finland from 1983–98, providing a much larger sample size than that of the CHDS or CPP (12). Furthermore, basic information on all citizens and elaborate data on pre-, peri- and neonatal periods for all births is recorded and the national registries documented all inpatient and outpatient diagnoses. Follow-up of virtually all of the schizophrenia cases in the country was made possible by Finland's low emigration rate, universal health care system and comprehensive psychiatric registries (13). Similar features are also present in studies of other national cohorts such as Denmark (14) and Sweden (15). These study design features allow for minimal selection bias and more complete case ascertainment. Using this design, findings can be replicated in other national birth cohorts.

The method of assessing for the presence of infection in birth cohort studies largely depends on the infection being examined. For instance, a clinical diagnosis of infection such as influenza, acquired from medical records, is less likely to be a false positive, compared to other infections due to the presence of characteristic symptoms. This would tend to decrease the likelihood of diagnostic misclassification. However, as mentioned above, influenza may not necessarily be identified in medical records in a birth cohort study. This limitation would tend to increase the chance of misclassifying individuals who are truly exposed as "unexposed". Due to the fact that serological studies offer the advantage of determining infection status even in the absence of symptoms or treatment, this method of studying birth cohorts would be particularly valuable for infections such as *Toxoplasma gondii* (*T. gondii*) and herpes simplex virus type 2 (HSV-2), which are often asymptomatic. Another potential study limitation is small sample sizes, which may lead to inadequate statistical power, as indicated by various birth cohort studies based on medical records that did not reveal an association between maternal infection, specifically influenza, and risk of schizophrenia in offspring (16,17). National, large birth cohort studies, such as the FIPS, offer the potential to obviate this limitation.

4.2.2.1 Birth Cohort Studies of Infection

As discussed earlier, researchers who conducted investigations in the CHDS (18,19) and CPP (20) utilized maternal sera biomarkers to investigate the association between maternal exposure to infections and subsequent schizophrenia risk in offspring. Analyses from the study of maternal influenza in the CHDS birth cohort revealed a threefold increase in risk for schizophrenia following exposure to influenza during the first half of pregnancy. Furthermore, for influenza exposure during the first trimester, the risk was increased sevenfold (18). Analyses from the study of maternal *T. gondii* exposure, based on antibody measures in the CHDS birth cohort, demonstrated a greater than twofold increased risk of schizophrenia in offspring (19). Additionally, a Danish cohort study utilized filter paper blood spots from newborns to determine significant associations between maternal infection status and schizophrenia risk in offspring. Analyses from the study of *T. gondii* in this cohort revealed an increased risk (odds ratio (OR) = 1.79) of schizophrenia in offspring of mothers exposed to the infection during pregnancy (21), replicating the finding in the CHDS cohort. Utilizing this same methodology, a Swedish birth cohort study also replicated these findings, indicating that higher *T. gondii* antibody levels were associated with higher subsequent risk (OR = 2.2) of schizophrenia (15). In the CPP cohort, analyses from the study of maternal exposure to *Toxoplasma gondii* produced mixed results. Although in an analysis of the Providence, Rhode Island cohort of the CPP, the association was not shown (20), a study utilizing a sample drawn from the Boston, Providence and Philadelphia cohorts of the CPP revealed an association between maternal antibody to *T.* gondii during pregnancy and increased risk of psychosis in offspring (22). Analyses from the studies of maternal HSV-2 exposure in the CPP cohort, however, did indicate an association between maternal exposure to this microbe and increased risk of schizophrenia in offspring (20,23). A further study of maternal HSV-2 exposure in the CHDS birth cohort did not replicate these findings (24). Additionally, analyses from the study of maternal HSV-2 exposure in the Swedish birth cohort were similarly unable to reveal an association between maternal exposure and subsequent schizophrenia in offspring (15). In the Finnish Prenatal Study of Schizophrenia (FIPS-S), we examined maternal exposure to HSV-2 and *Chlamydia trachomatis* (*C. trachomatis*) in offspring. Analyses from these studies of maternal exposure to HSV-2 and *C. trachomatis* did not indicate significant associations between biomarkers of either infection and subsequent development of schizophrenia (13). A Danish study, although similar to the FIPS-S in the fact that it was a nested case-control study of a national birth cohort, produced contrary findings, revealing a significant association between maternal exposure to HSV-2 and schizophrenia risk (incidence rate ratio (IRR) = 1.56) in offspring (14).

Maternal exposure to rubella virus and subsequent increased risk of schizophrenia in offspring has also been documented. In a follow-up of the Rubella Birth Defects Evaluation Project (RBDEP), we studied a cohort of subjects that were *in utero* during the rubella pandemic of 1964. The cohort's exposure to rubella virus was confirmed via both antibody measures and clinical examinations, increasing the diagnostic accuracy. Examination of this cohort revealed that over 20% of the offspring of mothers diagnosed clinically and serologically with rubella during pregnancy later developed schizophrenia and other schizophrenia spectrum disorders, representing a 10- to 15-fold increase in risk. Moreover, the rubella-exposed subjects that developed schizophrenia spectrum disorders were more likely than rubella-exposed controls to display a decline in IQ from childhood to adolescence in addition to increased premorbid neuromotor and behavioural abnormalities (25).

4.2.2.2 Birth Cohort Studies of Inflammatory Biomarkers

The fact that associations have been found between different maternal infections, discussed above, and subsequent schizophrenia in offspring supports the hypothesis of a common mechanism by which exposure to infection influences subsequent vulnerability to schizophrenia. One mechanism that is well known is the release of biomarkers of inflammation. Support for this hypothesis can be derived by quantifying maternal levels of inflammatory biomarkers of infection and subsequent development of schizophrenia in offspring. For instance, in the FIPS-S, we utilized maternal sera to examine the link between levels of C-reactive protein (CRP) and schizophrenia. Maternal CRP is a biomarker of inflammation resulting from infectious or non-infectious exposures. A significant association was found between increasing maternal CRP levels and schizophrenia in offspring (26). Other inflammatory markers, in addition to CRP, are pro- inflammatory cytokines (10). Studies have also linked fetal exposure to elevated maternal levels of the pro-inflammatory cytokines interleukin-8 (IL-8) (27) and tumour necrosis factor alpha (TNF-α) (28) with subsequent increased risk of schizophrenia and related psychotic disorders in offspring. Researchers have also associated elevated levels of anti-inflammatory Th2 cytokines in maternal sera with decreased vulnerability to the development of psychosis in offspring (29), providing further support for the hypothesis. The biological plausibility of associations between prenatal inflammatory biomarkers and offspring schizophrenia is also supported by a study (27) suggesting that elevated maternal levels of the pro-inflammatory cytokine IL-8 increase the risk of schizophrenia in offspring through structural neuroanatomic alterations in the regions of the brain commonly implicated in the development of this disorder (27). It is also possible, however, that individual infections have a direct impact on the neurodevelopmental trajectory that leads to increased vulnerability to schizophrenia in offspring and that cytokines serve merely as a marker of infection.

Taken together, the findings presented above support the hypothesis that maternal infection and inflammation are related to an elevated risk of schizophrenia among offspring. Ecologic studies, while less methodologically rigorous in this context, provided initial evidence in support of the hypothesis. The findings from birth cohort studies provided stronger evidence given individual-level data on the exposures, longitudinal follow-up and adjustment for confounders. Among birth cohort studies, those utilizing maternal biomarkers of exposure, in contrast to those based on medical reports of infection from medical records, are less prone to diagnostic misclassification given that many infections do not come to medical attention due to their being asymptomatic or to the individual choosing not to seek clinical treatment. Moreover, the use of maternal biomarkers of exposure are more likely to identify the specific type of infection, given that medical records' data are often analyzed with regard to broader categories of infection. Consequently, our view is that the strongest evidence of an association between maternal infection and inflammation can be derived from the use of maternal biomarkers, in contrast to other approaches.

4.2.2.3 Animal Models

In addition to birth cohort and ecological studies, animal models have also been utilized to provide further support for the association between prenatal infection and the brain and behavioural abnormalities frequently associated with schizophrenia. Epidemiologic studies, although valuable in their findings and implications, lack the ability to provide researchers with an understanding of the mechanisms that underlie prenatal exposure to infection and subsequent risk of schizophrenia. Animal model studies offer the advantage of allowing researchers to move beyond associations and into causal relationships, providing a deeper understanding of the biological processes. One limitation of these studies, however, is the fact that they rely on the assumption that neuropsychiatric phenotypes in animals can be generalized to human disorders (30). Inspired by the epidemiologic investigations reported above, studies of maternal immune activation in rodents, have evaluated the effect of poly(I: C), lipopolysaccharide and other immune stimulating molecules on brain structure, function and behaviour in offspring and have found intriguing relationships with phenotypes observed in schizophrenia (26,31). Lipopolysaccharide, a bacterial mimetic, and poly(I:C) a viral mimetic, induce virus-like responses when administered (32). Most studies have been conducted in rodents and have yielded valuable findings (30). Recently, investigators used a modified form of poly(I:C) in a study of pregnant rhesus monkeys. The viral mimic injected into the pregnant monkeys induced maternal immune activation and also revealed subsequent abnormal behaviours in offspring resembling those of schizophrenia in humans (33).

4.3 Childhood Infection

Multiple studies have linked serious childhood central nervous system (CNS) viral infections with the development of adult psychosis (34–35). Khandaker et al. found that childhood CNS infections such as mumps virus, coxsackie B5 virus, meningitis and tuberculosis were related to an increased risk of adult psychiatric illness, including schizophrenia and psychosis. The relationship between childhood CNS infections and adult psychiatric illness may be conferred by two mechanisms: the direct effect of specific pathogens and the secondary effect of inflammation on neurodevelopment. Childhood Epstein–Barr infection has been identified as a risk factor for psychotic experiences in adolescence in a population-based prospective serological study (36). Childhood infection has been shown to have an impact on later development of schizophrenia, regardless of other childhood adversity, parental history of psychiatric disorders or familial increased risk of infection (37).

4.4 Implications and Future Directions

Current and future investigations into the potential infectious causes of schizophrenia may inspire greater efforts toward preventative and treatment measures for the identified infections, especially in mothers that are exposed during pregnancy. Such efforts could have significant implications for the prevention of schizophrenia. One metric that has been used to evaluate the potential effect of prevention is the population attributable risk (PAR). The PAR refers to the proportion of subjects with schizophrenia in a population, or any other disease, that can be prevented if a given exposure is eliminated. In an example applicable to infection and schizophrenia, the PAR represents the proportion of schizophrenia patients that would not have developed schizophrenia if a specific maternal infection was not present. Brown and Derkits calculated the PAR corresponding to the effects of influenza, *T. gondii,* and genital/reproductive infections on schizophrenia from their own data and found that nearly one-third of schizophrenia cases in the pregnant population had the potential to be prevented if these infections were entirely eliminated (1). For influenza during the first half of pregnancy the OR was 3.0 and the attributable fraction was 14%. For *T. gondii* the OR was 2.6 and the attributable fraction was 13%. Lastly, for periconceptional genital/reproductive infection, the relative risk (RR) was 5.0 and the attributable fraction was 6%. Although the PAR might vary between populations, complete elimination of these infections may not be entirely realistic, and the results require further replication, this finding suggests that preventative measures could have an appreciable effect on reducing the incidence of schizophrenia in the population. Importantly, there are measures that are already being used to reduce the prevalence of these infections, including influenza vaccination, certain hygienic measures (for *T. gondii*), and antiviral medications and condom use for sexually transmitted infections (31).

Additionally, the integration of the reviewed studies, as well as future research, may lead to the development of a more thorough understanding of the potential interaction between genetic and environmental factors in the development of schizophrenia. For instance, it is possible that susceptibility genes increase the effect of exposure to infection on risk of schizophrenia. This is exemplified by a study that analyzed data from a large birth cohort. Among subjects with a family history of psychosis, the risk of schizophrenia was increased fivefold following prenatal exposure to pyelonephritis (38). Gene-environment interaction could also contribute to an increased risk of schizophrenia by an effect of infection on genes involved in the immune response. One such example is the modification of genes that encode major histocompatibility complex (MHC) class I proteins, molecules that play a substantial role in synaptic functioning and plasticity (39). If an individual is already genetically predisposed to decreased function of these MHC proteins, exposure to infection could result in a greater reduction of synaptic plasticity, which may play an important role in the development of schizophrenia (40).

To evaluate this hypothesis, Sekar et al. examined the variation in the MHC locus and its association with schizophrenia utilizing animal models (41). Specifically, this study implicated the two-complement component 4 (*C4*) genes in the development of schizophrenia. Although over 100 loci in the human genome have been linked to risk of schizophrenia, some of the strongest candidates are the genetic markers within the MHC locus, which plays a significant role in immunity. *C4* specifically is important to the classical complement cascade, an innate-immune-system pathway, the role of which is to eliminate pathogens. Intriguingly, the cascade is also known to play a role in synaptic "pruning", or the elimination of synapses in the brain, a key neurodevelopmental process. The study examined the *C4* alleles in mice in addition to analyzing variation in the MHC locus in humans. In mice, the *C4* protein was responsible for the elimination of synapses in the brain, therefore implying that excessive complement activity could be associated with the decreased number of synapses in the brains of schizophrenia patients. In another part of the study that analyzed variation in the MHC locus in humans, the researchers found that the different *C4* alleles impacted the expression of *C4A and C4B* in the brain. Schizophrenia risk was associated with each allele's effect on the expression of *C4A,* in particular. Genetic variation that increased the expression of *C4A* was associated most with increased risk of schizophrenia (41).

While genome-wide association studies (GWAS), or surveys that study genetic variants and their relationship to disease risk, are valuable, we recommend that future GWAS, rather than solely focusing on gene identification, also evaluate the influence of environmental factors and gene by environment interaction. One such method would be to scan the genomes specifically of populations exposed to a particular infection in order to identify susceptibility genes (1). Børglum et al. utilized this method in a study of all individuals born in Denmark since 1981 and diagnosed with schizophrenia up to 2010 and controls from the same national birth cohort (42). This served as the first GWAS to analyze the interaction between maternal cytomegalovirus infection (CMV) and offspring genotype and its impact on the risk of schizophrenia in those offspring. The gene CTNNA3, which had not previously been suggested as being associated with schizophrenia, was found to interact with CMV in predicting schizophrenia. Thus, this study emphasized the importance of studying the interaction between environmental factors and genotype (42).

In addition to an increased focus on gene-environment interaction, we recommend further investigation of epigenetic factors. Epigenetics refers to the heritable changes in gene expression that occur in the absence of an alteration in the actual DNA sequence, or genome. Epigenetics could represent one mechanism for gene-environment interaction, being that environmental exposures can alter the epigenome. Thus, epigenetic events could represent a plausible mechanism that relates environmental exposures during prenatal and postnatal development and subsequent alterations in gene expression later in life (39). Such epigenetic alterations could potentially play a role in risk of schizophrenia and other neuropsychiatric disorders (32). For example, prenatal exposure to an environmental factor such as smoking has been associated with epigenetic alterations and subsequent increased schizophrenia risk in offspring (12). Due to the heritability of the epigenetic alterations in gene expression, there is potential for transgenerational effects. This is exemplified in a study utilizing a mouse model of prenatal immune activation by poly(I:C) (32). The study revealed that pathological effects on brain and behaviour as a result of prenatal immune activation could be observed in multiple generations. The researchers also observed that the timing of prenatal immune activation during pregnancy could lead to different epigenetic effects and consequently different transgenerational effects (32). We wish to encourage further examination of epigenetic factors in both animal and human studies of schizophrenia.

Another point which remains unclear regards the role played by the type of infection. As mentioned previously (see 4.3 above), there are two relevant hypotheses. The first is that each type of infection has unique insidious properties and mechanisms that disrupt neurodevelopment. Rubella, for example, acts on the developing brain by crossing the placental barrier and infecting the fetus directly, causing widespread brain damage through inflammation and other processes. The second hypothesis is that there is a common mechanism between many or most infections, which accounts for the development of schizophrenia. This common mechanism may be the inflammatory response to these infections, such as to cytokines or acute phase reactants. As an example, influenza appears to disrupt neurological development through maternal inflammation rather than through direct effects on the brain (1).

4.5 Conclusions

As discussed in this chapter, a convergent literature has linked prenatal immune/infectious factors to the later development of schizophrenia in offspring. The earliest studies in this area of work, ecological studies, demonstrated the association between maternal exposure to naturally occurring epidemics in populations and subsequent risk of schizophrenia in offspring. Subsequent birth cohort studies have provided further methodologic advantages to ecological studies in their use of biomarkers of infection or available data to provide infection exposure status on individual pregnancies. Further improvements in the birth cohort design was made possible through the use of national samples, providing more complete ascertainment, less selection bias, and larger samples of subjects.

While ecological and birth cohort studies have revealed associations between maternal exposure to infection and subsequent increased risk of schizophrenia in offspring, the use of animal models provides the unique ability to investigate causal mechanisms. We believe that investigation into causal mechanisms should also include examining the interplay of prenatal factors, such as prenatal immunologic or infectious aetiologies and vulnerability genes. Furthermore, we recommend that future studies of prenatal infection and schizophrenia evaluate the interaction between the environment and the epigenome.

4.6 Acknowledgements

We would like to acknowledge the support of the National Institute of Mental Health, National Institute of Environmental Health Sciences and the Brain and Behavior Research Foundation.

References

1. Brown AS, Derkits EJ. Prenatal infection and schizophrenia: a review of epidemiologic and translational studies. *Am J Psychiatry*. 2010;167(3):261–80.

2. Mednick SA, Machon RA, Huttunen MO, Bonett D. Adult schizophrenia following prenatal exposure to an influenza epidemic. *Arch Gen Psychiatry*. 1988;45(2):189–92.

3. Barr CE, Mednick SA, Munk-Jorgensen P. Exposure to influenza epidemics during gestation and adult schizophrenia. A 40-year study. *Arch Gen Psychiatry*. 1990;47(9):869–74.

4. O'Callaghan E, Gibson T, Colohan HA, et al. Season of birth in schizophrenia. Evidence for confinement of an excess of winter births to patients without a family history of mental disorder. *Br J Psychiatry*. 1991;158:764–9.

5. Sham PC, O'Callaghan E, Takei N, et al. Schizophrenia following pre-natal exposure to influenza epidemics between 1939 and 1960. *Br J Psychiatry*. 1992;160:461–6.

6. Selten JP, Slaets JP. Evidence against maternal influenza as a risk factor for schizophrenia. *Br J Psychiatry*. 1994;164 (5):674–6.

7. Susser E, Lin SP, Brown AS, Lumey LH, Erlenmeyer-Kimling L. No relation between risk of schizophrenia and prenatal exposure to influenza in Holland. *Am J Psychiatry*. 1994;151(6):922–4.

8. Erlenmeyer-Kimling L, Folnegovic Z, Hrabak-Zerjavic V, et al. Schizophrenia and prenatal exposure to the 1957 A2 influenza epidemic in Croatia. *Am J Psychiatry*. 1994;151(10):1496–8.

9. Morgan V, Castle D, Page A, et al. Influenza epidemics and incidence of schizophrenia, affective disorders and mental retardation in Western Australia: no evidence of a major effect. *Schizophr Res*. 1997;26(1):25–39.

10. Canetta SE, Brown AS. Prenatal infection, maternal immune activation, and risk for schizophrenia. *Transl Neurosci*. 2012;3 (4):320–7.

11. Brown AS. Epidemiologic studies of exposure to prenatal infection and risk of schizophrenia and autism. *Dev Neurobiol*. 2012;72(10):1272–6.

12. Niemela S, Sourander A, Surcel HM, et al. Prenatal nicotine exposure and risk of

schizophrenia among offspring in a national birth cohort. *Am J Psychiatry.* 2016;173(8):799–806.

13. Cheslack-Postava K, Brown AS, Chudal R, et al. Maternal exposure to sexually transmitted infections and schizophrenia among offspring. *Schizophr Res.* 2015;166 (1–3):255–60.

14. Mortensen PB, Pedersen CB, Hougaard DM, et al. A Danish national birth cohort study of maternal HSV-2 antibodies as a risk factor for schizophrenia in their offspring. *Schizophr Res.* 2010;122 (1–3):257–63.

15. Blomström A, Karlsson H, Wicks S, et al. Maternal antibodies to infectious agents and risk for non-affective psychoses in the offspring – a matched case-control study. *Schizophr Bull.* 2012;140(1–3):25–30.

16. Crow TJ, Done DJ, Johnstone EC, et al. Schizophrenia and influenza. *Lancet.* 1991;338(8759):116–9.

17. Cannon M, Cotter D, Coffey VP, et al. Prenatal exposure to the 1957 influenza epidemic and adult schizophrenia: a follow-up study. *Br J Psychiatry.* 1996;168 (3):368–71.

18. Brown AS, Begg MD, Gravenstein S, et al. Serologic evidence of prenatal influenza in the etiology of schizophrenia. *Arch Gen Psychiatry.* 2004;61(8):774–80.

19. Brown AS, Schaefer CA, Queensberry CP, et al. Maternal exposure to toxoplasmosis and risk of schizophrenia in adult offspring. *Am J Psychiatry.* 2005;162 (4):767–73.

20. Buka SL, Tsuang MT, Torrey EF, et al. Maternal infection and subsequent psychosis among offspring. *Arch Gen Psychiatry.* 2001;58(11):1032–7.

21. Mortensen PB, Nørgaard-Pedersen B, Waltoft BL, et al. Toxoplasma gondii as a risk factor for early-onset schizophrenia: analysis of filter paper blood samples obtained at birth. *Biol Psychiatry.* 2007;61 (5):688–93.

22. Xiao J, Buka SL, Cannon TD, et al. Serological pattern consistent with infection with type I Toxoplasma gondii in mothers and risk of psychosis among adult offspring. *Microbes Infect.* 2009;11 (13):1011–8.

23. Buka SL, Cannon TD, Torrey EF, Yolken RH, CSGOtPOoSPD. Maternal exposure to herpes simplex virus and risk of psychosis among adult offspring. *Biol Psychiatry.* 2008;63 (8):809–15.

24. Brown AS, Schaefer CA, Queensberry CP, Shen L, Susser ES. No evidence of relation between maternal exposure to herpes simplex virus type 2 and risk of schizophrenia? *Am J Psychiatry.* 2006;163 (12):2178–80.

25. Brown AS, Cohen P, Harkavy-Friedmen J, et al. A.E. Bennett Research Award. Prenatal rubella, premorbid abnormalities, and adult schizophrenia. *Biol Psychiatry.* 2001;49(6):473–86.

26. Canetta S, Sourander A, Surcel HM, et al. Elevated maternal C-reactive protein and increased risk of schizophrenia in a national birth cohort. *Am J Psychiatry.* 2014;171(9):960–8.

27. Ellman LM, Deicken RF, Vinogradov S, et al. Structural brain alterations in schizophrenia following fetal exposure to the inflammatory cytokine interleukin-8. *Schizophr Res.* 2010;121(1–3):46–54.

28. Buka SL, Tsuang MT, Torrey EF, et al. Maternal cytokine levels during pregnancy and adult psychosis. *Brain Behav Immun.* 2001;15(4):411–20.

29. Allswede DM, Buka SL, Yolken RH, Torrey EF, Cannon TD. Elevated maternal cytokine levels at birth and risk for psychosis in adult offspring. *Schizophr Res.* 2016;172(1–3):41–5.

30. Meyer U, Feldon J, Fatemi SH. In-vivo rodent models for the experimental investigation of prenatal immune activation effects in neurodevelopmental brain disorders. *Neurosci Biobehav Rev.* 2009;33(7):1061–79.

31. Brown AS, Patterson PH. Maternal infection and schizophrenia: implications for prevention. *Schizophr Bull.* 2011;37 (2):284–90.

32. Weber-Stadlbauer U. Epigenetic and transgenerational mechanisms in infection- mediated neurodevelopmental disorders. *Transl Psychiatry*. 2017;7(5): e1113.

33. Bauman MD, Iosif AM, Smith SE, et al. Activation of the maternal immune system during pregnancy alters behavioral development of rhesus monkey offspring. *Biol Psychiatry*. 2014;75(4):332–41.

34. Khandaker GM, Zimbron J, Dalman C, Lewis G, Jones PB. Childhood infection and adult schizophrenia: a meta-analysis of population-based studies. *Schizophr Res*. 2012;139(1–3):161–8.

35. Dalman C, Allebeck P, Gunnell D, et al. Infections in the CNS during childhood and the risk of subsequent psychotic illness: A cohort study of more than one million Swedish subjects. *Am J Psychiatry*. 2008;165:(1):59–65.

36. Khandaker GM, Stochl J, Zammit S, Lewis G, Jones PB. Childhood Epstein-Barr Virus infection and subsequent risk of psychotic experiences in adolescence: A population-based prospective serological study. *Schizophr Res*. 2014;158(1–3):19–24.

37. Debost JC, Larsen JT, Munk-Olsen T, et al. Childhood infections and schizophrenia: The impact of parental SES and mental illness, and childhood adversities. *Brain Behav Immun*. 2019;81:341–7.

38. Clarke MC, Tanskanen A, Huttunen M, Whittaker JC, Cannon M. Evidence for an interaction between familial liability and prenatal exposure to infection in the causation of schizophrenia. *Am J Psychiatry*. 2009;166(9):1025–30.

39. Boulanger LM, Shatz CJ. Immune signalling in neural development, synaptic plasticity and disease. *Nature Rev Neurosci*. 2004;5:521.

40. Stephan KE, Baldeweg T, Friston KJ. Synaptic plasticity and dysconnection in schizophrenia. *Biol Psychiatry*. 2006;59 (10):929–39.

41. Sekar A, Bialas AR, de Rivera H, et al. Schizophrenia risk from complex variation of complement 4. *Nature*. 2016;530 (7589):177–83.

42. Borglum AD, Demontis D, Grove J, et al. Genome-wide study of association and interaction with maternal cytomegalovirus infection suggests new schizophrenia loci. *Mol Psychiatry*. 2014;19(3):325–33.

43. Brown AS. The environment and susceptibility to schizophrenia. *Prog Neurobiol*. 2011;93(1):23–58.

Chapter

5

The Role of Autoimmune Encephalitis in Immunopsychiatry and Lessons from Neuropsychiatric Systemic Lupus Erythematosus

Esha Abrol and Michael S. Zandi

5.1 Introduction

Neuropsychiatric symptoms in encephalitis and in lupus have been recognized and described for over 140 years, but we are only now in the twenty-first century finding reliable disease markers to categorize patients (1; 2). These markers have helped provide the first real world examples of precision medicine and bespoke therapies in brain autoimmunity. Autoimmune encephalitis, and N-methyl D-aspartate receptor (NMDAR) encephalitis in particular, currently lead the progress. The first realization that a systemic autoimmune disorder, systemic lupus erythematosus, affected the brain was that of Moriz Kapozi (1837–1902) in the 1870s. William Osler (1849–1919) described detailed case reports of young people with relapsing encephalopathies attributable to lupus (3). Lupus, like syphilis, is a great mimic. It has a range of subtle symptoms and can hide in plain sight. Brain involvement in lupus can be due to associated infarcts, sometimes with the added burden of the phospholipid syndrome; infection due to immune suppression agents or an intrinsic predisposition to infection; and a raised probability of developing autoimmune phenomena perhaps through auto-antibodies, cytokines and innate mechanisms, though exact mechanisms still remain elusive in the 2020s (4).

Autoimmune encephalitis predominantly refers to antibody-associated disorders of the brain, though some such as acute disseminated encephalomyelitis (ADEM) which is often triggered by a virus (including the novel SARS-CoV-2) are associated with cellular infiltration (5). In some conditions, immune cells infiltrate the brain, and in others, antibodies access the brain through a potentially disrupted blood-brain-barrier (BBB), and then have the potential to bind to cellular proteins on brain cells and cause dysfunction and disease. In some instances the antibodies block function (for example, NMDAR antibodies act in a similar manner to ketamine, blocking the receptor) or trigger inflammation (1).

Prior to 2001 it was thought that such disorders were rare and untreatable but following the discovery of two main classes of autoimmune encephalitis these syndromes are now recognized as some of the most treatable severe neurological and neuropsychiatric diseases. These were previously broadly termed 'potassium channel autoimmunity'. However, using radioimmunoassays to identify binding to specific protein complexes, we now know that they are associated with IgG antibodies binding to leucine rich glioma inactivated 1 (LGI1) or contactin-associated protein 2 (Caspr2), and can cause a relatively pure 'limbic' encephalitis with anterograde amnesia, affective and obsessional symptoms, faciobrachial dystonic seizures (LGI1 antibody encephalitis) or epilepsy with risk of long standing impairment of memory processes (6; 7). Cell based assays have also identified antibodies to synaptic proteins including most commonly the NMDA receptor (8). We have seen that such disorders are at least as common as infectious encephalitis (e.g., with herpes infection) (9), can be linked to prior-infection, to occult cancer (paraneoplastic) and are emerging as complications of cancer immunotherapies, for example, use of the checkpoint-inhibitors (10) and trials of novel multiple sclerosis immunotherapies e.g., daclizumab. Historically, people with auto-immune encephalitis may have been hidden among those with *encephalitis lethargica*, particularly the outbreak from 1915 which spread across the world (11), or other encephalopathies, and there may also be an overlap with those originally thought to have neuropsychiatric lupus.

Up to one in ten individuals with psychosis have been reported to have serum autoanti-bodies to brain antigens (12; 13). Though it should be noted that such antibodies have also been identified in one in twenty healthy participants and so do not make a diagnosis in themselves. Brain reactive antibodies have also been found to a lesser extent, and with less secure footing, in obsessive compulsive disorder and tic disorders and while these disorders may be associated epidemiologically with infection there is little evidence for a definite autoimmune encephalitis (14; 15; 16). Of note, old assays for instance for basal ganglia antibodies have been found in healthy individuals at high levels, and the original reports included some patients subsequently found to have NMDAR encephalitis, and so testing for basal ganglia antibodies by Western Blot is no longer recommended(17).

Empirical immune suppression, use of non-steroidal anti-inflammatory drugs (NSAIDS) and antibiotics are all associated with significant risk and should be avoided. If an auto-immune disorder of the brain is diagnosed (requiring more often than not MRI, EEG and lumbar puncture) then coordinated treatment along medical, psychological and psychiatric lines can be considered. A comprehensive clinical review with neurology and psychiatry services is required before making a diagnosis of autoimmunity in patients, particularly where there is potential harm from treatments. As a note of caution, we have seen patients in whom a presumed autoimmune diagnosis has been made, but in whom a neurodegenerative, genetic, metabolic or other disorder is eventually diagnosed. To assist in this, novel criteria to help diagnosis autoimmune psychosis have been proposed by Pollak and colleagues and await testing in populations (16). Spinal fluid testing for brain reactive antibodies after appropriate brain imaging is strongly encouraged, if supported by the clinical history and other examinations, though needs to be weighed up against the risks of lumbar puncture.

At the time of writing the novel coronavirus disease COVID-19 had been associated with encephalitis, encephalopathy and delirium, psychosis, anxiety and potential mental health implications with post-traumatic stress disorder (18; 19; 20).

What follows is an account of the two most common and important syndromes for psychiatrists, followed by a discussion of neuropsychiatric lupus. Of note, there are many emerging and new neuropsychiatric brain diseases with an immune association, which are individually rare. Further discussion of these rare disorders is beyond the scope of this

Table 5.1 Synaptic antigens associated with autoantibodies and clinical neuropsychiatric syndromes

Target	Syndrome
Frequently encountered in secondary care:	
N-methyl D-aspartate (NMDAR)	Psychosis, frontal and temporal cognitive changes, movement disorder and seizures
Leucine rich glioma inactivated 1 (LGI1)	Dense anterograde 'limbic' encephalitis with affective symptoms, faciobrachial dystonic seizures, ataxia and chorea also reported
Contactin associated protein 2 (Caspr2)	As LGI1 plus muscle cramps and sweating (neuromyotonia); higher rate of associated cancer
Glutamic acid decarboxylase (GAD)	Encephalitis, ataxia, seizures, stiff-person syndrome
Myelin associated glycoprotein (MOG), aquaporin 4 (AQ4)	Paediatric and adult encephalitis and neuromyelitis optica
Rare, even in tertiary settings:	
Gamma aminobutyric acid subunit A receptor (GABA(A)R)	Cognitive and affective symptoms
Dipeptidyl peptidase – like protein 6 (DPPX)	Myoclonus and brainstem features with gastrointestinal symptoms
AMPAR, GABA(B)R, neurexin 3alpha, mGlur1, IgLON5	A range of syndromes (rare) including status epilepticus to brainstem and sleep syndromes

chapter though they are listed in Table 5.1 as they represent differential diagnoses for the practicing psychiatrist or psychologist to be aware of.

5.2 N-Methyl D-Aspartate Receptor (NMDAR) Encephalitis

Perhaps Abigail and Betty in Salem had this disorder (21), and a few of those with encephalitis lethargica in the 1920s and 1930s may have done so (11), but we have only really understood and been able to make a definite diagnosis of this disorder since 2007. In 2007 Josep Dalmau and his team found IgG autoantibodies to the NR1 external domain of the brain-ubiquitous NMDAR in a group of young women with ovarian teratoma (22; 23). Translating this discovery from the lab to the clinic and following up a staining pattern of patients' serum on rat hippocampal neuropil preparations led back to a common clinical story. People with the disorder suffered headache and fever followed by changes in behaviour, sleep, mood, an encephalopathy, a psychotic syndrome characterized by auditory hallucinations and catatonia (24). Around two-thirds of patients present to psychiatrists or their general practitioner first. Seizures, coma, dysautonomia and rhythmic hyperkinetic movements may follow, as may prolonged (many months) intensive care admission. In some cases, psychotic symptoms can be indistinguishable from first-episode psychosis or early schizophrenia, and clinical diagnosis remains challenging. Tumours are uncommon but ovarian teratoma (in up to a third of young women with the disease) (25) and other cancers, for example Hodgkin lymphoma, do occur.

Most individuals with NMDAR encephalitis have a monophasic or relapsing immune disorder with potential similarities to myasthenia gravis, neuromyelitis optica or lupus which is also reflected in the choice of therapies with steroids and rituximab (a B-cell depleting agent). We now know that the incidence of NMDAR encephalitis is around 1.5 per million per year for the core disease (23). It is important to note that serum IgG antibodies to the NMDAR may be raised in healthy individuals and in themselves do not make a diagnosis. Furthermore, IgA and IgM antibodies are prevalent at around 10% in healthy individuals and cases of encephalitis or other neurological conditions and IgA and IgM testing is not recommended. A positive NMDAR antibody may also be a secondary phenomenon, for example to HIV, Hepatitis C (unpublished), and a range of other mimics where NMDAR encephalitis is not the diagnosis (26). Testing for the presence of IgG NMDAR antibodies in cerebrospinal fluid provides a more accurate measure of autoantibodies and helps exclude alternative disease pathologies in those with acute psychosis, including viral infection or malignant causes. Studies looking at the diagnostic accuracy of CSF IgG NMDAR antibodies and various proposed research criteria, for example of Graus and Pollak, are awaited.

Systematic review has shown that neuropsychological dysfunction is common and reported in >75% of patients. Cognitive impairments reported are diverse with variable severity reported during the acute, subacute, and recovery periods. Though despite this, in most cases (~75%) cognitive outcomes have ultimately been considered favourable (27). Impairments in overall intellectual functioning, language, attention, working memory and visuospatial processes are more common during the acute recovery period, though impairments in processing speed, episodic memory and features of executive functioning have been more consistently reported across time points. It is also worth noting that poorer neuropsychological outcomes are more commonly reported in patients where immunotherapy was delayed (p < 0.003) (27).

Pragmatic and organisational considerations with respect to completing brain imaging followed by spinal fluid examination for all individuals presenting to health services with acute psychosis remains a major challenge for health care systems globally, though there remains disparity and stigma. For example, an individual with one brain symptom (seizure) has a path of standard care that entails urgent MRI and detailed assessments and ongoing care; whereas those with another (psychosis) often fall in a path where investigation is felt not to be cost effective and care tends to follow a one-size-fits all approach. There are now criteria to help research in autoimmune encephalitis (28), and autoimmune psychosis (16), though individuals with alternative pathologies including HIV and prion disease (unpublished data) can fulfil these criteria early on so care must be taken in using such criteria for clinical diagnosis. The care of these patients also requires the use of full supportive care including anti-epileptic and antipsychotic medications when needed, and then often follows treatment algorithms developed for other immune disorders including lupus and vasculitis, with a range of therapies.

Therapies include first, corticosteroid use (e.g., prednisolone, which suppresses autoreactive inflammation at the cellular level and prevents antibody formation – though is associated with significant risk – cataracts, glaucoma, hypertension, gastric and duodenal ulceration, avascular necrosis, myopathy, listeria and other opportunistic infections). Further first line therapies include intravenous immunoglobulin, pooled blood product from donors, which are likely to modulate and suppress the adaptive immune system (with adverse effects of thrombosis, stroke, myocardial infarction, aseptic meningitis and renal failure, theoretical risk of prion disease), or plasma exchange (removal of circulating autoantibodies and humoral factors – risks of bleeding and infection related to dialysis line insertion, temporary effect). There are then second line therapies including cyclophosphamide (chemotherapy antiproliferative agent – associated with significant risk of opportunistic infection, bladder cancer, hair loss), steroid-sparing agents (azathioprine, mycophenolate – associated with malignancy, liver and bone marrow failure, rash). The next therapies are monoclonal antibody treatment with rituximab (B-cell depletion therapy which reduces B-cell help to autoreactive T cells, and reduces productions of eventual antibody producing cells – with adverse risk of infusion reactions, respiratory distress, opportunistic infection – including rarely of fatal progressive multifocal leukoencephalopathy and hypogammaglobulinemia resulting in a tendency for recurrent bacterial and other infections (29). In rare instances treatments that directly interfere with antibody producing cells (e.g., the boron containing bortezomib (30) which interferes with the turnover of plasma cells) can be tried, repurposed from myeloma, though at present there are no completed randomized controlled trials. Most of these treatments have been repurposed from rheumatology.

At the time of writing there is a placebo-controlled trial for patients with relatively isolated psychosis in whom NMDAR or related autoantibodies have been found, the SINAPPS2 trial (31). In this trial, patients with psychosis are screened for firm evidence of encephalitis (abnormal MRI, EEG or spinal fluid) that would make placebo therapy unacceptable. Individuals with no features to support a diagnosis of encephalitis but who have serum levels of autoantibodies to NMDAR, LGI1 or related antigens, are randomized to placebo versus intravenous immunoglobulin followed by placebo versus rituximab. Overall, patients with NMDAR encephalitis benefit from a coordinated approach with access to psychological services. Though there is currently no evidence base to support this, it is likely that a coordinated approach with access to medical diagnosis of reversible and treatable diagnoses, coupled with standard of care psychiatric therapy for those with psychosis and psychiatric symptoms, and then full access to rehabilitation leads to improved management and outcomes.

Patients with NMDAR encephalitis can also show other antibodies in the blood, for example, antibodies to thyroid peroxidase. Thyroid peroxidase autoantibodies are found commonly in the general population, other immune disorders including multiple sclerosis and in thyroiditis associated with a steroid responsive encephalopathy, often termed Hashimoto's encephalopathy. However, it remains more likely in Hashimoto's encephalopathy, that this antibody is an immune association and not directly pathogenic, and that cases of NMDAR encephalitis were previously labelled Hashimoto's encephalopathy.

The social challenges and holistic approach to rehabilitation of an individual dealing with the burden, and stigma, of multiple brain processes (neuropsychiatric symptoms, seizures, cognitive impairment) requires frequent specialist follow up and integration with local services. We can still learn a lot from the historical examples of Felix Stern, Josephine Bicknell Neal and the Matheson Commission and the legal challenges to improve access to treatment and care for encephalitis lethargica in the 1930s and 1940s, for these core issues in the care of those with complex neuropsychiatric brain diseases have not substantially changed.

The outstanding questions in the field include: 1) how to make a bespoke and accurate diagnosis, as serum and CSF autoantibodies alone are likely to lead to false-negative and positive diagnoses; 2) how to measure active brain inflammation reliably to determine who needs augmentation of immune therapy and who needs a focus on rehabilitation and conventional psychiatric care; and 3) how to develop safer and more tolerable treatments for patients.

5.3 Leucine Rich Glioma-Inactivated 1 (LGI1) Encephalitis

This form of autoimmune encephalitis deserves special attention as it can present with psychosis or mania, in older adults, with a dramatic anterograde amnesia with accelerated forgetting. There are often brief seizures that can be hard to detect clinically (faciobrachial dystonic seizures). There is an emerging association with affective symptoms (32). This is a form of limbic encephalitis and represents the most common form of what was previously termed potassium channel antibody encephalopathy or encephalitis (33) or voltage gated potassium channel (VGKC) antibody encephalitis. Of note, VGKC antibody testing is no longer recommended due to the high false-negative intracellular antibody detection rate (34), and instead, testing with direct cell-based assays for LGI1 and the related Caspr2 is recommended. Patients with Caspr2 antibodies are more likely to have an underlying tumour, and bespoke screening of individuals in a minimally invasive way for occult tumours underlying a paraneoplastic syndrome is advised. Thymoma is a common tumour association, as seen in the first reported cases in 2001 (35). There is also an interesting emerging story in the parallel worlds of mutations in these receptors or proteins and resultant autoimmunity, for instance LGI1 mutations are associated with nocturnal epilepsy (36), and Caspr2 gene *CNTNAP2* mutations with an autism like disorder (37).

5.4 Neuropsychiatric Systemic Lupus Erythematosus (NPSLE)

Systemic lupus erythematosus (SLE) is often thought of as a diverse autoimmune disorder with symptoms which range from a characteristic malar rash and arthritis, to life-threatening multi-organ failure. This systemic autoimmune disease has the potential to teach us about mechanisms of autoantibody associated neuropsychiatric symptoms, varying from affective disorders to rarer psychotic syndromes.

Whilst SLE can affect all ethnic groups, geographic regions and ages, it has a preponderance for women (Female:Male ratio of 9:1) of child-bearing age (15 to 45 years) and of Afro-Caribbean ethnicity (Afro-Caribbean:Caucasian ratio of 3:1). The precise aetiology of SLE remains unclear, with many roads leading to the syndrome, including dysregulation of innate immune mechanisms, for example, type 1 interferons, dysregulated adaptive immune responses, particularly overactivity of B cells, and through relaxation of checkpoint breaks perhaps selected through evolutionary pressures (38). Up to 180 different autoantibodies have been linked to SLE (39), though their exact role in the disease remains unclear and most are likely to be epiphenomena. The most characteristic of these are autoantibodies reactive with double stranded DNA (dsDNA), and anti-nuclear antibodies (ANA). Some antibodies to dsDNA may also bind to extracellular epitopes of a range of proteins, including the NR2 subunits of the NMDAR (40) – though these appear to be a distinct process to those NMDAR antibodies seen in NMDAR encephalitis. Also, NR2 antibodies as measured by ELISA do not correlate with neurological disease and are not part of current clinical practice.

NPSLE research criteria from the American College of Rheumatology (41) has identified 19 discrete syndromes (12 CNS, 7 PNS) (Table 5.2). Though in recent years there has been a renewed focus on distinguishing 'focal' versus 'diffuse' NPSLE symptoms. Some manifestations, for instance lupus myelopathy or optic neuropathy, are now found to be either focal

Table 5.2 Central and peripheral nervous system manifestation adapted from the American College of Rheumatology neuropsychiatric SLE case definitions 1999 ('The American College of Rheumatology nomenclature and case definitions for neuropsychiatric lupus syndromes', 1999)

Central nervous system manifestations	Peripheral nervous system manifestations
Aseptic Meningitis	Acute Inflammatory Demyelinating Polyradiculoneuropathy
Acute Confusional State	Autonomic Disorders
Anxiety Disorder	Cranial Neuropathy
Cerebrovascular Disease	Mononeuropathy
Cognitive Dysfunction	Myasthenia Gravis
Demyelinating Syndrome	Plexopathy
Headache	Polyneuropathy
Movement Disorder (consider phospholipid syndrome, infarcts, autoimmune encephalitis)	
Mood Disorders	
Myelopathy (AQ4 and MOG antibody testing required)	
Psychosis (consider autoimmune encephalitis)	
Seizures (consider autoimmune encephalitis)	

vascular manifestations, or lupus associated neuromyelitis optica (with aquaporin 4 auto-antibodies)(42).

When appropriately diagnosed and managed aggressively with immunosuppressive and other agents specific to the presentation (e.g., antipsychotics for psychosis), the long-term outcome can be favourable. However, compared to SLE without neuropsychiatric manifestations, risk of poor outcome remains elevated, especially for NPSLE manifestations such as seizures and stroke where there is an eight-fold increased mortality compared to non-NP SLE (43).

5.4.1 Biomarkers in NPSLE and Obstacles

Although progress has been made over the past three decades, NPSLE diagnosis remains largely subject to the bias of clinical assessment (based on the 19 ACR case definitions for NPSLE syndromes shown in Table 5.2). Despite efforts to make these definitions and exclusions comprehensive, interpretation of the definition of NPSLE remain heterogeneous globally, and reports of its prevalence range widely; from 18% in studies which underestimate the criteria, to as high as 91% in studies which are overinclusive and include common or 'minor' manifestations such as headache (44; 45; 22). As a result, the true prevalence of NPSLE is largely unknown. Moving forward, identifying objective markers such as imaging, serological, or CSF correlates is necessary. In the meantime, there are attribution criteria based on longitudinal studies of the systemic lupus international collaborating clinics (SLICC) group papers (46) that try to minimize false attribution of neuropsychiatric symptoms to active SLE. Currently known biomarkers are non-specific for NPSLE and implicate inflammatory proteins, inflammatory cytokines, microglial activation, ischaemia, oxidative stress, mitochondrial dysfunction and BBB dysfunction.

Our current knowledge about NPSLE is restricted by retrospective studies, with small sample sizes, which traditionally exclude severe NP manifestations (severe depression, psychosis, suicidality). The diagnostic criteria are also a limiting factor with widespread agreement that the all-encompassing term 'NPSLE' is not clinically useful and nor is it useful for research purposes. It is necessary for future studies to divide up this diverse group in order to move forward in our understanding of the immunological basis of different neuropsychiatric manifestations of SLE.

Psychiatric symptoms in SLE include psychoses, mood disorders, cognitive dysfunction, acute confusional state (delirium) and anxiety disorders, all not attributable to another cause or primary psychiatric disorder. They are common, present in at least half of patients with SLE (47) depending on the criteria used. Some groups argue that as psychiatric disorders do not correlate with SLE disease activity and there is no evident cumulative organ damage, they are likely the consequence of concurrent psychosocial stressors rather than primary SLE disease (47). However, as many current studies exclude patients with severe psychiatric symptoms (requiring hospitalisation, electroconvulsive therapy, severe depression, psychosis) such conclusions are unreliable.

5.4.2 Lupus Psychosis

Lupus psychosis refers to a discrete psychotic episode (as per *Diagnostic and Statistical Manual 4*) not attributable to primary psychotic disorder, substance- or drug-induced psychotic disorder (e.g., antimalarial drugs), metabolic or psychological mediated reactions. Understanding pathogenic mechanisms underlying lupus psychosis has the potential to inform our understanding of the immunological basis of psychotic disorders generally.

Lupus psychosis is a rare manifestation, with a reported prevalence ranging from 1.9 to 29.8% depending on the criteria used, which consistently presents early, either in the year prior to, or within three years of SLE diagnosis (45). In small studies, with treatment, lupus psychosis rarely recurs during long-term follow up (48). No reliable biomarker or antibody association has been found for this complication, though in-depth study of cases can reveal some similarities with cases of autoimmune encephalitis. Additionally, autoimmune and infective encephalitis can occur in individuals with SLE. Conversely the inflammatory state in SLE has provided insight into new mechanisms in immunopsychiatry and safe therapies. Formal randomized controlled trials of biologic therapies, for example, Rituximab, and other immune dampening treatments are warranted in NPSLE and lupus psychosis, however these presentations are often excluded from existing trials due to the diversity in aetiopathogenesis and challenging treatments (49; 50).

5.4.3 Interferon Signature

Active SLE is associated with a raised expression of genes related to interferon-α (51). Shiozawa and colleagues (52) demonstrated raised interferon-α in the CSF of 5/6 patients with lupus psychosis, but not 11 other patients with NPSLE, or 28 SLE controls. This finding provides evidence for interferon-α in lupus psychosis, as demonstrated in other disorders such as Hepatitis B where interferon-α treatment induces dose-related, reversible psychiatric symptoms with EEG changes mimicking viral encephalitis (53; 54; 55; 56). It is likely

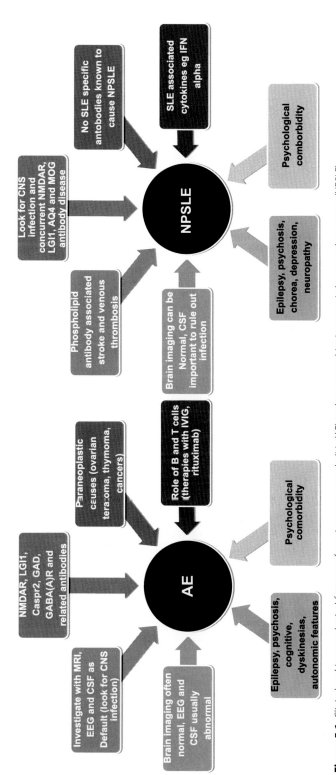

Figure 5.1 Clinical and immunological features of autoimmune encephalitis (AE) and neuropsychiatric systemic lupus erythematosus (NPSLE).

therefore that there are cytokine and other neurochemical mechanisms beyond brain-targeting autoantibodies that can affect neuropsychiatric symptoms in SLE.

5.5 Implications and Future Directions

We have seen how advances in molecular diagnosis of some individuals with common neuropsychiatric symptoms (psychosis, amnesia) has enabled the study of disease processes and improved patient outcomes. Neurologists have based their own trials of immune suppression on the greater precedents in rheumatology and autoimmunity and there are many lessons from lupus that are applicable to immunopsychiatry. It is important for psychiatrists to be aware of neurological and other systemic symptoms which overlap between autoimmune encephalitis and psychotic disorders in order to prompt early diagnosis and intervention. With advances in genetics and precision medicine we are entering an opportune time to tackle, perhaps in small increments at first, immunopsychiatric disease (Figure 5.1).

References

1. Crisp SJ, Kullmann DM, Vincent A. Autoimmune synaptopathies. *Nat Rev Neurosci*. 2016; 17:103–17.

2. Hanly JG, Urowitz MB, Gordon C, et al. Neuropsychiatric events in systemic lupus erythematosus: a longitudinal analysis of outcomes in an international inception cohort using a multistate model approach. *Ann Rheum Dis*. 2020;79:356–62.

3. Smith CD, Cyr M. The history of lupus erythematosus. From Hippocrates to Osler. *Rheum Dis Clin North Am*. 1988;14:1–14.

4. McGlasson S, Wiseman S, Wardlaw J, Dhaun N, Hunt DPJ. Neurological disease in lupus: toward a personalized medicine approach. *Front Immunol*. 2018;9:1146.

5. Koralnik IJ, Tyler KL. COVID-19: a global threat to the nervous system. *Ann Neurol*. 2020;88:1–11.

6. Irani SR, Michell AW, Lang B, et al. Faciobrachial dystonic seizures precede LGI1 antibody limbic encephalitis. *Ann Neurol*. 2011; 69:892–900.

7. Miller TD, Chong TT-J, Aimola Davies AM, et al. Focal CA3 hippocampal subfield atrophy following LGI1 VGKC-complex antibody limbic encephalitis. *Brain*. 2017;140:1212–9.

8. Dalmau J. NMDA receptor encephalitis and other antibody-mediated disorders of the synapse: the 2016 Cotzias Lecture. *Neurology*. 2016;87:2471–82.

9. Gable MS, Sheriff H, Dalmau J, Tilley DH, Glaser CA. The frequency of autoimmune N-methyl-D-aspartate receptor encephalitis surpasses that of individual viral etiologies in young individuals enrolled in the California Encephalitis Project. *Clin Infect Dis*. 2012;54:899–904.

10. Williams TJ, Benavides DR, Patrice K-A, et al. Association of autoimmune encephalitis with combined immune checkpoint inhibitor treatment for metastatic cancer. *JAMA Neurol*. 2016;73:928–33.

11. Zandi M. Encephalitis Lethargica: a dying fall. *Brain*. 2019;142(9):2888–91. https://doi.org/10.1093/brain/awz228

12. Deakin J, Lennox BR, Zandi MS. Antibodies to the N-methyl-D-aspartate receptor and other synaptic proteins in psychosis. *Biol Psychiatry*. 2014;75:284–91.

13. Lennox BR, Palmer-Cooper EC, Pollak T, et al. Prevalence and clinical characteristics of serum neuronal cell surface antibodies in first-episode psychosis: a case-control study. *Lancet Psychiatry*. 2017;4:42–8.

14. Singer HS, Hong JJ, Yoon DY, Williams PN. Serum autoantibodies do not differentiate PANDAS and Tourette syndrome from controls. *Neurology*. 2005;65:1701–7.

15. Edmiston E, Ashwood P, Van de Water J. Autoimmunity, autoantibodies, and autism spectrum disorder. *Biological Psychiatry*. 2017;81:383–90.

16. Pollak TA, Lennox BR, Müller S, et al. Autoimmune psychosis: an international consensus on an approach to the diagnosis and management of psychosis of suspected autoimmune origin. *Lancet Psychiatry*. 2020 Jan;7(1):93–108. doi:10.1016/S2215-0366(19)30290-1. Epub 2019 Oct 24. Review. Erratum in: Lancet Psychiatry. 2019 Dec;6(12):e31.

17. Dale RC, Irani SR, Brilot F, et al. N-methyl-D-aspartate receptor antibodies in pediatric dyskinetic encephalitis lethargica. *Ann Neurol*. 2009 Nov;66(5):704–9. doi:10.1002/ana.21807

18. Paterson RW, Brown RL, Benjamin L, et al. The emerging spectrum of COVID-19 neurology: clinical, radiological and laboratory findings. *Brain*. 2020;143 (10):3104–20.

19. Ellul M, Benjamin L, Singh B, et al. Neurological Associations of COVID-19. Rochester, NY: Social Science Research Network; 2020 [cited 2020 May 11]. https://papers.ssrn.com/abstract=3589350

20. Rogers JP, Chesney E, Oliver D, et al. Psychiatric and neuropsychiatric presentations associated with severe coronavirus infections: a systematic review and meta-analysis with comparison to the COVID-19 pandemic. *The Lancet Psychiatry*. 2020; 0 [cited 2020 May 20]. www.thelancet.com/journals/lanpsy/article/PIIS2215-0366(20)30203-0/abstract

21. Tam J, Zandi MS. The witchcraft of encephalitis in Salem. *J Neurol*. 2017;264:1529–31.

22. Dalmau J, Erdem T, Haiyan W, et al. Paraneoplastic anti-N-methyl-D-aspartate receptor encephalitis associated with ovarian teratoma. *Ann Neurol*. 2007 Jan;61 (1):25–36.

23. Dalmau J, Armanque T, Planaguma J, et al. An update on anti-NMDA receptor encephalitis for neurologists and psychiatrists: mechanisms and models. *Lancet Neurol*. 2019 Nov;18(11):1045–57.

doi:10.1016/S1474-4422(19)30244-3. Epub 2019 Jul 17. Review.

24. Al-Diwani A, Handel A, Townsend L, et al. The psychopathology of NMDAR-antibody encephalitis in adults: a systematic review and phenotypic analysis of individual patient data. *Lancet Psychiatry*. 2019;6:235–46.

25. Matute C, Palma A, Serrano-Regal MP, et al. N-methyl-D-aspartate receptor antibodies in autoimmune encephalopathy alter oligodendrocyte function. *Ann Neurol*. 2020;87:670–6.

26. Zandi MS, Paterson RW, Ellul MA, et al. Clinical relevance of serum antibodies to extracellular N-methyl-D-aspartate receptor epitopes. *J Neurol Neurosurg Psychiatry*. 2015 Jul;86(7):708–13. doi:10.1136/jnnp-2014-308736. Epub 2014 Sep 22.

27. McKeon GL, Robinson GA, Ryan AE, et al. Cognitive outcomes following anti-N-methyl-D-aspartate receptor encephalitis: A systematic review. *J Clin Exp Neuropsychol*. 2018;40:234–52.

28. Graus F, Titulaer MJ, Balu R, et al. A clinical approach to diagnosis of autoimmune encephalitis. *Lancet Neurol*. 2016 Apr;15 (4):391–404. doi:10.1016/S1474-4422(15) 00401-9. Epub 2016 Feb 20. Review.

29. Nepal G, Shing YK, Yadav JK, et al. Efficacy and safety of rituximab in autoimmune encephalitis: a meta-analysis. *Acta Neurol Scand*. 2020;142(5):449–59.

30. Keddie S, Crisp SJ, Blackaby J, et al. Plasma cell depletion with bortezomib in the treatment of refractory N-methyl-d-aspartate (NMDA) receptor antibody encephalitis. Rational developments in neuroimmunological treatment. *Eur J Neurol*. 2018;25:1384–8.

31. Lennox BR, Tomei G, Vincent S-A, et al. Study of immunotherapy in antibody positive psychosis: feasibility and acceptability (SINAPPS1). *J Neurol Neurosurg Psychiatry*. 2019;90:365–7.

32. Dodich A, Cerami C, Iannaccone S, et al. Neuropsychological and FDG-PET profiles in VGKC autoimmune limbic encephalitis. *Brain Cogn*. 2016;108:81–7.

33. Vincent A, Buckley C, Schott JM, et al. Potassium channel antibody-associated encephalopathy: a potentially immunotherapy-responsive form of limbic encephalitis. *Brain*. 2004 Mar;127(Pt 3): 701–12. Epub 2004 Feb 11.

34. Lang B, Makuch M, Moloney T, et al. Intracellular and non-neuronal targets of voltage-gated potassium channel complex antibodies. *J Neurol Neurosurg Psychiatry*. 2017 Apr;88(4):353–61. doi:10.1136/jnnp-2016-314758. Epub 2017 Jan 23.

35. Buckley C, Oger J, Clover L, et al. Potassium channel antibodies in two patients with reversible limbic encephalitis. *Ann Neurol*. 2001 Jul;50(1):73–8.

36. Ottman R, Winawer MR, Kalachikov S, et al. LGI1 Mutations in Autosomal Dominant Partial Epilepsy with Auditory Features. *Neurology*. 2004;62(7):1120–6.

37. Canali G, Goutebroze L. CNTNAP2 heterozygous missense variants: risk factors for autism spectrum disorder and/ or other pathologies? *J Exp Neurosci*. 2018 12:1179069518809666.

38. Langefeld CD, Ainsworth HC, Graham DSC, et al. Transancestral mapping and genetic load in systemic lupus erythematosus. *Nature Communications*. 2017;8:16021.

39. Ho R, Thiaghu C, Ong H, et al. A meta-analysis of serum and cerebrospinal fluid autoantibodies in neuropsychiatric systemic lupus erythematosus. *Autoimmun. Rev*. 2016;15:124–38.

40. DeGiorgio LA, Konstantinov KN, Lee SC, et al. A subset of lupus anti-DNA antibodies cross-reacts with the NR2 glutamate receptor in systemic lupus erythematosus. *Nat Med*. 2001 Nov;7 (11):1189–93.

41. ACR Ad Hoc committee on neuropsychiatric lupus nomenclature. The American College of Rheumatology nomenclature and case definitions for neuropsychiatric lupus. *Arthritis Rheum*. 1999;42:599–608.

42. Kleiter I, Gahlen A, Borisow N, et al. Neuromyelitis optica: evaluation of 871 attacks and 1,153 treatment courses. *Ann Neurol*. 2016;79(2):206–16.

43. Ahn G, Kim D, Won S, et al. Prevalence, risk factors, and impact on mortality of neuropsychiatric lupus: a prospective, single-center study. *Lupus*. 2018;27:1338–47.

44. Hanly JG. Diagnosis and management of neuropsychiatric SLE. *Nat Rev Rheumatol*. 2014;10:338–47.

45. Hanly JG, Li Q, Su L, et al. Psychosis in systemic lupus erythematosus: results from an international inception cohort study. *Arthritis & Rheumatology* (Hoboken, NJ). 2019;71:281–9.

46. Hanly JG, Urowitz MB, Su L, et al. Prospective analysis of neuropsychiatric events in an international disease inception cohort of patients with systemic lupus erythematosus. *Ann. Rheum. Dis*. 2010;69:529–35.

47. Hanly J, Su L, Urowitz M, et al. Mood disorders in systemic lupus erythematosus: results from an international inception cohort study. *Arthritis Rheumatol*. 2015;67:1837–47.

48. Pego-Reigosa JM, Isenberg DA. Psychosis due to systemic lupus erythematosus: characteristics and long-term outcome of this rare manifestation of the disease. *Rheumatology (Oxford)*. 2008 47:1498–502.

49. Bertsias GK, Ioannidis JPA, Aringer M, et al. EULAR recommendations for the management of systemic lupus erythematosus with neuropsychiatric manifestations: report of a task force of the EULAR standing committee for clinical affairs. *Ann Rheum Dis*. 2010;69:2074–82.

50. Fanouriakis A, Kostopoulou M, Alunno A, et al. 2019 update of the EULAR recommendations for the management of systemic lupus erythematosus. *Annals of the Rheumatic Diseases*. 2019;78:736–45.

51. Bennett L, Palucka AK, Arce E, et al. Interferon and granulopoiesis signatures in systemic lupus erythematosus blood. *J Exp Med*. 2003;197(6):711–23.

52. Shiozawa S, Kuroki Y, Kim M, Hirohata S, Ogino T. Interferon-alpha in lupus

psychosis. *Arthritis Rheum.*
1992;35:417–22.

53. Davis GL, Esteban-Mur R, Rustgi V, et al.
Interferon alfa-2b alone or in combination
with ribavirin for the treatment of relapse
of chronic hepatitis C. International
Hepatitis Interventional Therapy Group.
N Engl J Med. 1998;339:1493–9.

54. Moulin M du, Nürnberg P, Crow YJ,
Rutsch F. Cerebral vasculopathy is
a common feature in Aicardi–Goutières

syndrome associated with SAMHD1
mutations. *PNAS.* 2011;108:E232.

55. McGlasson S, Jury A, Jackson A, Hunt D.
Type I interferon dysregulation and
neurological disease. *Nature Reviews
Neurology.* 2015;11:515–23.

56. Murakami Y, Ishibashi T, Tomita E, et al.
Depressive symptoms as a side effect of
Interferon-α therapy induced by induction
of indoleamine 2,3-dioxygenase 1.
Scientific Reports. 2016;6:29920.

Chapter

6

Effectiveness of Immunotherapies for Psychotic Disorders

Rachel Upthegrove and Bill Deakin

6.1 Why Might Anti-Inflammatory Agents Work in Psychosis?

There is consistent evidence that psychosis is associated with a degree of peripheral immune activation. Many studies and meta-analyses report increased circulating concentrations of pro-inflammatory cytokines including IL-6, IL-1β and TNF-α together with acute phase proteins, such as CRP in patients with psychosis compared with controls. Meta-analysis confirms increased circulating IL-6 and other inflammatory markers in medication-naïve first-episode psychosis (FEP) (1), and in the CSF of schizophrenia patients compared with controls (2). Longitudinal studies show an association between elevated IL-6/CRP in childhood/adolescence and risk of psychotic symptoms or diagnosis of schizophrenia in adulthood (3,4). Genetic analysis shows that possession of a functional variant in the *IL-6 R* gene (Asp358Ala, rs2228145), which is known to reduce the activity of IL-6, is also associated with decreased risk of psychosis (5). This suggests that the association of raised IL-6 with psychosis may be causal and not due to reverse causality or residual confounding, i.e., the effect of a factor associated with psychosis that also by chance increases levels of this cytokine. However, Mendelian randomization analysis also suggests that elevated CRP levels may be protective for schizophrenia (6), in contrast to observational studies consistently reporting higher CRP levels in patients with the illness compared with controls (7). Divergent results for two known pro-inflammatory markers raises questions about potential mechanisms though which immune dysfunction may influence brain and behaviour to increase the risk of psychotic disorders. One explanation is that genetically predicted levels of low CRP may predispose to infections, which in turn, may increase schizophrenia risk through immune and non-immune mechanisms (6,8).

There are three major caveats to the peripheral cytokine evidence; (i) specificity: the same abnormalities have been described in depression, (ii) degree of immune dysregulation: the increased levels in comparison with controls are rarely in the pathological range and (iii) increases appear to be continuously distributed with inconsistent evidence for a discrete subpopulation of psychosis with raised cytokine levels. These factors may indicate a transdiagnostic inflammatory component of pathogenesis to both depression and psychotic disorders. However, the demonstration of causality requires that treatments that reduce circulating cytokines are therapeutically effective in relation to their ability to normalize peripheral cytokine activation – the topic of this review.

It is possible that peripheral immune activation is not directly pathogenic but rather an indicator or a predisposing factor for inflammation in the brain. IL-6 is a key mediator in the innate immune pathway relevant to brain function, with ability to cross the blood-brain barrier (BBB) and importantly to increase its permeability (9). IL-6 is released from monocytes and T lymphocytes in response to pro-inflammatory mediators such as IL-1β and TNF-α. IL-6 increases CRP and local inflammatory mediators including nitric oxide and chemokines leading to recruitment of circulating immune cells into the brain and activation of microglia (10), the resident macrophages of the brain. Activated microglia can contribute to an inflammatory neurotoxic mix of cytokines, chemokines, leukotrienes, metalloproteinases and reactive oxygen and nitrogen species (ROS, RNS) in experimental systems and probably do so in many neuroinflammatory disorders. Astrocytes, oligodendroglia and neurones themselves can respond to, and secrete inflammatory messengers.

Whether such changes occur in the brain in psychosis is not known. Despite 150 years of cellular and molecular pathological studies in human post-mortem brain, there is no diagnostic or subtype selective signature of psychosis. Quantitative changes in the number of inflammatory cellular elements or molecular markers in psychosis have so far proved inconsistent. The recent development of Positron Emission Tomography (PET) imaging of radioligand binding to molecular markers of inflammatory cell activation offers a way forward by enabling assessments in living symptomatic patients free of potentially confounding effects of antipsychotic drug treatment. The sole radioligand target so far is the translocator protein (TSPO) which is overexpressed by activated microglia but probably also by other cell types. Nevertheless, most studies report no increases or reductions of TSPO in schizophrenia (11). This does not exclude a role of microglia in an inflammatory pathogenesis of schizophrenia as they have a number of potentially pathogenic phenotypes not captured by TSPO binding. The field is young and a number of radioligands are in development that have the promise of clarifying the role of inflammatory cells in psychiatric illness.

Peripheral inflammation can trigger the formation of ROS by microglia as part of the defence against infectious agents. Glutathione (GSH) is the main redox buffer mechanism in the brain and it can be detected in vivo using magnetic resonance spectroscopy (MRS). A recent meta-analysis of 18 studies reported a small but statistically significant depletion of glutathione in anterior cingulate cortex in active psychosis suggesting an active production of ROS and possibly reflecting a response to neuroinflammation (12). Circulating or central IL-6 can have direct effect on neuronal function. IL-6 signal transduction pathways (MAPK) that decrease the function of vesicular monoamine transportation (VMAT2), with impact on monoamines such as dopamine. IL-6 can also affect the glutamate (Glu) system by activation of indoleamine 2,3 dioxygenase (IDO) which then catabolizes tryptophan into kynurenine and downstream quinolic acid (QUIN). Kynurenic acid acts as an antagonist to Glu receptors and QUIN can directly activate the n-methyl-d-aspartate receptor (NMDAR) and increase excitotoxicity (9). See Figure 6.1.

Thus, there are a number of potential mechanistic pathways on which repurposed and new molecules could act to influence an inflammatory pathway to psychotic illnesses. As yet, however, it has not been possible to delineate a biomarker profile that identifies a subgroup of patients with a likely immunological pathogenesis.

6.2 Evidence of Effectiveness of Neuroprotective Antibiotics

6.2.1 Minocycline

Negative symptoms remain the most difficult to treat in psychosis, and impact significantly on impaired quality of life and social functioning (13). The duration of untreated illness and repeated episodes, predict greater negative symptoms and this suggests that an active process is at play in acute phases of illness, that results in negative symptoms, and that

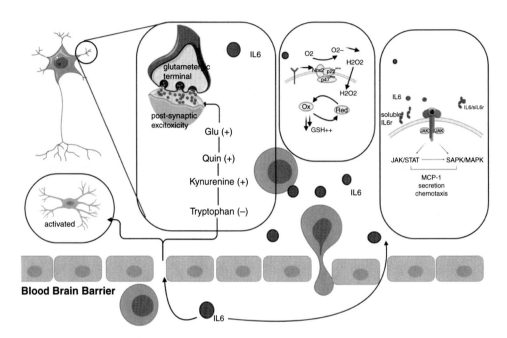

Figure 6.1 Schematic overview of potential mechanisms for immune actions relevant to psychosis. (Upthegrove 2020, unpublished).

this is taking hold early in the course of illness (14). This has led to interest in directly targeting neuroprotection and early treatment to prevent the development of negative symptoms, particularly as no current medication is effective. Even clozapine's efficacy for negative symptoms is marginal, and thus this remains an area of significant unmet need.

Minocycline is a tetracycline antibiotic that has well-known neuroprotective properties, and may stop the activation of resting state to activated microglia (15). Preliminary evidence from clinical trials suggested that post-stroke and Parkinson's disease may be helped by minocycline (16,17). In psychosis, there is evidence of dendritic loss and loss of astroglia and oligodendroglial cells that support neuronal function. Subtle loss of grey matter occurs early, before transitions to psychosis and is progressive, in unmedicated patients transitioning to psychosis and in early phases of first episode (18). Thus, the indication that minocycline may lessen grey-matter loss via impairing the actions of activated microglia. Minocycline also acts on glutamatergic pathways that have long been implicated in the pathogenesis of schizophrenia. Phencyclidine and ketamine block NMDA function and reproduce predominantly the negative symptoms of schizophrenia in healthy volunteers (19) and minocycline's potential action here has also been demonstrated in animal models (20,21).

There have been three large double-blind randomized placebo-controlled trials (RCT) of minocycline for the treatment of schizophrenia. A two-centre study in Brazil and Pakistan was concluded in 2014 with 94 people diagnosed with schizophrenia on stable medication who completed 12 months add-on treatment with placebo or minocycline (22). Minocycline-treated patients showed greater improvement on total positive and negative symptom scale

(PANSS) score, and this was mainly because the negative syndrome score improved more in those taking minocycline. Positive symptom subscale scores showed a smaller, trend significant minocycline effect. The study's results also suggest that improvement in negative symptoms continues up to 12 months. A second RCT was carried out in Tel Aviv (23) in 70 relapsed patients. After stabilisation on second-generation antipsychotic drugs, they were randomized to placebo or minocycline in a 1:2 ratio. Significant treatment effects on negative but not positive symptoms were detectable at the first rating at three months.

These studies provided proof of concept for the Benefits of Minocycline on Negative Symptoms in Psychosis (BeneMin) study, a 12-month definitive trial, which recruited 207 patients within 5 years of diagnosis of schizophrenia spectrum disorder from early psychosis and community services in the UK. Patients were randomly assigned by automated per-muted blocks algorithm, stratified by pharmacy, to receive minocycline (200 mg per day for two weeks, then 300 mg per day) or matching placebo, as adjunct to antipsychotic treatment. BeneMin assessed both clinical outcomes (PANSS negative symptoms) and biomarker outcomes including grey-matter volume, dorsolateral prefrontal cortex activation during a working memory task, and plasma concentration of IL-6. However, in BeneMin, the effects of minocycline were largely negative. The primary clinical outcomes improved over the 12 months study period and were not different in minocycline or placebo groups. Biomarker outcomes did not change over time and were not affected by minocycline (24). At this stage of illness (within five years onset of first treatment) there was no evidence of a persistent progressive neuropathic or inflammatory process on which minocycline could have acted to reduce negative symptoms. Post hoc subset analysis did not reveal any evidence that minocycline had effects in those with greater circulating CRP or IL-6 concentrations for example in 129 patients with IL-6 concentrations >0.5 pg/ml. The negative result of the BeneMin study was recently corroborated by a further large and negative study in 200 patients with long-standing psychosis with marked positive and negative symptoms (25). It is possible that minocycline might have beneficial effects in a subgroup of the schizophrenia spectrum for example in those with at risk mental states or with treatment-resistant symptoms.

The BeneMin study concluded that further trials of minocycline in early psychosis are not warranted without clearer evidence of an inflammatory process against which minocycline has proven efficacy. In a recent study from China, groups of 25 patients who received 100 mg or 200 mg/day of minocycline may have improved more than those on placebo because the patient group had greater baseline levels of IL-6, IL-1B and TNF-α than a healthy control group (26). Any future studies need also to beware the possibility that microglial responses can be beneficial; a recent study reported that although minocycline reduced PET evidence of microgliosis after brain trauma, cognitive performance worsened and CSF levels of neurofilamnet-1, a marker of neurodegeneration, increased (27). Minocycline is generally well tolerated but rare side effects include vestibular and gastrointestinal disturbance, yeast infection and cutaneous symptoms including pigmentation and urticaria. Therefore, in the absence of clear evidence of effective-ness, minocycline cannot be recommended in routine practice.

6.3 Non-Steroidal Anti-Inflammatory Agents (NSAIDs)

NSAIDs work by inhibiting cyclo-oxygenase (COX) enzymes, which are responsible for the production of prostaglandins. COX-1 is constitutively expressed in most tissues, and elevated activity is implicated in inflammatory disorders. In the central nervous system

(CNS) COX-2 is involved in synaptic activity, particularly glutamate transmission, cytokine metabolism and an essential component of inflammatory pathways including microglial activation (9). Common side effects from longer term use include gastrointestinal erosion, renal and hepatic insufficiency (28).

6.3.1 Aspirin

Aspirin is an NSAID agent that irreversibly inhibits COX-1 and modifies activity of COX-2. It therefore suppresses the production of prostaglandins and other key messengers in the inflammatory process. Although aspirin does not easily cross the BBB, it is known to suppress the HPA stress response. Trials have largely been small and few in numbers. Somner et al.'s review of anti-inflammatory treatments in schizophrenia reported on two studies that investigated aspirin (1,000 mg per day) as an adjunct to antipsychotic treatment in schizophrenia; aspirin had a weak/moderate benefit over placebo (effect size 0.3) (29). A later study from Iran reported significantly greater improvement in groups of 20 patients receiving aspirin at 350 mg or 500 mg than those on placebo. However, the initial group mean PANSS scores (respectively 147, 135, 111) indicate an exceptionally ill group with major baseline differences none of whom dropped out during the four week trial (30).

6.3.2 Celecoxib

Celecoxib is a COX-2 inhibitor, which may reduce the synthesis of pro-inflammatory cytokines or bring the type-1 and type-2 immune responses back into balance and may prevent neuronal death induced by kainic acid (31). Yokota suggested additional actions outside of the COX-2 pathway may be indicated in patients with schizophrenia, as no up regulation of COX-2 hippocampal expression was seen compared to healthy controls or patients with Alzheimer's disease (32). In their meta-analysis of eight randomized controlled trials, Zengh et al. (33), concluded that celecoxib is a safe and effective adjunct to antipsychotic therapy, particularly in first-episode schizophrenia. However, two of the positive studies were reported only as conference abstracts and overall evidence was limited. A 2016 narrative review of randomized clinical trials concluded that the beneficial effects of celecoxib are mostly evident in the early stages of schizophrenia (34). However, there are negative trials including Rapaport et al. 2005 (35), who augmented antipsychotic medication with celecoxib in continuously unwell patients with schizophrenia and a negative meta-analysis conducted by Sommer et al. in 2013 (29). In summary, the existing celecoxib trials vary a great deal with regards to quality, study design, inclusion criteria including demographic and clinical features, illness stage, data analyses and country of origin. This may explain the current lack of clarity in results. A comprehensive Cochrane review of celecoxib plus standard care in schizophrenia is currently registered and due to report in 2021 (36).

6.4 Antibody Immunotherapy

Monoclonal antibodies were developed from the mid-1990s able to target inflammatory pathways, cancer cells and atherosclerosis. Monoclonal antibodies against cytokines such as TNF-α (e.g., infliximab, adalumumab), IL-6/IL-6 R (e.g., tocilizumab, siltuximab) are used particularly for rheumatoid arthritis and other systemic inflammatory conditions (37). Side effects of monoclonal antibodies vary but include hypothyroidism, nephrolithiasis, hepatic disorders, pancytopenia and Stevens–Johnson syndrome. These medications are currently investigated in experimental medicine studies to better elucidate mechanisms and therapeutic potential for psychiatric indications. A small recent trial of tocilizumab, an anti-IL-6 R monoclonal antibody (mAb), in stable patients with established schizophrenia who were not selected for any evidence of inflammation, found no evidence of benefit (38).

There is evidence that selection of immune active patients is possible and may allow more specific targeting. In a recent trial of 60 patients, the antidepressant response to infliximab was related to higher CRP levels at baseline, response was only seen in those with a baseline CRP of greater than 5 mg/l, and TNF-α concentrations were significantly higher in infliximab responders vs non-responders (39). Currently, a number of RCTs are testing anti-cytokine mAbs for depression based on patients with evidence of inflammation including the *Insight* study led by Khandaker and colleagues (40). However, RCTs of immune-modulating agents in psychosis based on a specific patient group characterized by illness stage, symptom profile and evidence of immune activation are lacking. Weikert et al. are in the process of a randomized controlled trial of Catakunimab, which acts on IL-1β in adult patients with schizophrenia or schizoaffective disorder (Universal trial number: U1111-1166–6037). Upthegrove, Khandaker et al. will investigate the mechanistic effect of tocilizumab in a stratified sample of participants with FEP in a trial expected to begin in 2021 (personal communication).

6.5 Immunosuppressants

6.5.1 Methotrexate and Azathioprine

Low dose methotrexate is commonly used as an anti-inflammatory and immunosuppressive drug to treat conditions such as rheumatoid arthritis and psoriasis, and as a cancer treatment. Methotrexate's mode of action in inflammatory disorders is poorly understood. It restores the pro-anti–inflammatory cytokine balance and this is thought to involve a restoration of regulatory T cell function (41). At much higher doses, methotrexate is used as an antiproliferative agent in cancer chemotherapy. Subsequent effects of higher doses can include life-threatening immune suppression, and at lower oral doses renal and hepatic toxicity and neurological toxicity (42).

Given the evidence of possible autoimmune mechanisms in schizophrenia, Chaudhry et al. completed a double-blind 12-week randomized controlled trial in participants with schizophrenia spectrum disorders of low dose (10 mg) methotrexate given weekly, in addition to treatment as usual, over 12 weeks. All participants took folate supplements. Forty-seven participants were randomized to placebo and 45 to methotrexate with respectively 39 and 37 completing 12 weeks of treatment. PANSS positive subscale scores improved by 2.5 more than those on placebo (p = 0.023; ANOVA co-varying for baseline) but PANNS negative scores did not differ between groups (43,44).

The possibility of effectiveness of an immune suppressant mechanism also resonates with two anecdotal case reports that report stem cell marrow transplantation in one case, which was associated with a permanent cure of a chronic schizophrenic illness (45) and in another case, transmitted a severe illness from an affected donor to previously well and middle-aged recipient (46).

Azathioprine was developed as a chemotherapy medication and subsequently used as an immunosuppressive agent for the treatment of Crohn's disease, ulcerative colitis, rheumatoid arthritis, other immune related disorders and to prevent transplant rejection. It also suppresses purine synthesis. Azathioprine is activated in several steps to two active metabolites. One pilot study in 1997 demonstrated clinical improvement in 2 out of 11 patients with chronic resistant schizophrenia co-prescribed azathioprine at 150 mg per day for 7 weeks (47). No further trials have been registered or reported.

6.6 Antioxidants

Schizophrenia can be characterized by a pro-oxidative as well as pro-inflammatory state. See Figure 6.1. During normal oxidative metabolism, radicals are produced, and antioxidants are present to regulate and balance this in a mechanism termed redox homeostasis. Radicals are highly reactive species that play an important role in signalling and adaptation, but left unchecked, will contribute to a status of 'oxidative stress'. This may lead to cell injury (lipid peroxidation, protein carboxylation and DNA damage) or death (48). Together with the low incidence of side effects and general tolerance, this knowledge has led to a number of trials of agents focussing on antioxidants to be proposed.

6.6.1 N-Acetylcysteine

N-acetylcysteine (NAC) has anti-inflammatory properties that include the inhibition of IL-6, TNF-α and IL-1β, all key actors in the innate inflammatory pathway. NAC is also the main precursor of GSH, and this may be neuroprotective in improving oxidative stress buffering in psychosis, as detailed in Section 6.1. This action is the basis of its clinical use to prevent liver toxicity after paracetamol overdose. NAC also influences synaptic glutamate content through the glutamate-cysteine transporter. Despite its novel actions, few studies have assessed the influence of NAC addition to antipsychotic medication. Berk et al. used NAC or placebo with atypical antipsychotics in 140 subjects with chronic schizophrenia, in a double-blind RCT and showed no effect of NAC at 8 weeks but significant difference in negative symptoms and general symptoms at 24 weeks (49). Farokhnia et al. (2013) used NAC or placebo in addition to risperidone in 42 people with established schizophrenia who were experiencing acute exacerbation of symptoms. This small double-blind RCT showed significant difference also in negative and general symptoms on PANSS at eight weeks (50). Russell et al. have an ongoing large multisite Australian RCT of NAC in schizophrenia with data collection due to be completed in 2019 (51).

6.6.2 Polyunsaturated Fatty Acids

Polyunsaturated Fatty Acids (PUFAs) are essential to the BBB development, fluidity, and permeability (52). It is hypothesized that treatment with omega-3 PUFAs such as eicosapentaenoic acid, may reduce the amount of unhelpful omega-6 PUFAs in cell membranes and this in turn would lead to a decreased synthesis of prostaglandins by COX enzymes. Omega-3 also reduces activated pro-inflammatory actors such as cytokines, monocytes, macrophages and microglia.

There have been a number of trials of omega-3 in schizophrenia, FEP and in the clinical high risk (CHR) state for psychosis. A recent systematic review in schizophrenia had a total sample of 167 subjects and meta-analysis showed no evidence for the effect of omega-3 augmentation on positive or total symptoms (53). In a randomized double-blind controlled trial of first-episode received omega-3 or placebo in addition to antipsychotic medication over 12 weeks. While there was no difference in the primary outcome (symptom change scores) those in the active treatment arm received lower average dose of antipsychotic medication (54). In CHR groups, one trial reported a clear benefit of omega-3 in preventing the transition to psychosis both in the short (55) and longer term follow up (56). However, this was not replicated in the larger, multicentre, double-blind placebo-controlled NEUROAPRO-E study, which showed no significant difference in transition rates (57).

6.6.3 Statins

Fluvastatin, simvastatin and atorvastatin have been shown to block effects of the pro-inflammatory cytokine IL-6 in vitro. IL-6 induces monocyte chemoattractant protein (MCP-1), a chemokine that plays an important role in the monocyte/macrophage chemotaxis and JAK/STAT pathway involved in inflammation. See Figure 6.1. Statins suppress MCP-1 expression (58). In relation to inflammation affecting the brain, simvastatin has been shown to have a neuroprotective effect in preventing loss of cortical grey matter in patients with multiple sclerosis (59). However, Vincenzi et al. conducted a randomized placebo-controlled trial of adjunctive pravastatin in psychosis over 12 weeks with results showing an effect on lipids but not on clinical symptoms (60). Ghanizadeh et al. completed a double-blind randomized controlled trial of lovastatin in schizophrenia over eight weeks, with no effect on primary endpoint of clinical rating of psychosis symptoms (61). In contrast, simvastatin added to TAU was associated with a small overall improvement on PANSS negative symptom scores in a 2 × 2 study that included the 5HT3 receptor antagonist ondansetron and placebo in 300 participants (62,63).The small improvements were probably not clinically significant and those treated with the combination of ondansetron and simvastatin showed no benefit over placebo, possibly due to a greater side-effect burden. Begemann et al. are concluding a randomized controlled trial of simvastatin in recent-onset schizophrenia (within three years) in a multisite double-blind design – positive and negative symptoms score together with inflammatory markers will be the primary end point (64).

Therefore, in keeping with the evidence of PUFAs, no clear signal for efficacy of statins for treating symptoms of psychosis has yet emerged. Statins do have some rare side effects that would need to be weighted in any decision for their wider use, including hepatic dysfunction, myositis and peripheral neuropathy. Furthermore, statins have the potential to affect CNS function in many ways such as their influence on neurosteroids and cell signalling pathways; and there is presently no evidence that statins benefit psychosis through an anti-inflammatory mechanism. Nevertheless statins may have an important role in treating and preventing metabolic dysfunction in schizophrenia (65) which may relate to a potential pro-inflammatory pathway that is common to both psychosis and metabolic dysfunction (66).

6.7 Summary and Next Steps

While innate immune targets could be important for novel therapeutic options in schizophrenia, RCTs of anti-inflammatory agents in psychosis to date have been limited in number of trials and scale, and have yielded mixed results. This may simply reflect a need for larger replication studies, but also potentially because of a non-specific choice of patient group. Adjunct treatment with aspirin, omega-3, NAC, statins and Cox-2 inhibitors appear to have no clear signal or limited evidence at the group level in schizophrenia (32,33). Side effects from these interventions may range from mild and infrequent (e.g., NAC) to potentially more significant (monoclonal antibodies and immunosuppressants). Caution must therefore be taken when making any treatment recommendations based on current evidence. Knowledge must build on the most robust evidence to date, for example the BeneMin study, a large sufficiently powered high quality RCT that found no benefit from add-on minocycline in early phases of established schizophrenia (34). There are no randomized control trials of anti-inflammatory drugs that have used inflammatory markers or other strategies to preselect potentially responsive patients based on evidence of immune dysfunction. However, there is yet no validated or a priori profile of peripheral cytokines or other markers that could be justified as a stratifier. Similarly, there is no clearly defined inflammatory clinical subgroup although some studies have focused on early psychosis as a time when inflammation may be driving the development of psychosis.

RCTs of immune-modulating agents in psychosis based on targeted, personalized patient selection criteria that include evidence of an inflammatory state in psychosis are essential but are in their infancy. The Optimization of Treatment and Management of Schizophrenia in Europe (OPTiMiSE) is a cohort study that will validate stratification clustering based on clinical symptoms and treatment response, but also include additional information from inflammatory markers (67). They have found that patients characterized by the most severe symptoms (including positive, negative and general physiopathology) had the highest levels of IL-7, IL-15, IL-17, IFN-γ and TNF-α and propose that clustering methods aimed at reducing clinical heterogeneity may also reduce biological heterogeneity (68). Our own study Psychosis Immune Mechanism Stratified Medicine Study (PIMS) aims to identify a phenotypic profile and stage of psychosis related to elevated IL-6 and related pro-inflammatory cytokines advanced data science, including machine learning, to inform a stratified experimental trial of tocilizumab. These are two much needed first steps to both advance the field and allow immunology and psychosis to catch up with targeted interventions and match the advances seen in cancer and inflammatory disorders.

In terms of clinical practice, given the lack of replicated findings and key uncertainties, together with their known side-effect profile, the use of anti-inflammatory medication is not currently recommended for the treatment or prevention of psychosis in routine clinical practice (69).

Key Points

- Primary evidence suggests the innate immune pathway could be an important, novel target for new therapies
- Further evidence of the relevance of peripheral markers of immune dysfunction to brain changes seen in in psychosis would increase the certainty of a causal pathway and give vital information about more refined targets
- Mixed evidence from trials of various repurposed agents may be the result of a lack of targeting to those with evidence of active immune dysfunction
- New studies are needed that provide evidence for how to stratify participants in future trials, and what stage of symptom profile should be targeted

References

1. Upthegrove RN, Manzanares-Teson NM Barnes, NM. Cytokine function in medication-naive first episode psychosis: a systematic review and meta-analysis. *Schizophrenia Research*. 2014;155 (1–3):101–8.

2. Wang AK, Miller BJ. Meta-analysis of cerebrospinal fluid cytokine and tryptophan catabolite alterations in psychiatric patients: comparisons between schizophrenia, bipolar disorder, and depression. *Schizophr Bull*. 2018;44(1):75–83.

3. Khandaker GM, Pearson RM, Zammit S, et al. Association of serum interleukin 6 and C-reactive protein in childhood with depression and psychosis in young adult life: a population-based longitudinal study. *JAMA Psychiatry*. 2014;71(10):1121–8.

4. Metcalf SA, Jones PB, Nordstrom T, et al. Serum C-reactive protein in adolescence and risk of schizophrenia in adulthood: A prospective birth cohort study. *Brain Behav Immun*. 2017;59:253–9.

5. Khandaker GM, Zammit S, Burgess S, et al. Association between a functional interleukin 6 receptor genetic variant and risk of depression and psychosis in a population-based birth cohort. *Brain, Behavior, and Immunity*. 2018;69:264–72.

6. Hartwig FP, Borges MC, Horta BL, et al. Inflammatory biomarkers and risk of schizophrenia: a 2-sample Mendelian randomization study. *JAMA Psychiatry*. 2017;74(12):1226–33.

7. Miller BJ Culpepper N, Rapaport, MH. C-reactive protein levels in schizophrenia: a review and meta-analysis. *Clin Schizophr Relat Psychoses*. 2014;7(4):223–30.

8. Khandaker GM. Commentary: causal associations between inflammation, cardiometabolic markers and schizophrenia: the known unknowns. *International Journal of Epidemiology*. 2019;48(5)1735.

9. Upthegrove R, Barnes NM. The immune system and schizophrenia: an update for clinicians. *Advances in Psychiatric Treatment*. 2014;20(2):83–91.

10. Khandaker GM, Dantzer, R. Is there a role for immune-to-brain communication in schizophrenia? *Psychopharmacology (Berl)*. 2016;233(9):1559–73.

11. Notter T, Coughlin JM, Gschwind T, et al. Translational evaluation of translocator protein as a marker of neuroinflammation in schizophrenia. *Molecular Psychiatry*. 2018;23(2):323.

12. Das TK, Javadzadeh A, Dey A, et al. Antioxidant defense in schizophrenia and bipolar disorder: a meta-analysis of MRS studies of anterior cingulate glutathione. *Progress in Neuro-Psychopharmacology and Biological Psychiatry*. 2019;91:94–102.

13. Barnes TR, Leeson VC, Mutsatsa SH, et al. Duration of untreated psychosis and social function: 1-year follow-up study of first-episode schizophrenia. *The British Journal of Psychiatry*. 2008;193(3): 203–9.

14. Boonstra N, Klaassen R, Sytema S, et al. Duration of untreated psychosis and negative symptoms – a systematic review and meta-analysis of individual patient data. *Schizophrenia Research*. 2012;142 (1–3):12–19.

15. Chen M, Ona VO, Li M, et al. Minocycline inhibits caspase-1 and caspase-3 expression and delays mortality in a transgenic mouse model of Huntington disease. *Nature Medicine*. 2000;6(7):797

16. Lampl Y, Boaz M, Gilad R, et al. Minocycline treatment in acute stroke: an open-label, evaluator-blinded study. *Neurology*. 2007;69(14):1404–10.

17. Gordon PH, Moore DH, Miller RG, et al. Efficacy of minocycline in patients with amyotrophic lateral sclerosis: a phase III randomised trial. *The Lancet Neurology*. 2007;6(12):1045–53.

18. Takahashi T, Wood SJ, Yung AR, et al. Progressive gray matter reduction of the superior temporal gyrus during transition to psychosis. *Archives of General Psychiatry*. 2009;66(4):366–76.

19. Deakin JW, Lees J, McKie S, et al. Glutamate and the neural basis of the subjective effects of ketamine: a pharmaco–magnetic resonance imaging study.

Archives of General Psychiatry. 2008; 65(2):154–64.

20. Olney JW, Farber, NB. Glutamate receptor dysfunction and schizophrenia. *Archives of General Psychiatry.* 1995;52(12):998–1007.

21. Zhang L, Shirayama Y, Iyo M, et al. Minocycline attenuates hyperlocomotion and prepulse inhibition deficits in mice after administration of the NMDA receptor antagonist dizocilpine. *Neuropsychopharmacology.* 2007; 32(9):2004.

22. Chaudhry IB, Hallak J, Husain N, et al. Minocycline benefits negative symptoms in early schizophrenia: a randomised double-blind placebo-controlled clinical trial in patients on standard treatment. *Journal of Psychopharmacology.* 2012;26 (9):1185–93.

23. Levkovitz Y, Mendlovich S, Riwkes S, et al. A double-blind, randomized study of minocycline for the treatment of negative and cognitive symptoms in early-phase schizophrenia. *Journal of Clinical Psychiatry.* 2010;71(2):138.

24. Deakin B, Suckling J, Barnes TRE, et al. The benefit of minocycline on negative symptoms of schizophrenia in patients with recent-onset psychosis (BeneMin): a randomised, double-blind, placebo-controlled trial. *The Lancet Psychiatry.* 2018;5(11):885–94.

25. Zhang L, Zheng H, Wu R, et al. Minocycline adjunctive treatment to risperidone for negative symptoms in schizophrenia: association with pro-inflammatory cytokine levels. *Progress in Neuropsychopharmacology and Biological Psychiatry.* 2018;85:69–76.

26. Zhang L, Zheng H, Wu R, et al. The effect of minocycline on amelioration of cognitive deficits and pro-inflammatory cytokines levels in patients with schizophrenia. *Schizophrenia Research.* 2019;212:92–8.

27. Scott G, Zetterberg H, Jolly A, et al. Minocycline reduces chronic microglial activation after brain trauma but increases neurodegeneration. *Brain.* 2018;141 (2):459–71.

28. Jones R, Tait, C. Gastrointestinal side-effects of NSAIDs in the community. *The British Journal of Clinical Practice.* 1995;49(2):67–70.

29. Sommer IE, van Westrhenen R, Begemann MJH, et al. Efficacy of anti-inflammatory agents to improve symptoms in patients with schizophrenia: an update. *Schizophrenia Bulletin.* 2013;40 (1):181–91.

30. Attari A, Mojdeh A, Soltani F, et al. Aspirin inclusion in antipsychotic treatment on severity of symptoms in schizophrenia: A randomized clinical trial. *Iranian Journal of Psychiatry and Behavioral Sciences.* 2017;11(1):e5848.

31. Akhondzadeh S, Tabatabaee M, Amini H, et al. Celecoxib as adjunctive therapy in schizophrenia: a double-blind, randomized and placebo-controlled trial. *Schizophrenia Research.* 2007;90 (1–3):179–85.

32. Yokota O, Terada S, Ishihara T, et al. Neuronal expression of cyclooxygenase-2, a pro-inflammatory protein, in the hippocampus of patients with schizophrenia. *Progress in Neuropsychopharmacology and Biological Psychiatry.* 2004;28(4):715–21.

33. Zheng W, Cai DB, Yang XH, et al. Adjunctive celecoxib for schizophrenia: a meta-analysis of randomized, double-blind, placebo-controlled trials. *Journal of Psychiatric Research.* 2017;92:139–46.

34. Marini S, De Berardis D, Vellante F, et al. Celecoxib adjunctive treatment to antipsychotics in schizophrenia: a review of randomized clinical add-on trials. *Mediators of Inflammation.* 2016. https:// doi.org/10.1155/2016/3476240

35. Rapaport MH, Delrahim KK, Bresee J, et al. Celecoxib augmentation of continuously ill patients with schizophrenia. *Biological Psychiatry.* 2005;57(12):1594–6.

36. Kotecha A, Upthegrove R. Celecoxib plus standard care for people with schizophrenia. *Cochrane Database of Systematic Reviews.* 2018;(12):CD009205. doi:10.1002/14651858.CD009205.pub2

37. Suzuki M, Kato C, Kato A. Therapeutic antibodies: their mechanisms of action and the pathological findings they induce in toxicity studies. *Journal of Toxicologic Pathology*. 2015;28(3):133–9.

38. Girgis RR, Ciarleglio A, Choo T, et al. A randomized, double-blind, placebo-controlled clinical trial of tocilizumab, an interleukin-6 receptor antibody, for residual symptoms in schizophrenia. *Neuropsychopharmacology*. 2018;43(6):1317–23.

39. Raison CL, Rutherford RE, Woolwine BJ, et al. A randomized controlled trial of the tumor necrosis factor antagonist infliximab for treatment-resistant depression: the role of baseline inflammatory biomarkers. *JAMA Psychiatry*. 2013;70(1):31–41.

40. Khandaker GM, Khandaker GM, Oltean BP, et al. Protocol for the insight study: a randomised controlled trial of single-dose tocilizumab in patients with depression and low-grade inflammation. *BMJ Open*. 2018;8(9):e025333.

41. Cribbs AP, Kennedy A, Penn H, et al. Methotrexate restores regulatory T cell function through demethylation of the FoxP3 upstream enhancer in patients with rheumatoid arthritis. *Arthritis & Rheumatology*. 2015;67(5):1182–92.

42. Cronstein B. The antirheumatic agents sulphasalazine and methotrexate share an anti-inflammatory mechanism. *Rheumatology*. 1995;34(suppl_2):30–2.

43. Chaudhry IB, Husain N, ur Rahman R, et al. A randomised double-blind placebo-controlled 12- week feasibility trial of methotrexate added to treatment as usual in early schizophrenia: study protocol for a randomised controlled trial. *Trials*. 2015;16(1):9.

44. Chaudhry IH, Husain MO, Khoso AB, et al. A randomised clinical trial of methotrexate points to possible efficacy and adaptive immune dysfunction in psychosis. *Transl Psychiatry*. (in press) 2020.

45. Miyaoka T, Wake R, Hashioka S, et al. Remission of psychosis in treatment-resistant schizophrenia following bone marrow transplantation: a case report. *Frontiers in Psychiatry*. 2017;8:174.

46. Sommer I, van Bekkum DW, Klein H, et al. Severe chronic psychosis after allogeneic SCT from a schizophrenic sibling. *Bone Marrow Transplantation*. 2015;50 (1):153–4.

47. Levine J, Gutman J, Feraro R, et al. Side effect profile of azathioprine in the treatment of chronic schizophrenic patients. *Neuropsychobiology*. 1997;36 (4):172–6.

48. Mahadik SP, Evans D, Lal H. Oxidative stress and role of antioxidant and omega-3 essential fatty acid supplementation in schizophrenia. *Prog Neuropsychopharmacol Biol Psychiatry*. 2001;25(3):463–93.

49. Berk M, Copolov D, Dean O, et al. N-acetyl cysteine as a glutathione precursor for schizophrenia – a double-blind, randomized, placebo-controlled trial. *Biological Psychiatry*. 2008;64(5):361–8.

50. Farokhnia M, Azarkolah A, Adinehfar F, et al. N-acetylcysteine as an adjunct to risperidone for treatment of negative symptoms in patients with chronic schizophrenia: a randomized, double-blind, placebo-controlled study. *Clinical Neuropharmacology*. 2013;36 (6):185–92.

51. Rossell SL, Francis PS, Galletly C, et al. N-acetylcysteine (NAC) in schizophrenia resistant to clozapine: a double-blind randomised placebo-controlled trial targeting negative symptoms. *BMC Psychiatry*. 2016;16(1):320.

52. Fusar-Poli P, Berger, G. Eicosapentaenoic acid interventions in schizophrenia: meta-analysis of randomized, placebo-controlled studies. *Journal of Clinical Psychopharmacology*. 2012;32 (2):179–85.

53. Bozzatello P, Brignolo E, Grandi E, et al. Supplementation with omega-3 fatty acids in psychiatric disorders: a review of literature data. *Journal of Clinical Medicine*. 2016;5(8):67.

54. Berger GE, Proffitt TM, McConchie M, et al. Ethyl-eicosapentaenoic acid in

first-episode psychosis: a randomized, placebo-controlled trial. *Journal of Clinical Psychiatry*. 2007;68(12):1867–75.

55. Amminger GP, Schäfer MR, Papageorgiou K, et al. Long-chain ω-3 fatty acids for indicated prevention of psychotic disorders: a randomized, placebo-controlled trial. *Archives of General Psychiatry*. 2010;67(2):146–54.

56. Amminger GP, Schäfer MR, Schlögelhofer M, et al. Longer-term outcome in the prevention of psychotic disorders by the Vienna omega-3 study. *Nature Communications*. 2015;6(1):1–7.

57. McGorry PD, Nelson B, Markulev C, et al. Effect of ω-3 polyunsaturated fatty acids in young people at ultrahigh risk for psychotic disorders: the NEURAPRO randomized clinical trial. *JAMA Psychiatry*. 2017;74 (1):19–27.

58. Jougasaki M, Ichiki T, Takenoshita Y, et al. Statins suppress interleukin-6-induced monocyte chemo-attractant protein-1 by inhibiting Janus kinase/signal transducers and activators of transcription pathways in human vascular endothelial cells. *British Journal of Pharmacology*. 2010;159 (6):1294–303.

59. Chataway J., Schuerer N, Alsanousi A, et al. Effect of high-dose simvastatin on brain atrophy and disability in secondary progressive multiple sclerosis (MS-STAT): a randomised, placebo-controlled, phase 2 trial. *The Lancet*. 2014;383(9936):2213–21.

60. Vincenzi B, Stock S, Borba CP, et al. A randomized placebo-controlled pilot study of pravastatin as an adjunctive therapy in schizophrenia patients: effect on inflammation, psychopathology, cognition and lipid metabolism. *Schizophrenia Research*. 2014;159(2–3):395–403.

61. Ghanizadeh A, Rezaee Z, Dehbozorgi S, et al. Lovastatin for the adjunctive treatment of schizophrenia: a preliminary randomized double-blind placebo-controlled trial. *Psychiatry Research*. 2014;219(3):431–5.

62. Chaudhry IB, Husain N, Drake R, et al. Add-on clinical effects of simvastatin and ondansetron in patients with schizophrenia stabilized on antipsychotic treatment: pilot study. *Therapeutic Advances in Psychopharmacology*. 2014;4 (3):110–16.

63. Deakin JF, Husain N, Parker AJ, et al. Efficacy of ondansetron and simvastatin on cognition and negative symptoms in established schizophrenia. *Neuropsychopharmacology*. 2014;39: S355–6.

64. Begemann MJ, Schutte MJ, Slot MI, et al. Simvastatin augmentation for recent-onset psychotic disorder: A study protocol. *BBA Clinical*. 2015;4:52–8.

65. Blackburn R, Osborn D, Walters K, et al. Statin prescribing for people with severe mental illnesses: a staggered cohort study of 'real-world' impacts. *BMJ Open*. 2017;7 (3):e013154.

66. Perry BI, Upthegrove R, Thompson A, et al. Dysglycaemia, inflammation and psychosis: findings from the UK ALSPAC birth cohort. *Schizophrenia Bulletin*. 2018;45(2):330–8.

67. Leucht S, Winter-van Rossum I, Heres S, et al. The optimization of treatment and management of schizophrenia in Europe (OPTiMiSE) trial: rationale for its methodology and a review of the effectiveness of switching antipsychotics. *Schizophrenia Bulletin*. 2015;41(3): 549–58.

68. Martinuzzi E, Barbosa S, Daoudlarian D, et al. Stratification and prediction of remission in first-episode psychosis patients: the OPTiMiSE cohort study. *Translational Psychiatry*. 2019;9(1):20.

69. Barnes TR, Drake R, Paton C, et al. Evidence-based guidelines for the pharmacological treatment of schizophrenia: Updated recommendations from the British Association for Psychopharmacology. *Journal of Psychopharmacology*. 2020 Jan;34(1):3–78.

Inflammation, Sickness Behaviour and Depression

Golam Khandaker, Alessandro Colasanti and
Neil Harrison

7.1 Introduction

The association between infections and changes in mood, motivation and cognition including induction of lethargy, irritability, impaired concentration and memory, lowering of mood, decreased social activity, anhedonia and somnolence has been known for centuries (1). However, it was only in the late 1980s when it was realized that these behavioural changes are the same regardless of the infecting organism (2; 3), and that sickness behaviours represent a critical component of the *host* response to infection. Indeed, it is now clear that pro-inflammatory cytokines such as interleukin (IL)-1 and tumour necrosis factor-α (TNF-α) that play a central role in coordinating peripheral immune response also play a critical role in triggering systemic responses to infection including fever and sickness behaviours through direct and indirect actions on the brain (4).

Sickness behaviours are a *normal* response to infection in the same way that subjective, behavioural and autonomic fear responses are a normal response to threats from external predators. By coordinating behavioural, autonomic and endocrine responses with peripheral immune responses, sickness behaviours facilitate a rapid motivational reorientation (5) that prioritizes mobilization of whole-body resources to fighting the infection. Typically, these sickness responses are mild and short-lived and resolve with successful eradication of the infectious agent. However, if the host immune response is prolonged, for example due to autoimmune diseases such as rheumatoid arthritis (6), during sustained therapeutic use of interferon-alpha (IFN-α) (7) or perhaps also through obesity and chronic non-infectious threats such as stress (8; 9), persistent activation of the mechanisms underpinning sickness behaviours can result in the emergence of true major depressive symptoms and episodes (10).

Depression itself is a complex, heterogeneous disorder with a multifactorial aetiology that remains poorly understood. Historically, dominant biological models of depression have implicated brain neurotransmitters, particularly the brain serotonergic system, as a central causative mechanism (11). However, this is being increasingly challenged by biological models whose focus extends well beyond classical neurotransmitters including inflammatory models of depression where the peripheral and central immune system are thought to play critical roles. Over the past two decades, evidence implicating the immune system in the neurobiology of depression has increased dramatically (12). Various strands of evidence have contributed to this, though three key areas have been critical to the emergence of the immune theory of depression: 1) discovery that acute inflammatory challenges induce 'sickness behaviours' that show a remarkably similar phenomenology to symptoms of depression; 2) chronic inflammation, e.g., through repeat therapeutic administration of the pro-inflammatory cytokine IFN-α, commonly precipitates bona fide major depressive episodes; and 3) epidemiological data demonstrating raised pro-inflammatory cytokines in depressed individuals and those at risk of developing depression, and high comorbidity of depression in patients with chronic immune mediated inflammatory disorders (IMIDs), such as rheumatoid arthritis and Crohn's disease.

Further convergent findings include direct and indirect evidence of increased molecular markers of inflammation in the brains of patients with major depressive disorder (MDD) (13; 14), longitudinal epidemiological evidence that inflammation precedes emergence of depression (15, 16), and evidence that some conventional antidepressant drugs show immune-modulatory properties (17) and similarly, some anti-inflammatory therapies have antidepressant properties (18). However, the most important stimulus for the rapid growth of the immune theory of depression, and emergence of immunopsychiatry more broadly, was the observation that inflammation readily induces sickness behaviours, and when chronic, bona fide depressive episodes (19). This discovery has facilitated preclinical and human experimental medicine studies that have provided solid evidence that the relationship between inflammation and depression is not purely spurious and that inflammation could be the cause rather than the consequence of depression. All these discoveries are at the origin of new mechanistic insights that have the potential of facilitating development of novel immune targeted antidepressant therapies.

7.1.1 Sickness Behaviour

Sickness represents a highly regulated strategy aimed at prioritizing whole-body resources to fighting the infecting agent and promoting recovery (3). Importantly, despite widespread use of the term 'sickness behaviour', sickness responses actually encompass systemic physiological changes (including fever, neuroendocrine and autonomic changes including activation of the hypothalamic-pituitary axis, HPA, and alterations in glycemia), and discrete changes in mood, motivation and cognition in addition to specific changes in behaviour. Physiological components e.g., fever, typically serve to accelerate host biochemical and cellular responses to the infecting organism while creating an environment unfavourable for microbial proliferation (20). However, this comes with a substantial metabolic cost (21), which is further exacerbated by accompanying malaise, anorexia and adipsia aimed at minimizing risk of further exposure to the infecting organism. Conceptually, many of the behavioural and subjectively experienced components of sickness serve either to conserve energy or minimize further exposure to the infecting organism/ other threats. For example, feelings of lethargy and fatigue, lowering of mood, anhedonia, reduced reward sensitivity and reduced grooming and sexual/reproductive activity all serve to conserve energy enabling the limited metabolic resources to be reprioritized to fighting the infection. At the same time, heightened sensitivity to pain and punishment, anxiety, social withdrawal and decreased novelty exploration serve to minimize risk of further exposure to pathogens/other risks to bodily integrity. Interestingly, sickness also impairs some aspects of learning and memory (particularly temporal lobe dependent memory processes) such as context-dependent fear learning (22) yet leaves others such as cue-based learning (22) and procedural (motor-skill) learning intact (23). It may also favour interoception-based learning such as conditioned taste aversion that have an insula-based mechanism (24). Sickness also disrupts sleep (25) potentially through disruption of the physiological role of brain cytokines in initiating local sleep onset (26).

This complex set of sickness-associated behavioural changes was first characterized experimentally in rodents, though similar techniques have subsequently been used to show that they are highly conserved in vertebrates (27) and invertebrates. In rodents, studies have typically used sterile injections of lipopolysaccharide (LPS) (also known as endotoxin) or poly(I:C), to mimic Gram-negative bacterial or viral infections respectively, or manipulation of pro- e.g., IL-1, IL-6, TNF-α, or anti-inflammatory e.g., IL-10 or insulin-like growth factor-I (IGF-I) cytokine signalling pathways. Studies in humans require the use of less-potent inflammatory challenges such as low-dose LPS, typhoid and other vaccinations, as well as some pro-inflammatory cytokines such as IFN-α that are used therapeutically e.g., in the treatment of hepatitis C viral infection. These approaches which trigger and/or manipulate components of the host innate immune response (in the absence of a true infection), have comprehensively demonstrated that the complete set of physiological, behavioural and subjective sickness responses result from host immune responses rather than the infectious agent per se (4).

Taking an evolutionary perspective, acute infections represent one of the most serious risks to an organism and are frequently associated with substantial mortality or long-term morbidity. Sickness responses constitute a survival-oriented adaptive response that rapidly shunts energy resources towards fighting the infection and wound healing while simultaneously minimizing risk of attack from predators and limiting within group spread. Ancestrally, integration of behavioural and systemic inflammatory physiological responses such as fever and HPA changes, provided an evolutionary advantage in the highly pathogenic environment in which early humans evolved (3; 28). In this context where outcomes were potentially grave, a highly sensitive system tuned to react to relatively minor threats or even cues signalling potential threat (i.e., high rates of false alarms) was evolutionarily advantageous (the fire alarm hypothesis) (29). However, in the modern human environment where relatively minor threats e.g., psychological stress and obesity, are common and medical intervention mitigate the risk associated with infections, chronic activation of sickness mechanisms can result in substantial morbidity. This is also readily observed across a range of common inflammatory disorders such as the IMIDs e.g., rheumatoid arthritis and Crohn's disease, and metabolic disorders such as diabetes mellitus and obesity where sickness symptoms and depression are common and show a rising incidence even before formal diagnosis (30).

7.1.2 Similarities between Sickness and Depression

As initially pointed out by Yirmiya (31), symptoms of sickness and clinical depression are remarkably similar phenomenologically (see Figure 7.1). For example, sickness symptoms such as anorexia, weight loss, fatigue, lethargy, sleep disturbance, hyperalgesia and psychomotor retardation correspond closely to the vegetative/somatic symptoms dimension of depression. Sickness symptoms such as anhedonia, low mood, anxiety and difficulty concentrating also constitute some of the core cognitive/affective symptoms of depression. However, there are also some phenomenological differences between sickness and depression. For example, malaise, a core symptom of sickness rarely occurs in depression, while pyrexia appears to be a sickness specific phenomenon. Furthermore, depression is not always accompanied by anorexia, indeed many individuals presenting with atypical depression demonstrate hyperphagia. Finally, though sickness behaviour is an acute, time-limited, adaptive response, clinical depression typically shows an insidious onset and often,

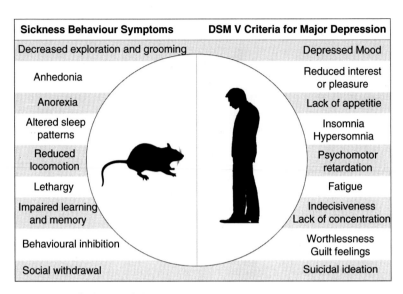

Sickness Behaviour Symptoms	DSM V Criteria for Major Depression
Decreased exploration and grooming	Depressed Mood
Anhedonia	Reduced interest or pleasure
Anorexia	Lack of appetitie
Altered sleep patterns	Insomnia Hypersomnia
Reduced locomotion	Psychomotor retardation
Lethargy	Fatigue
Impaired learning and memory	Indecisiveness Lack of concentration
Behavioural inhibition	Worthlessness Guilt feelings
Social withdrawal	Suicidal ideation

Figure 7.1 Comparison of sickness and depression symptoms.

a chronic relapsing-remitting course which is characterized in some cases by sensitization and progression (32).

Sickness-like symptoms are common concomitants of various chronic inflammatory diseases. For example, fatigue and hyperalgesia are central subjective complaints in conditions such as multiple sclerosis (MS) and rheumatoid arthritis, that frequently present with comorbid long-lasting and difficult to treat depression. Indeed, the similarities between vegetative symptoms of depression and inflammation-associated sickness symptoms can confound assessment of depression in patients suffering simultaneously from both (33). This has stimulated growing interest in the identification of clinical features that distinguish 'idiopathic' depression from depressive syndromes associated with underlying medical illness. For example, while the factor structure of depression in MS appears identical to that of idiopathic depression, the contribution of individual symptoms to overall severity differs between these groups. For example, in MS fatigue and irritability make a greater contribution to overall depression severity, while in idiopathic depression, anhedonia makes a stronger contribution (34). Phenotypic characterization of depression associated with psoriatic arthritis has also revealed multiple dimensions of depression such as anhedonia, cognitive dysfunction and alexithymia, that are differentially associated with pain (35). In the context of interferon-induced depression, phenotypic characteristics overlap with idiopathic depression (36), however greater expression of psychomotor retardation and weight loss has been reported (36). Whale and colleagues (37), have also reported a different factor structure in IFN-α-induced depression, which is characterized by a tighter covariance between depressive and anxiety symptoms than typically observed in idiopathic depression.

7.1.3 Communicating the State of the Immune System to the Brain

Use of immune challenges in rodents has shown that peripheral inflammation is rapidly communicated to the brain via parallel neural, humoral and cellular interoceptive pathways

(4; 38; Figure 7.2). Interestingly, though these pathways were originally characterized in the context of sickness behaviours, it seems increasingly likely that they serve a far broader role, akin to an additional sense, immunoception, tuned to the state of the immune system. This broader conceptualization, emphasizes the immune system's function as a diffuse chemosensory system that allows the brain to continually monitor immune responses throughout the body (39; 40). It also accords with the concept of a wider interoceptive sense ascribed to visceral projections to the insula, which is tuned to all aspects of the internal physiological state of the body (41; 42), and implicated in a range of psychiatric disorders, particularly depression and anxiety (43).

Early studies identified a neurally mediated pathway mediated by visceral afferent (sensory) fibres that travel in autonomic nerves such as the vagus (44). Here, cytokines such as IL-1, IL-6 and TNF-α (as well as other inflammatory mediators) released by

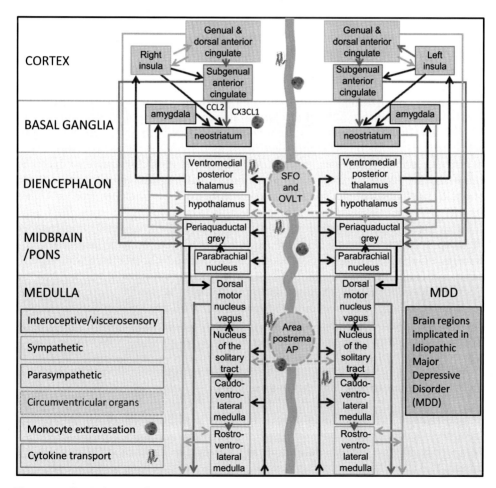

Figure 7.2 Circuit diagram illustrating visceral, humoral, and cellular interoceptive signalling pathways and the major points of interaction. AP, area postrema; CCL2, chemokine (C-C motif) ligand 2; CXCL1, chemokine (C-X3-C motif) ligand 1; OVLT, organum vasculosum laminae terminalis; SFO, subfornical organ. Shaded areas highlight brain regions implicated in the aetiology of idiopathic MDD. (A black and white version of this figure will appear in some formats. For the colour version, please refer to the plate section.)

activated immune cells rapidly activate visceral afferent fibres that project to the nucleus tractus solitarius in the brain stem (45) in a similar manner to signalling of other visceral (interoceptive) processes. The importance of this pathway to rodent sickness responses was further illustrated by vagotomy studies which resulted in a significant reduction (though not complete absence) of sickness responses following peripheral immune challenge (46). Higher projections of this pathway to a viscerosensory network of brain structures including the parabrachial nucleus, hypothalamic nuclei, central amygdala, insula and bed nucleus of the stria terminalis facilitate the integration of peripheral inflammatory responses with central homeostatic (e.g., fever, cortisol release) and behavioural sickness responses (44). Brain imaging studies have reported activation of a similar network of structures following inflammatory challenges in humans (47; 48; 49).

The brain can also sense humoral (blood borne) inflammatory mediators via areas such as the sensory circumventricular organs. These regions are located in the walls of the third and fourth ventricle, and have a specially modified blood-brain barrier (BBB) together with dense receptor expression that facilitates detection of low concentrations of circulating factors including inflammatory mediators (4; 50). Some of these mediators e.g., IL-6 and IFN-α can also directly enter the central nervous system (CNS) in small amounts through active transport mechanisms (51). Inflammation-induced changes in body temperature which result from action of IL-6 at the hypothalamus and local release of prostaglandin E2 provide a good example of this mechanism (which is not affected by vagotomy) (52).

The immune system also communicates with the brain through cellular pathways, particularly monocyte trafficking. In healthy rodents, this occurs at a low level. However, it increases markedly following severe and prolonged stress that negatively impacts the integrity of the BBB (particularly in stress-responsive brain regions) where it appears to play a role in amplifying behavioural stress responses (9). Recently, cytokines such as IL-4 and interferon-gamma released by lymphocytes residing in the meninges have also been shown to regulate aspects of social behaviour in rodents which is disrupted during impairment of the adaptive immune system (53). Cellular mechanisms have yet to be demonstrated in humans, though brain imaging data associating circulating monocyte levels with impaired functional connectivity within brain emotional regulation networks in youth exposed to multiple socioeconomic stressors suggest a potential role (54).

Within the brain, transduction of inflammatory signals also involves another immune cell type: microglia (specialized brain macrophages). Similar to peripheral macrophages, microglia exist in multiple morphological and functional states. In their healthy 'resting' state, microglia continuously extend and retract multiple branched ramifications to sample their local environment (55). In addition to their surveillance role, 'resting' microglia are also implicated in pruning dendrites in a complement C3 dependent manner (56), indicating a potentially critical role in healthy learning and memory. On detection of diverse 'danger signals', microglia rapidly adopt a variety of 'activated' states, in which they show changes in morphometry (both increases and decreases in ramifications) and shifts in secretory profile that can alter local neuronal and endothelial function (57). This shift to an activated state can occur in response to danger signals occurring within the brain e.g., ischaemia, as well as danger signals occurring within the body (including peripheral inflammation), and even exposure of the whole organism to repeated environmental stresses (58).

During systemic inflammation, microglial activation likely occurs through activation of immune-brain communication pathways that involve passage of cytokines across the

BBB (59), release of prostaglandin E2 by perivascular and endothelial cells in response to intravascular inflammation (60) or entry of stress-sensitive monocytes into the CNS (58). It can also occur as a consequence of sustained activity of glutamatergic neurons within stress-responsive regions where activity-dependent release of ATP can lead to microglial activation through purinergic receptors such as P2X7 (9). In rodents, systemic inflammation results in rapid activation of microglia within the circumventricular organs, meninges, and choroid plexus, which release TNF-α and trigger a cascade of microglial activation that spreads across the brain (61). Use of translocator protein (TSPO) PET which is sensitive to microglial activation state both in the cerebral white (62) and grey matter (63) has illustrated a similar pattern of widespread microglial activation within 3–4 hours of endotoxin-induced peripheral inflammation in humans (64).

7.2 Human Studies Investigating Associations between Inflammation, Sickness and Depression

Human studies investigating the relationship between inflammation, sickness behaviours and depression have typically adopted two complementary approaches: 1) experimental approaches that use acute and chronic immune challenges/inhibitors of peripheral immune activity to investigate effects on brain and behaviour; and 2) epidemiological approaches that investigate cross-sectional, longitudinal and genetic associations between peripheral inflammatory markers and symptoms/diagnoses of depression.

7.2.1 Experimental Approaches

Experimental approaches using a variety of short-lived inflammatory challenges in healthy human participants have been used to understand how inflammation acts on the brain to rapidly induce individual components of sickness behaviour. Immune challenges used have ranged from vaccines (65) or inhaled antigens which induce mild increases in inflammatory cytokines (similar to those observed in patients with depression), to low-dose LPS which induce more robust pro-inflammatory responses (66; 67). Together these types of study have confirmed the cognitive, motivational and mood lowering effects of acute inflammation previously reported in rodents (68). As discussed in more detail throughout this section, combining these challenges with diverse neuroimaging approaches has led to the identification of a discrete set of brain regions which are particularly susceptible to peripheral inflammation in humans. Use of a range of neuroimaging techniques providing complementary information on metabolic activity, tissue microstructure and neurochemistry has also provided a deeper mechanistic insight into how these regions generate key components of sickness. Together, these studies have revealed that many of the cognitive processes and brain structures underpinning sickness behaviours are also implicated in the aetiology of depression.

However, sickness symptoms are typically short-lived and acute challenge studies cannot determine whether sustained activation of their underlying mechanisms would ultimately lead to the emergence of bona fide depressive symptoms or syndromes. Furthermore, though invaluable in generating hypotheses about why some people are more susceptible to the motivationally impairing effects of inflammation, clarification of why only a subgroup of chronically inflamed patients develop true depressive episodes, how anti-inflammatory therapies improve depressive symptoms or whether inflammation also modulates these processes in depression cohorts requires studies in clinical populations.

As discussed later in this section cross-sectional studies in MDD cohorts as well as longitudinal studies in patients initiating pro- or anti-inflammatory treatments such as IFN-α for hepatitis C or anti-TNF-α therapies for inflammatory arthritis are beginning to address these questions. They are also revealing that acute effects of pro-/anti-inflammatory therapies on structures such as the amygdala and ventral striatum (that are critical to inflammation-associated mood and motivational impairment) can also predict the later emergence/resolution of true depressive symptoms (10; 65).

7.2.1.1 Fatigue

Fatigue is one of the most readily induced features of sickness and is reported following even mild inflammatory challenges. It is also one of the most common and functionally impairing features of chronic inflammatory disorders such as rheumatoid arthritis. Numerous experimental studies have now investigated the neural basis of inflammation-induced fatigue and broader subjective symptoms of malaise and with a few exceptions (discussed at the end of this section) have localized these subjectively experienced feelings to changes within the insula cortex (47; 49; 69; 70). As highlighted in Section 7.1.3, the insula represents the cortical projection of a neurally mediated interoceptive pathway that has been shown to be sensitive to peripheral inflammation in both rodent and human studies. More broadly, the insula is widely acknowledged to serve as viscerosensory cortex, and to underpin brain representations of diverse visceral stimuli. Progressive integration and re-representation of these interoceptive signals along the posterior-to-anterior axis of the insula is proposed to provide increasingly complex representations of interoceptive signals which ultimately become able to enter awareness i.e., consciously accessible (41), and provide an anatomical substrate for Jamesian theories of emotion where visceral and somatic feelings of the body form the foundation of emotional experience (71).

This conceptualization was based on neuroanatomical considerations as well as direct electrical stimulation of the insula in awake humans undergoing neurosurgical mapping which elicit a variety of visceral sensations (72). In addition, lesions to the insula and visceral deafferentation (pure autonomic failure) have been associated with diminished emotional arousal (73) and emotional reactivity respectively (74). Insula activity has also been associated with subjective experiences as diverse as feelings of coolness, itch and intensity of dynamic exercise in neuroimaging studies (41). Altered insula activity and interoceptive processing is also a key feature of MDD (see 43 for a review). Together, these studies emphasize the importance of this interoceptive pathway projecting to insula in the central communication of visceral information including peripheral inflammation. They also highlight the likely importance of the insula in translating these interoceptive signals into subjective experiences which in the context of inflammation include fatigue and malaise.

Interestingly, projections of this interoceptive pathway to the insula appear less important in mediating subjective fatigue-related responses to inflammation induced using IFN-α (65; 75). This suggests that visceral afferents are unlikely to be the only pathway mediating inflammation-induced fatigue (76). Preclinical studies show that peripheral injection of IFN-α rapidly activates IFN-sensitive genes in the brain, particularly within subcortical areas and the cerebellum (77). Furthermore, IFN-α is rapidly observed within the cerebrospinal fluid (CSF) following peripheral administration (78), suggesting that direct actions on basal ganglia may play a greater role in precipitating subjective experiences of fatigue, or impaired effort (79; 80).

7.2.1.2 Motivational Change

Impairments in reward-related behaviour are core features of the reorientation of priorities that characterizes both inflammation-induced sickness behaviour (2) and depression (81). During inflammation, this reorientation enables the organism to redirect resources to clearing the infecting agent. However, if inflammation is prolonged it may predispose to the development of MDD (4).

A mature human and non-human literature has firmly established the importance of dopaminergic signalling in the ventral striatum for mammalian reward-related processing (82). Central to this are midbrain dopaminergic cells which encode a reward prediction error signal (the mismatch between expected and received rewards) (83). Projections of these cells to the ventral striatum and subsequently medial prefrontal areas enable the value of different available options to be continually updated and bias behavioural choices to maximize long-term future rewards. Though details are beyond the scope of the current chapter, application of a variety of reward learning algorithms have proven to be a powerful way of modelling this dopaminergic prediction error signal and its influence on behaviour (84). They have also allowed interrogation of brain imaging data to identify how pharmacological manipulations alter reward prediction error signals within discrete brain regions (85).

Both MDD (86) and inflammatory challenges (87; 88) reduce ventral striatal responses to reward outcomes. Inflammation has also been linked to reduced ventral striatal reactivity to cues predicting rewards (89). During experimental inflammation, reduced ventral striatal responses to reward cues and outcomes correlate with induced anhedonia (87; 89). Application of computational models has also demonstrated that patients with MDD show reduced encoding of reward prediction error in the striatum and midbrain (86). Furthermore, this correlates with severity of anhedonic (diminished interest or pleasure in response to stimuli that were previously perceived as rewarding) symptoms suggesting that abnormal encoding of prediction errors may result in anhedonia by altering the learning and salience of rewarding events (86).

Application of similar learning models to experimental inflammation studies has shown an association with acute impairments in sensitivity to rewards compared to punishments (90), likely through opposing actions on ventral striatal reward and right anterior insula punishment prediction error encoding. In this study, inflammation reduced striatal reward prediction error encoding, similar to results reported in MDD (86). It was also associated with a reduced propensity to choose rewarded options but enhanced avoidance of punished ones. A similar reduction in striatal reward prediction error has been reported on this task using the dopamine D2 receptor antagonist haloperidol (85) suggesting that effects of inflammation on striatal prediction errors were likely mediated by actions on dopamine signalling. Supporting this, inflammation has been linked to altered nucleus accumbens dopamine efflux in rodents (91) and disrupted presynaptic dopamine synthesis/release in humans (87). After an LPS challenge, monkeys also exhibit significantly lower cerebrospinal fluid concentrations of the dopamine metabolite homovanillic acid (78).

The other interesting finding from this study was that inflammation significantly *increased* sensitivity to punishment. This was captured as a significant increase in the subjective (negative) value of punishment, i.e., punishments were experienced as being more potent after inflammation (90). This behavioural change was also associated with greater encoding of negative punishment prediction error in the right anterior insula. Increasing punishment prediction error is one way to increase the subjective value of punishment and may serve as the mechanism through which the insula drives this improvement in avoidance behaviour during inflammation. Furthermore, this mechanism is in alignment with theories proposing that brain areas like the insula which are involved with affective representations are causally involved in choice behaviours (41; 42; 85), particularly in the context of potential losses (92). Impaired punishment sensitivity has also been reported in patients with selective insula lesions (93).

Overall, these findings suggest that relative sensitivity to rewards compared to punishments is state-dependent, and can be flexibly adjusted to enhance loss minimization in the context of serious threats such as an infection. Interestingly, evidence for common neural mechanisms mediating motivational change and anhedonia in MDD and inflammation have been further strengthened by a study in unmedicated MDD patients showing that decreased connectivity between the ventral striatum and ventromedial prefrontal cortex (vmPFC) also mediates observed associations between raised C-reactive protein (CRP) and anhedonia (94).

7.2.1.3 Psychomotor Retardation

Psychomotor retardation is defined as a slowing-down of thought and physical movements. It is readily induced by even relatively mild inflammatory challenges (95) and is a cardinal feature of depression (96).

In humans, mild peripheral inflammation has been shown to attenuate substantia nigra reactivity during performance of both simple and more cognitively demanding button-press tasks (95). In this study, inflammation-induced changes in IL-6 also correlated with motor slowing across both simple and more cognitively demanding conditions suggesting an action on low-level processes, which conforms with effects reported in rodents. Furthermore, changes in both IL-6 and substantia nigra reactivity predicted inter-individual differences in sensitivity to the motor impairing effects of inflammation. This association between IL-6 and poorer performance on simple and choice movement time tasks has also been replicated in MDD patients (97).

These findings are noteworthy as the substantia nigra is the major source of dopamine in the brain and plays a critical role in the facilitation of movement (98). Projections to the striatum also modulate sensorimotor processing in response to stimulus salience (99) and have been linked to the reduction in novelty salience that is also observed during inflammation (100). Lower levels of striatal dopamine transporter are associated with slower motor reactions in healthy elderly humans (101), and decreased striatal presynaptic dopamine function is reported in depressed patients presenting with psychomotor retardation (102). The importance of the dorsal striatum to psychomotor retardation associated with MDD and inflammation is further strengthened by demonstration of a link between plasma and CSF levels of CRP, left basal ganglia glutamate (the other major neurochemical input to the striatum) and psychomotor slowing in untreated depressed patients (103).

Together, these data support a central role for bottom up dopaminergic (substantia nigra) and cortical top-down glutamatergic inputs into the dorsal striatum in both inflammation- and MDD-associated psychomotor retardation. During infection, psychomotor slowing may serve to minimize energy expenditure and conserve heat, thereby enhancing immune function. Convergent findings in inflammation and MDD-associated psychomotor retardation suggest that chronic activation of these mechanisms may differentiate MDD patients presenting with predominant psychomotor retardation or impulsivity/anxiety symptoms.

7.2.1.4 Social Behaviours

Social disconnection or withdrawal is one of the most noticeable features of sickness in animals (3; 9) and central to the phenomenology of human depression (104). Inflammation-induced social withdrawal contributes to the development of depression (105) and is sensitive to pharmacological modulation by antidepressant treatment (31). This observation stimulated interest in the study of mechanisms underlying inflammation-induced disruption of social behaviours, as it enables a precise understanding of crucial intermediate neurobiological mechanisms relevant to the relationship between inflammation and depression.

In seminal human studies by Eisenberger and colleagues, LPS was shown to induce feelings of social disconnection expressed as both a desire to withdraw socially and feelings of social isolation/disconnection (106). These were proposed to represent potentially dissociable effects on motivational processes (desire to 'be alone'), and processes involved in social cognition and social perception. In support of this, during performance of a Cyberball task, LPS induced IL-6 correlated with increased activity within a network of brain areas implicated in social processing, such as dorsomedial PFC, posterior superior temporal sulcus (pSTS), dorsal anterior cingulate (dACC) and insula (107). Though this relationship was observed across all participants only in women did it significantly mediate associations between inflammation and depressed mood. Women also reported stronger feelings of social disconnection and depressed mood after LPS despite lack of enhanced cytokine response (108). These findings highlighted the importance of considering the role of inflammation in mechanisms underlying women's greater reactivity to interpersonal stressors and higher vulnerability to develop MDD (109), although their interpretation should take into close consideration the possible interference effect of gendered norms with respect to engagement in neuropsychological computerized tasks (110).

Another study demonstrated that experimental inflammation also impaired participants' performance on a test of theory of mind (111), which evaluated how accurately participants could identify another's emotional state by looking only at their eyes. This leads to intriguing speculations about the possibility that inflammation deeply affects social processes central to our ability to correctly infer others mental and emotional states. It is also consistent with neuroimaging evidence showing that brain regions 'activated' by experimentally induced inflammation, such as the pSTS and medial PFC (107), are strongly implicated in social cognition tasks that involve extracting socially meaningful information and inferring another's mental state (112).

7.2.1.5 Mood Change and Depression

Studies investigating the effects of inflammation on mood show a more complex picture – likely reflecting the importance of interactions between multiple brain regions such as the amygdala, subgenual cingulate cortex (sACC), ventral striatum, insula and socially sensitive areas e.g., STS, to the generation and regulation of mood. These studies have typically used emotional face paradigms that are known to modulate activity in these areas and/or approaches that allow functional connections between these regions to be assessed.

The first of these studies used a simple connectivity approach to show that inflammation-associated changes in overall mood modulated activity within the sACC and its functional connectivity to the amygdala, nucleus accumbens and medial PFC, and STS, (regions central to the processing of emotional stimuli, reward and socially salient information respectively) (189). Interestingly, inflammation-induced increases in IL-6 also scaled with reductions in the connection strength of the sACC to each of these regions. This study is noteworthy as many of the key areas identified are implicated in the aetiology of depression and have subsequently been shown to mediate discrete effects of inflammation on reward and social processing as illustrated in previous sections.

For example, the sACC is recognized as a key node in functional and anatomical models of mood regulation (113) and the coordination of emotional processing. It is also strongly implicated in the pathophysiology of MDD (114). Depression-associated increases in sACC activity have also been shown to reverse with successful depression treatment regardless of whether these treatments target pharmacological (115, 114), physical (116) or psychological processes (115). Recruitment of the sACC in inflammation-induced mood change suggests that inflammation-associated changes in mood involves a network of brain regions similar to those implicated in idiopathic depression.

Another key component of this network is the amygdala. Heightened amygdala reactivity to negatively valanced emotional stimuli is a reliable finding (117; 118) in depression, and has even been proposed to mediate the characteristic mood-congruent processing bias (119). It also has value in predicting therapeutic response to CBT (120), normalizes following successful treatment with selective serotonin reuptake inhibitors (119) and serves as a physiological vulnerability marker for relapse in patients in remission (119). Other studies have investigated the effects of more potent inflammatory challenges on resting brain functional connectivity networks. Together, these have revealed a rapid and widespread reduction in the functional coupling of the amygdala, insula and cingulate cortices to multiple brain networks involved in affective-emotional, motivational and cognitive-modulatory processes (121).

Interestingly, a recent study sought to address the question of whether acute effects of inflammation on amygdala reactivity predisposes to the later development of major depressive symptoms and conversely whether anti-TNF-α therapy can reverse this process. By prospectively recruiting patients about to start IFN-α therapy for hepatitis C and those initiating anti-TNF-α therapy for inflammatory arthritis then scanning them immediately before and 4–24 hours their first treatment dose, the investigators showed that both IFN-α and anti-TNF-α significantly modulated amygdala reactivity. In particular, IFN-α acutely enhanced amygdala responses to sad (compared with neutral) faces and anti-TNF-α conversely decreased amygdala reactivity across emotional valence. More importantly, these changes in amygdala reactivity significantly predicted interferon-induced increases in depressive symptoms four weeks later and anti-TNF-α-associated decreases in depressive symptoms at 24 hours suggesting that actions of systemic inflammation on amygdala emotional reactivity play a mechanistic role in inflammation-associated depressive symptoms (10). In further support of this, correlation between the circulating inflammatory marker CRP and amygdala reactivity has been reported in a cross-sectional MDD study (122).

7.2.1.6 Sleep

Sleepiness and disrupted sleep are common complaints in many inflammatory disorders. Sleep disturbance is also an important risk factor for depression and associated with an increased risk of developing inflammatory disease and all-cause mortality (123). It also increases susceptibility to infections during exposure to airborne viruses (124). Studies in population-based samples have revealed a robust association of sleep disturbance with the markers of systemic inflammation CRP and IL-6 (25). While these and other studies have suggested that sleep disruption increases inflammation, accumulating evidence from experimental studies indicate that a reverse direction of causality is also possible: a single injection of typhoid vaccine impaired sleep time and efficiency (125). Underlying mechanisms include the sleep-regulating activity of pro-inflammatory cytokines (particularly IL-1 and TNF-α), and reciprocal dynamic interactions between peripheral and central cytokines potentiating their effects on sleepiness, duration of non-REM sleep and slow wave power (26). Some of these effects rely on intact vagal neurotransmission suggesting a role for neural interoceptive pathways in mediating the effects of inflammation on sleep (126).

7.2.1.7 Memory

Processes that are central to learning and memory, i.e., synaptic plasticity, neurogenesis and long-term potentiation (LTP), are closely orchestrated by microglia activity and pro-inflammatory cytokines. This regulatory function is intended to serve a neural circuitry remodelling role under physiological conditions. However, in the presence of systemic inflammation this positive regulatory function is disrupted, leading to memory impairment. Memory impairment is typically mild and tends to self-resolve with recovery from inflammation, however prolonged and severe inflammation can lead to an acceleration of age-related cognitive decline (127) and in some cases even to persistent cognitive impairment (128) .

The hippocampus and other medial temporal lobe (MTL) structures appear particularly vulnerable to inflammatory pathology, as also demonstrated by post-mortem reports of microglia activation and neuroinflammatory pathology in demyelinating disease. This may reflect the higher BBB permeability of these regions (129), and their pro-inflammatory cytokine receptor expression leading to heightened humoral pro-inflammatory signalling (130; 131). Furthermore, their direct connectivity to the insula implicates hippocampal and parahippocampal regions in neural interoceptive signalling pathways (132).

Studies in rodents demonstrated increased IL-1 expression within the MTL (133) after experimental induction of peripheral inflammation. Consistent with these findings, experimental inflammatory challenges in humans caused an acute but reversible impairment of spatial, verbal and non-verbal declarative memory (134; 135). Importantly, chronic inflammation has been linked to reduced hippocampal volume (136). This indicates a likely important role for chronic inflammation of MTL structures in the pathophysiology of depression, considering that depression is specifically associated to both chronically raised inflammatory markers and reduced hippocampal volume (137; 138), and that episodic memory impairment is a common cognitive deficit in depression (139; 140). Future studies will need to disentangle the exact molecular mechanisms through which sustained inflammatory stimuli lead to persistent changes in MTL structure and function and identify potential therapeutic targets for dampening and reversing these processes.

7.2.2 Clinical and Epidemiological Approaches

7.2.2.1 Studies of Depressed Patients and Controls

Cohort studies demonstrate that depression is a pro-inflammatory state associated with elevated concentrations of CRP and inflammatory cytokines such as IL-1, IL-6, TNF-α in peripheral blood and in CSF. Patients also show a decrease in concentrations of anti-inflammatory cytokines such as IL-4 and IL-10. However, this evidence comes from meta-analyses of case-control studies comparing large numbers of patients with non-depressed controls (141; 142; 143; 144) and not all patients with depression display evidence of peripheral inflammation. Recently, a meta-analysis reported that about a quarter of patients with depression (27%) have elevated peripheral blood CRP levels (>3mg/L) (145). Furthermore, compared to matched controls, depressed patients were about 50% more likely to have elevated CRP, regardless of the CRP threshold used to define inflammation (>1, >3 or >10mg/L) (145). Another meta-analysis suggests that increased inflammatory markers in depressed patients at group level, compared with controls, is likely to be due to a right shift of concentrations of inflammatory markers in all cases rather than very high levels in a subgroup (146). In this regard, the relationship between CRP and depression is conceptually akin to that between systolic blood pressure and cardiovascular disease.

While evidence from these case-control studies is consistent regarding increased inflammation in depression, they cannot confirm the direction of association, i.e., whether inflammation is a cause or consequence of illness (reverse causation). Demonstrating a temporal relationship between risk factor/exposure and a disease outcome is important for establishing causality. In recent years, this issue has been addressed by a number of epidemiological longitudinal cohort studies.

7.2.2.2 Evidence for Causality from Longitudinal Cohort Studies

Longitudinal studies can address the issue of reverse causation by measuring exposure (inflammation) before the outcome (depression). Accumulating evidence from longitudinal studies now suggests that inflammation precedes depression, so it could be a cause rather than simply be a consequence of illness. This evidence comes from longitudinal cohort studies from the UK (e.g., ALSPAC, Whitehall II) and Netherlands (e.g., Rotterdam, NESDA) among others (15; 16; 147; 148). In the Avon Longitudinal Study of Parents and Children (ALSPAC), a general population-representative birth cohort from the city of Bristol and surrounding areas in England, levels of circulating IL-6 and CRP were measured in over 5,000 children at age 9, and assessments for depression and psychosis were conducted at age 18 (16). Higher IL-6 levels in childhood were associated with increased risks for depression (and psychosis) subsequently in early-adulthood in a linear, dose-response fashion (16) (see Figure 7.3). Evidence for this association remained after controlling for potential confounding by age, sex, ethnicity, body mass index, socioeconomic status, maternal depression and childhood psychological and behavioural problems preceding the measurement of IL-6 (16). This is one of the first evidence from human population samples that inflammation precedes the emergence of depression.

Similarly, results from the UK Whitehall II cohort, a prospective study based on a large sample of civil servants from London, reported that elevated IL-6 and CRP at baseline were associated with increased cognitive symptoms of depression at follow-up (15). In the Netherlands Study of Depression and Anxiety (NESDA) cohort bidirectional longitudinal associations were found between depression and IL-6 levels (147). No associations were found for CRP. However, in the English Longitudinal Study of Ageing (ELSA) higher baseline levels of CRP were associated with increased depressive symptoms at follow-up, but not the other way around (149).

Longitudinal studies also suggest that inflammation is associated with subsequent persistent depressive symptoms. For instance, in the Dutch Rotterdam cohort higher CRP

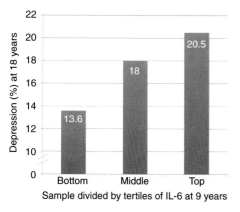 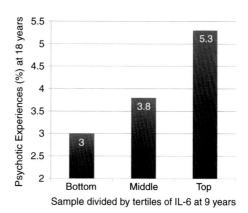

Figure 7.3 Longitudinal association between serum IL-6 level at age 9 and risk of depression and psychotic experiences at age 18 in the ALSPAC birth cohort.
Footnote: Cases of depression and psychotic experiences at age 18 in the ALSPAC birth cohort grouped by serum IL-6 levels at age 9. Cut-off values for the top and bottom thirds of the distribution of IL-6 values in the total sample (cases and non-cases combined) were 1.08 and 0.57pg/mL, respectively. Figure adapted from Khandaker et al. *JAMA Psychiatry.* 2014;71:1121–8.

levels in childhood were associated with persistent depressive symptoms in older adults (148). Similarly, in the ALSPAC cohort elevated IL-6 levels in childhood were associated with persistent depressive symptoms during adolescence and early-adulthood (150).

Most existing longitudinal studies have used one measurement of IL-6/CRP to index inflammation, so effects of persistent inflammation on depression risk at the population level is unclear. This is largely because of data availability as large population samples with repeated blood tests in the same individuals over a long period are scarce. An exception is the ALSPAC birth cohort where serum CRP levels were measured three times during childhood at ages 9, 15 and 18 years. These data were used to identify four distinct population subgroups based on the temporal pattern of CRP (151). The groups with persistently elevated CRP and increasing levels of CRP during adolescence had an increased risk of severe depression subsequently in adulthood, compared with those with persistently low CRP (151).

7.2.2.3 Evidence for Causality from Genetic Studies

Emerging evidence from genetic studies particularly Mendelian randomization (MR) also suggest that previously reported associations between IL-6, CRP and depression are likely to be causal, rather than solely attributable to reverse causation or residual confounding. MR is a genetic epidemiological design that aims to address reverse causation and residual confounding by using genetic variants regulating levels/activity of a biomarker as proxies (152; 153). It can address reverse causation because genetic variants are fixed at conception, so the exposure must precede any disease outcome. It also addresses residual confounding because genetic variants segregate at random during meiosis, so are unrelated to potential confounding by socioeconomic, lifestyle or other factors. Therefore, demonstrating associations of genetic variants related to IL-6 and CRP with depression would strongly support that these associations have a causal basis.

Using the MR approach, a genetic variant in the *IL-6 R* gene known to reduce inflammation has been shown to be protective for depression (154). The *IL-6 R* functional variant Asp358Ala (rs2228145 A>C) impairs *IL-6 R* classical signalling by reducing cell surface expression of *IL-6 R* (155). Carriers of the 'anti-inflammatory' minor Asp358Ala allele had lower circulating CRP levels and a decreased risk of depression (155). Similarly, another MR study based on a much larger sample of over 367,000 individuals including over 14,000 cases of depression from the UK Biobank cohort reported evidence for potential causal associations of IL-6 and CRP with depression (156).

7.2.2.4 Evidence from Randomized Controlled Trials (RCTs)

RCTs of anti-inflammatory drugs have been crucial for our understanding of the potential role of inflammation in depression. In addition to testing therapeutic efficacy, RCTs are among the strongest and most widely accepted tools in medicine for establishing causality of association. A large number of RCTs of anti-inflammatory drugs of various kinds as treatments for depression have been conducted, and many are ongoing. These will be discussed in depth in Chapter 11. Here, we briefly discuss key evidence, which largely supports a role of inflammation in depression.

The largest evidence base is for non-steroidal anti-inflammatory drugs (NSAIDs) particularly COX-2 inhibitors given as add-on to antidepressants or as monotherapy. These RCTs suggest that adding NSAIDs along with antidepressants could offer an additional benefit for depressive symptoms over antidepressants alone. The pooled effect size for antidepressant effect is around 0.8 for NSAIDs add-on treatment and 0.3 for NSAIDs monotherapy according to two recent large meta-analyses of such RCTs (157; 158). More precise evidence for a role of inflammation has come from RCTs of anti-cytokine drugs as these drugs are highly specific with regards to their mechanism of action. Various monoclonal antibodies and cytokine inhibitors are now established treatments for chronic inflammatory physical illness such as rheumatoid arthritis, inflammatory bowel disease and psoriasis. A meta-analysis of RCTs of anti-cytokine drugs in patients with chronic inflammatory physical illness suggests that these drugs improve depressive symptoms (effect size around 0.4), independently of improvements in physical illness (18), supporting a causal role for inflammatory cytokines in depression. These findings were confirmed in a subsequent meta-analysis (159).

However, thus far all three RCTs of novel anti-cytokine drugs conducted solely in patients with depression have been 'negative' (160; 161; and NCT02473289). Some of this has been attributed to patient selection criteria used. Not all patients with depression have evidence of inflammation, and so immunotherapies are unlikely to be useful for all patients with the illness. Currently, a number of ongoing RCTs are using more refined inclusion criteria to enhance selection of patients most likely to benefit from immunotherapy, e.g., elevated CRP levels +/– presence of inflammation-related symptoms, specific genotype or evidence of microglia activation; for example (162). These studies would further add to our understanding of the role of inflammation in depression.

7.2.2.5 Association with Specific Symptoms

There is a great deal of phenotypic heterogeneity in the depression syndrome. We have already mentioned that symptoms of depression can be broadly classified as *somatic* (e.g., fatigue, sleep problems) which are akin to sickness behaviour, and *psychological* (e.g., hopelessness, excessive/inappropriate guilt). It is well known that many different combinations of symptoms are possible all meeting the ICD-10/DSM-5 criteria for depression. However, it is likely that different symptoms or symptom dimensions are underpinned by distinct pathophysiological mechanisms.

Emerging evidence indicates that inflammation may be particularly relevant for somatic symptoms. Elevated serum CRP levels are associated with somatic symptoms (e.g., fatigue, impaired sleep, activity levels), but not with psychological symptoms in the general population (163) and in depressed patients (164). In the ALSPAC birth cohort, higher IL-6 levels in childhood were associated with both somatic and psychological symptom dimension scores in early-adulthood (165). However, at the symptom level, IL-6 was associated with fatigue, sleep disturbances, concentration difficulties and diurnal mood variation particularly (all so-called somatic symptoms) out of 19 individual symptoms of depressive and anxiety (165).

Atypical features of depression, particularly increased appetite or weight gain, have been reported to be associated with elevated CRP levels and with genetic predisposition for obesity, suggesting that these symptoms may be underpinned by immuno-metabolic alterations (166). Consistent with this evidence, young adults with depression *plus* elevated CRP (>3mg/L) were found to have increased cardiometabolic risk factors, e.g., higher BMI, triglycerides levels and insulin insensitivity (167).

7.3 Potential Mechanisms Linking Inflammation to Depression

Within the brain, pro-inflammatory cytokines and/or activated microglia alter diverse biological processes implicated in the aetiology of depression, including actions on neurotransmitters such as the monoamines and glutamate, cortisol signalling and the HPA, sleep circuits (26) and a variety of processes such as long-term potentiation, neurogenesis and homeostatic synaptic scaling (168) that are critical to neuroplasticity. Here we highlight some of the key mechanisms.

7.3.1 Neurotransmitters

One area that has received particular attention is the action of pro-inflammatory cytokines on neurotransmitters, particularly the monoamines. As illustrated in Figure 7.3, numerous pro-inflammatory cytokines have been shown to alter key enzymes in the tryptophan metabolic pathway in preclinical studies. This includes activation of Indoleamine-2-3-dioxygenase (IDO) which shunts tryptophan away from serotonin production into the kynurenic pathway (169) as well as the enzymes kynurenine monooxygenase (KMO) and kynurenine aminotransferase which regulate the balance of kynurenic acid (KYNA) to quinolinic acid (QUIN) in astrocytes and microglia respectively (see 170 for an excellent review). These actions serve to reduce the availability of serotonin. However, perhaps more importantly, they also alter the ratio of the metabolites KYNA to QUIN, which have been shown to have important inhibitory (neuroprotective) and excitatory (neurotoxic) actions on NMDA-type glutamate receptors respectively (169). Translational support for these mechanisms also comes from studies of patients treated with IFN-α which increases tryptophan metabolism through the kynurenine pathway (indexed by an increased kynurenine to tryptophan ratio) (171). In this population alterations in this ratio also correlate with changes in clinical depression and anxiety scores (172). Increased serum kynurenine is also commonly reported in studies of depressed patients (170). Furthermore, elevated QUIN has been reported in the CSF of suicide attempters (173) and in microglia within the subgenual cingulate of severely depressed individuals (174).

Inflammatory cytokines also alter glutamatergic signalling pathways in a number of other important ways including by decreasing the expression of the glutamate transporter and glutamine synthetase enzyme (which converts glutamate to glutamine) in astrocytes. Interestingly, administration of the NMDA receptor antagonist ketamine prior to LPS in rodents has been shown to inhibit the usual depressogenic effects of LPS. Mechanistically, this appears to occur by blocking the agonist activity of QUIN on the NMDA receptor (importantly ketamine did not block microglial activation itself). Together, these findings suggest a potential mechanism linking the inflammation and glutamate hypotheses of depression (175).

In addition to their effects on serotonin and glutamatergic signalling, pro-inflammatory cytokines can also reduce the synthesis, release and reuptake of dopamine (Figure 7.3). These actions appear to be at least partially mediated via actions on the redox-sensitive cofactor tetrahydrobiopterin (BH4) which is required for the function of both phenylalanine hydroxylase (which catalyses the synthesis of tyrosine from phenylalanine) and tyrosine hydroxylase (which catalyses the subsequent conversion of tyrosine to L-3,4-dihydroxyphenylalanine: L-DOPA). During inflammation, increases in reactive and inducible oxygen species can reduce BH4 availability and consequently impair dopamine synthesis (176; 177). Pro-inflammatory cytokines can also reduce expression of the monoamine transporter, which is required to produce dopaminergic vesicles (178), and reduce reuptake of dopamine into presynaptic terminals (177). Human neuroimaging studies support a particular sensitivity of dopamine-rich brain areas to peripheral inflammation. For example, inflammation-induced changes in substantia nigra activity have been linked to psychomotor slowing (95) and impairments in novelty responding (100) and changes in the ventral striatum to anhedonia (79) and reduced reward sensitivity (89; 90). IFN-α has also been shown to impair striatal dopamine turnover using F-DOPA PET (87). Interestingly, the limited clinical data currently available also suggest that selective dopamine-reuptake inhibitors may be more efficacious than SSRIs in patients with depression in the context of raised CRP (179)

7.3.2 Neurogenesis

Over recent years, neurogenesis (a process that predominantly occurs in the dentate gyrus of the hippocampus) has been increasingly implicated in the aetiology of depression (180). For example, in rodents, stress-induced decreases in dentate neurogenesis play an important causal role in precipitating depressive episodes (180). Serotonin and SSRIs can also both attenuate this process. In humans, reduced hippocampal volume is among the most robust findings in the depression neuroimaging literature (138). It is therefore noteworthy that both the anti-inflammatory stress-associated hormone cortisol and pro-inflammatory cytokines can potently inhibit neurogenesis.

At first sight it may seem paradoxical that pro-inflammatory cytokines and the anti-inflammatory cortisol have both been associated with inhibition of neurogenesis and further, that elevations of both co-occur in depression (181). However, though acute increases in cortisol are rapidly normalized by negative feedback on central glucocorticoid receptors in health, dysfunction of the glucocorticoid receptor (known as glucocorticoid resistance) impairs this process in depression (182). Furthermore, pro-inflammatory cytokines such as IL-1 actively contribute to this glucocorticoid resistance by impairing the translocation of the glucocorticoid

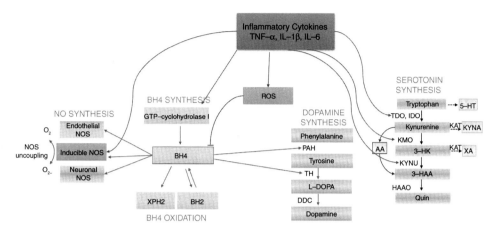

Figure 7.4 Actions of pro-inflammatory cytokines on neurotransmitters synthesis and metabolic pathways.
Adapted from: 170; and 177

receptor from the cytoplasm to the nucleus. Cortisol acting through multiple pathways, including activation and upregulation of the GR-stimulated gene, serum and glucocorticoid-inducible kinase 1 (SGK1), is one of the most potent inhibitors of neurogenesis. Interestingly, elevated SGK1 is itself linked to depression (181).

In addition to actions mediated via actions on cortisol, pro-inflammatory cytokines can themselves impair neurogenesis (183). For example, in rodents, cognitive impairments induced by systemic LPS are associated with both increases in hippocampal cytokines (IL-1 and TNF-α), and reductions in brain-derived neurotrophic factor (BDNF) (a key modulator of neurogenesis) and hippocampal neurogenesis (184). Studies using various methods to block CNS cytokine e.g., with IL-1 receptor knock-out mice, infusion of IL-1 receptor antagonist (IL-1ra) or injection of IL-1ra secreting neural progenitor cells into the hippocampus support the possibility that effects on neurogenesis are mediated by IL-1. Interestingly, though effects of IL-1 on neurogenesis are mediated by activation of NFκB in vitro (185), release of glucocorticoids may be required for IL-1 effects on the brain during stress in vivo (186).

Together, these and other studies illustrate that the serotonin hypothesis of depression as originally conceived is too narrow to account for the wealth of pathological changes associated with depression. Though pro-inflammatory cytokines do modulate monoaminergic processes, they also engage a wealth of other processes including some such as neural plasticity, stress responses, neurogenesis and sleep that are fundamental to healthy brain function. As these processes are further understood they will undoubtedly offer novel therapeutic opportunities and renewed hope for the many patients in whom conventional antidepressants provide only limited benefit.

7.4 Concluding Remarks and Future Directions

As discussed in this chapter, there is a striking overlap between sickness and depression symptoms, notably vegetative/somatic symptoms such as fatigue, sleep disturbance, which are common to both. Immune activation in humans rapidly induces depression-like symptoms and alters sensitivity to emotionally valenced stimuli and to rewards and punishments. It also rapidly activates a network of brain areas that are very similar to those associated with stress and depression. Furthermore, when inflammation is chronic it readily induces bona fide depressive episodes. However, there is considerable between-person variability in sensitivity to inflammatory challenge. For instance, only ⅓ of individuals chronically treated with interferon develop full blown depression even though the vast majority develop sickness symptoms. Early evidence suggests that inter-individual differences in sensitivity of stress (i.e., HPA) (187), reward (ventral striatum) (65) and emotion (amygdala) (10) circuits to inflammation may be important in this regard. However, more work needs to be done to further understand this and interaction with other risk factors, both environmental and genetic, seems likely.

Notable environmental risk factors include psychological stress, particularly early-life adversity, which is associated with both a higher risk of depression and increased concentrations of circulating inflammatory markers (188). Understanding what determines risk of depression following immune activation would be important not only for further mechanistic insights, but also for developing effective targeted strategies for treatment and prevention of inflammation-related depression.

Preclinical studies particularly evidence from rodents have advanced our understanding of the potential mechanisms through which peripheral inflammation communicates with the brain and contributes to the development of depression, and the role of specific processes within the brain. This evidence points to key roles for actions of inflammation on stress-sensitive neural circuits, IDO and kynurenine pathway, dopamine synthesis and neural plasticity mechanisms including hippocampal neurogenesis. Actions of cytokines entering the brain, microglia and/or monocytes recruited to the brain are implicated in many of these processes. Further work is needed to identify potential treatment targets for engagement and validation in animal models and ultimately in humans. Experimental medicine studies will have a vital role to play in this regard.

The wealth of epidemiological evidence confirms that depression is a pro-inflammatory state associated with increased concentrations of inflammatory cytokines in peripheral blood. Population-based longitudinal studies and genetic MR studies strongly suggest that associations of IL-6, CRP with depression are likely to be causal rather than solely explained by reverse causation or residual confounding. Furthermore, evidence from RCTs of anti-inflammatory drugs including NSAIDs and novel anti-cytokine drugs suggests that these drugs improve depressive symptoms, further suggesting a role of inflammation in the pathogenesis of depression.

Inflammation is a clinically relevant phenotype as it is associated with poor response to antidepressants and physical multimorbidity notably cardiometabolic disease. However, inflammation is unlikely to be relevant for all patients with depression as evidence of inflammation is present in only a subset of patients – *not everyone* – with depression. From a translational point of view, which patients may benefit from immunotherapy is now a key question for the field. Further work is needed to understand the characteristics of inflammation-related depression, which would inform patient selection in future RCTs of immunotherapies for depression. Depending on the answer to some of the key questions discussed in this chapter, a future is conceivable where, guided by tests to inform a more personalized treatment choice, some patients are treated with immunotherapies. This would be a giant leap for our understanding of the causes of serious mental illness, and a great improvement from the current one-size-fits-all approach to the monoaminergic pharmacological treatments for depression.

References

1. Dantzer R, Bluthe R, Castanon N, et al. Cytokines, sickness behavior, and depression. In Ader, R, ed. *Psychoneuroimmunology* (4th ed.). Academic Press, New York; 2007;281–318.

2. Hart, BL. Behavior of sick animals. *Vet Clin North Am Food Anim Pract.* 1987;3:383–91.

3. Hart, BL. Biological basis of the behavior of sick animals. *Neurosci Biobehav Rev.* 1988;12:123–37.

4. Dantzer R, O'Connor JC, Freund GG, Johnson RW, Kelley KW. From inflammation to sickness and depression: when the immune system subjugates the brain. *Nat Rev Neurosci.* 2008;9:46–56.

5. Miller NE. Some psychophysiological studies of motivation and of the behavioral effects of illness. *Bull Br Psychol Soc.* 1964;17:1–20.

6. Matcham F, Rayner L, Steer S, Hotopf M. The prevalence of depression in rheumatoid arthritis: a systematic review and meta-analysis, *Rheumatology.* 2013;52 (12):2136–48.

7. Mattson K, Niiranen A, Iivanainen M, et al. Neurotoxicity of interferon. *Cancer Treat Rep.* 1983;67:958–61.

8. André C, Dinel AL, Ferreira G, Layé S, Castanon N. Diet-induced obesity progressively alters cognition, anxiety-like behavior and lipopolysaccharide-induced depressive-like behavior: focus on brain indoleamine 2,3-dioxygenase activation. *Brain Behav Immun.* 2014;41:10–21.

9. Wohleb ES, McKim DB, Sheridan JF, Godbout JP. Monocyte trafficking to the brain with stress and inflammation: a novel axis of immune-to-brain communication that influences mood and behavior. *Front Neurosci.* 2014;8:447.

10. Davies KA, Cooper E, Voon V, et al. Interferon and anti-TNF therapies differentially modulate amygdala reactivity which predicts associated bidirectional changes in depressive symptoms. *Mol Psychiatry.* 2020. https://doi.org/10.1038/s41380-020-0790-9

11. Bullmore E. *The Inflamed Mind: A Radical New Approach to Depression.* Short Books, London; 2018.

12. Krishnadas R, Cavanagh J. Depression: an inflammatory illness? *J Neurol Neurosurg Psychiatry.* 2012;83:495–502.

13. Hercher C, Turecki G, Mechawar N. Through the looking glass: examining neuroanatomical evidence for cellular alterations in major depression. *J Psych Res.* 2009;43(11):947–61.

14. Setiawan E, Wilson AA, Mizrahi R, et al. Role of translocator protein density, a marker of neuroinflammation, in the brain during major depressive episodes. *JAMA Psychiatry.* 2015;72:268–75.

15. Gimeno D, Kivimäki M, Brunner EJ, et al. Associations of C-reactive protein and interleukin-6 with cognitive symptoms of depression: 12-year follow-up of the Whitehall II study. *Psychol Med.* 2009;39 (3):413–23.

16. Khandaker GM, Pearson RM, Zammit S, Lewis G, Jones PB. Association of serum interleukin 6 and C-reactive protein in childhood with depression and psychosis in young adult life: a population-based longitudinal study. *JAMA Psychiatry.* 2014;71:1121–8.

17. Sacre S, Jaxa-Chamiec A, Low CMR, Chamberlain G, Tralau-Stewart C. Structural modification of the antidepressant Mianserin suggests that its anti-inflammatory activity may be independent of 5-Hydroxytryptamine receptors. *Frontiers in Immunology.* 2019;10:1167.

18. Kappelmann N, Lewis G, Dantzer R, Jones PB, Khandaker GM. Antidepressant activity of anti-cytokine treatment: a systematic review and meta-analysis of clinical trials of chronic inflammatory conditions. *Mol Psychiatry.* 2018;23 (2):335–43.

19. Musselman DL, Lawson DH, Gumnick JF, et al. Paroxetine for the prevention of depression induced by high-dose interferon alfa. *N Engl J Med.* 2001;344:961–6.

20. Kluger MJ. Temperature regulation, fever, and disease. *Int Rev Physiol.* 1979;20:209–51.

21. Evans SS, Repasky EA, Fisher DT. Fever and the thermal regulation of immunity: the immune system feels the heat. *Nat Rev Immunol.* 2015;15:335–49.

22. Yirmiya R, Goshen I. Immune modulation of learning, memory, neural plasticity and neurogenesis. *Brain Behav Immun.* 2011;25:181–213.

23. Harrison NA, Doeller CF, Voon V, Burgess N, Critchley HD. Peripheral inflammation acutely impairs human spatial memory via actions on medial temporal lobe glucose metabolism. *Biol Psychiatry.* 2014;76:585–93.

24. Dunn LT, Everitt BJ. Double dissociations of the effects of amygdala and insular cortex lesions on conditioned taste aversion, passive avoidance, and neophobia in the rat using the excitotoxin ibotenic acid. *Behavioral Neuroscience.* 1988;102(1):3–23.

25. Irwin MR, Olmstead R, Carroll JE. Sleep disturbance, sleep duration, and inflammation: a systematic review and meta-analysis of cohort studies and experimental sleep deprivation. *Biol Psychiatry.* 2016;80:40–52.

26. Krueger JM, Rector DM, Roy S, et al. Sleep as a fundamental property of neuronal assemblies. *Nat Rev Neurosci.* 2008;9:910–19.

27. Dantzer R, Kelley KW. Twenty years of research on cytokine-induced sickness behavior. *Brain Behav Immun.* 2007;21:153–60.

28. Miller AH, Raison CL. The role of inflammation in depression: from evolutionary imperative to modern treatment target. *Nat Rev Immunol.* 2016;16(1):22–34.

29. Dantzer R. Cytokine-induced sickness behaviour: a neuroimmune response to activation of innate immunity. *Eur J Pharmacol.* 2004;50:399–411.

30. Marrie R, Walld R, Bolton J, et al. Rising incidence of psychiatric disorders before diagnosis of immune-mediated inflammatory disease. *Epidemiology and Psychiatric Sciences.* 2019;28(3):333–42.

31. Yirmiya R. Behavioral and psychological effects of immune activation: implications for 'depression due to a general medical condition'. *Cur Opin Psychiatry.* 1997;10(6):470–6.

32. Maes M, Berk M, Goehler L, et al. Depression and sickness behavior are Janus-faced responses to shared inflammatory pathways. *BMC Med.* 2012;10:66.

33. Minden, SL, Feinstein, A, Kalb, RC. Evidence-based guideline: assessment and management of psychiatric disorders in individuals with MS: report of the Guideline Development Subcommittee of the American Academy of Neurology. *Neurology.* 2014;82(2):174–81.

34. Hasselmann H, Bellmann-Strobl J, Ricken R, et al. Characterizing the phenotype of multiple sclerosis-associated depression in comparison with idiopathic major depression. *Mult Scler.* 2016;22(11):1476–84.

35. Mathew AJ, Chandran V. Depression in psoriatic arthritis: dimensional aspects and link with systemic inflammation. *Rheumatol Ther.* 2020;7(2):287–300.

36. Capuron L, Fornwalt FB, Knight BT, et al. Does cytokine-induced depression differ from idiopathic major depression in medically healthy individuals?. *J Affect Disord.* 2009;119(1–3):181–5.

37. Whale R, Fialho R, Field AP, et al. Factor analyses differentiate clinical phenotypes of idiopathic and interferon-alpha-induced depression. *Brain Behav Immun.* 2019;80:519–24.

38. Savitz J, Harrison NA. Interoception and inflammation in psychiatric disorders. *Biol Psychiatry Cogn Neurosci Neuroimaging.* 2018;3:514–24.

39. Blalock JE. The immune system as a sensory organ. *J Immunol.* 1984;132(3):1067–70.

40. Kipnis J. Immune system: the "seventh sense". *J Exp Med.* 2018;215(2):397–98.

41. Craig, AD. How do you feel? Interoception: the sense of the physiological condition of the body. *Nat Rev Neurosci.* 2002;3:655–66.

42. Critchley HD, Harrison NA. Visceral influences on brain and behavior. *Neuron.* 2013;77(4):624–38.

43. Khalsa SS, Adolphs R, Cameron OG, et al. Interoception and mental health: a roadmap. *Biol Psychiatry: Cog Neuro and Neuroim.* 2018;3(6):501–13.

44. Wan W, Wetmore L, Sorensen CM, Greenberg AH, Nance DM. Neural and biochemical mediators of endotoxin and stress-induced c-fos expression in the rat brain. *Brain Res Bull.* 1994;34:7–14.

45. Goehler LE, Relton JK, Dripps D, et al. Vagal paraganglia bind biotinylated interleukin-1 receptor antagonist: a possible mechanism for immune-to-brain communication. *Brain Res Bull.* 1997;43:357–64.

46. Bluthé RM, Walter V, Parnet P, et al. Lipopolysaccharide induces sickness behaviour in rats by a vagal mediated mechanism. *C R Acad Sci III.* 1994;317 (6):499–503.

47. Harrison NA, Brydon L, Walker C, et al. Neural origins of human sickness in interoceptive responses to inflammation. *Biol Psychiatry.* 2009;66:415–22.

48. Hannestad J, Subramanyam K, Dellagioia N, et al. Glucose metabolism in the insula and cingulate is affected by systemic inflammation in humans. *J Nucl Med.* 2012;53:601–7.

49. Harrison NA, Cooper E, Dowell NG, et al. Quantitative magnetization transfer imaging as a biomarker for effects of systemic inflammation on the brain. *Biol Psychiatry.* 2015b;78:49–57.

50. Gross PM. Morphology and physiology of capillary systems in subregions of the subfornical organ and area postrema. *Can J Physiol Pharmacol.* 1991;69:1010–25.

51. Banks WA. From blood-brain barrier to blood-brain interface: new opportunities for CNS drug delivery. *Nat Rev Drug Discov.* 2016;15:275–92.

52. Luheshi GN, Bluthé R-M, Rushforth D, et al. Vagotomy attenuates the behavioural but not the pyrogenic effects of interleukin-1 in rats. *Autonomic Neuroscience.* 2000;85:127–32.

53. Filiano A, Xu Y, Tustison N, et al. Unexpected role of interferon-γ in regulating neuronal connectivity and social behaviour. *Nature.* 2016;535:425–9.

54. Nusslock R, Brody GH, Armstrong CC, et al. Higher peripheral inflammatory signaling associated with lower resting-state functional brain connectivity in emotion regulation and central executive networks. *Biol Psychiatry.* 2019;86(2):153–62. doi:10.1016/j.biopsych.2019.03.968

55. Nimmerjahn A, Kirchhoff F, Helmchen F. Resting microglial cells are highly dynamic surveillants of brain parenchyma in vivo. *Science.* 2005;308:1314–18.

56. Schafer DP, Lehrman EK, Kautzman AG, et al. Microglia sculpt postnatal neural circuits in an activity and complement-dependent manner. *Neuron.* 2012;74:691–705.

57. Prinz M, Priller J. Microglia and brain macrophages in the molecular age: from origin to neuropsychiatric disease. *Nat Rev Neurosci.* 2014;15:300–12.

58. Weber MD, Godbout JP, Sheridan JF. Repeated social defeat, neuroinflammation, and behavior: monocytes carry the signal. *Neuropsychopharmacology.* 2017;42:46–61.

59. Rivest S. Regulation of innate immune responses in the brain. *Nat Rev Immunol.* 2009;9:429–39.

60. Saper CB, Romanovsky AA, Scammell TE. Neural circuitry engaged by prostaglandins during the sickness syndrome. *Nat Neurosci.* 2012;15:1088–95.

61. Laflamme N, Rivest S. Toll-like receptor 4: the missing link of the cerebral innate immune response triggered by circulating gram-negative bacterial cell wall components. *FASEB J.* 2001;15:155–63.

62. Colasanti A, Guo Q, Muhlert N, et al. In vivo assessment of brain white matter

inflammation in multiple sclerosis with (18)F-PBR111 PET. *J Nucl Med.* 2014;55 (7):1112–18.

63. Colasanti A, Guo Q, Giannetti P, et al. Hippocampal neuroinflammation, functional connectivity, and depressive symptoms in multiple sclerosis. *Biol Psychiatry.* 2016;80(1):62–72.

64. Sandiego CM, Gallezot JD, Pittman B, et al. Imaging robust microglial activation after lipopolysaccharide administration in humans with PET. *Proc Natl Acad Sci USA.* 2015;112:12468–73.

65. Dowell NG, Cooper EA, Tibble J, et al. Acute changes in striatal microstructure predict the development of interferon-alpha induced fatigue. *Biol Psychiatry.* 2016;79(4):320–8.

66. Harrison NA. Brain structures implicated in inflammation-associated depression. *Curr Top Behav Neurosci.* 2017;31:221–48.

67. Lasselin J, Lekander M, Benson S, Schedlowski M, Engler H. Sick for science: experimental endotoxemia as a translational tool to develop and test new therapies for inflammation-associated depression. *Mol Psych.* 2020 Sep 1. https://doi.org/10.1038/s41380-020-00869-2

68. Reichenberg A, Yirmiya R, Schuld A, et al. Cytokine-associated emotional and cognitive disturbances in humans. *Arch Gen Psychiatry.* 2001;58:445–52.

69. van den Heuvel MP, Pol HEH. Exploring the brain network: a review on resting-state fMRI functional connectivity. *Eur Neuropsychopharm.* 2010;20:519–34.

70. Lekander M, Karshikoff B, Johansson E, et al. Intrinsic functional connectivity of insular cortex and symptoms of sickness during acute experimental inflammation. *Brain Behav Immun.* 2016 Aug;56:34–41.

71. James W. What is an emotion? In Calhoun C, Solomon RC eds. *What is an Emotion?* Oxford University Press: New York; 1984;125–42. (Original work published 1890).

72. Penfield W, Faulk ME. The insula: further observations on its function. *Brain.* 1955;78:445–70.

73. Berntson GG, Norman, GJ, Bechara A, et al. The insula and evaluative processes. *Psychol Sci.* 2011;22:80–6.

74. Chauhan B, Mathias CJ, Critchley HD. Autonomic contributions to empathy: evidence from patients with primary autonomic failure. *Auton Neurosci.* 2008;140:96–100.

75. Capuron L, Pagnoni G, Demetrashvili MF, et al. Basal ganglia hypermetabolism and symptoms of fatigue during interferon-alpha therapy. *Neuropsychopharmacology.* 2007;32:2384–92.

76. Treadway MT, Cooper JA, Miller AH. Can't or won't? Immunometabolic constraints on dopaminergic drive. *Trends Cogn Sci.* 2019;23(5):435–48.

77. Wang J, Campbell IL, Zhang H. Systemic interferon-α regulates interferon stimulated genes in the central nervous system. *Mol Psychiatry.* 2008;13:293–301.

78. Felger JC, Alagbe O, Hu F, et al. Effects of interferon-alpha on rhesus monkeys: a nonhuman primate model of cytokine-induced depression. *Biol Psychiatry.* 2007;62:1324–33.

79. Haroon E, Woolwine BJ, Chen X, et al. IFN-alpha-induced cortical and subcortical glutamate changes assessed by magnetic resonance spectroscopy. *Neuropsychopharmacology.* 2014;39:1777–85.

80. Dowell NG, Bouyagoub S, Tibble J, et al. Interferon-alpha-induced changes in NODDI predispose to the development of fatigue. *Neuroscience.* 2019;403:111–17.

81. Huys QJ, Pizzagalli DA, Bogdan R, Dayan P. Mapping anhedonia onto reinforcement learning: a behavioural meta-analysis. *Biol Mood Anxiety Disord.* 2013;3:12.

82. Schultz W, Apicella P, Scarnati E, Ljungberg T. Neuronal activity in monkey ventral striatum related to the expectation of reward. *J Neurosci.* 1992;12:4595–610.

83. Schultz W. Predictive reward signal of dopamine neurons. *J Neurophysiol.* 1998;80:1–27.

84. Dayan P, Abbott L. *Theoretical neuroscience: computational and mathematical modelling of neural systems.* The MIT Press, Cambridge, MA; 2001.

85. Pessiglione M, Seymour B, Flandin G, Dolan RJ, Frith CD. Dopamine-dependent prediction errors underpin reward-seeking behaviour in humans. *Nature.* 2006;442:1042–5.

86. Gradin VB, Kumar P, Waiter G, et al. Expected value and prediction error abnormalities in depression and schizophrenia. *Brain.* 2011;134:1751–64.

87. Capuron L, Pagnoni G, Drake DF, et al. Dopaminergic mechanisms of reduced basal ganglia responses to hedonic reward during interferon alfa administration. *Arch Gen Psychiatry.* 2012;69:1044–53.

88. Pizzagalli DA, Holmes AJ, Dillon DG, et al. Reduced caudate and nucleus accumbens response to rewards in unmedicated individuals with major depressive disorder. *Am J Psychiatry.* 2009;166:702–10.

89. Eisenberger NI, Berkman ET, Inagaki TK, et al. Inflammation-induced anhedonia: endotoxin reduces ventral striatum responses to reward. *Biol Psychiatry.* 2010a;68:748–54.

90. Harrison NA, Voon V, Cercignani M, et al. A neurocomputational account of how inflammation enhances sensitivity to punishments versus rewards. *Biol Psychiatry.* 2016;80:73–81.

91. Borowski T, Kokkinidis L, Merali Z, Anisman H. Lipopolysaccharide, central in vivobiogenic amine variations, and anhedonia. *Neuroreport.* 1998;9:3797–802.

92. Paulus MP, Rogalsky C, Simmons A, Feinstein JS, Stein MB. Increased activation in the right insula during risk-taking decision making is related to harm avoidance and neuroticism. *Neuroimage.* 2003;19:1439–48.

93. Palminteri S, Justo D, Jauffret C, et al. Critical roles for anterior insula and dorsal striatum in punishment-based avoidance learning. *Neuron.* 2012;76:998–1009

94. Felger JC, Li Z, Haroon E, et al. Inflammation is associated with decreased functional connectivity within corticostriatal reward circuitry in depression. *Mol Psychiatry.* 2015;21:1358–65.

95. Brydon L, Harrison NA, Walker C, Steptoe A, Critchley HD. Peripheral inflammation is associated with altered substantia nigra activity and psychomotor slowing in humans. *Biol Psychiatry.* 2008;63:1022–9.

96. Zung WW, Richards CB, Short MJ. Self-rating depression scale in an outpatient clinic. Further validation of the SDS. *Arch Gen Psychiatry.* 1965;13:508–15.

97. Goldsmith DR, Haroon E, Woolwine BJ, et al. Inflammatory markers are associated with decreased psychomotor speed in patients with major depressive disorder. *Brain Behav Immun.* 2016a;56:281–8.

98. Graybiel AM, Aosaki T, Flaherty AW, Kimura M. The basal ganglia and adaptive motor control. *Science.* 1994;265:1826–31.

99. Bunzeck N, Duzel E. Absolute coding of stimulus novelty in the human substantia nigra/VTA. *Neuron.* 2006;51:369–79.

100. Harrison NA, Cercignani M, Voon V, Critchley HD. Effects of inflammation on hippocampus and substantia nigra responses to novelty in healthy human participants. *Neuropsychopharmacology.* 2015a,40.831–8.

101. van den Biggelaar AH, Gussekloo J, de Craen AJ, et al. Inflammation and interleukin-1 signaling network contribute to depressive symptoms but not cognitive decline in old age. *Exp Gerontol.* 2007;42:693–701.

102. Martinot M, Bragulat V, Artiges E, et al. Decreased presynaptic dopamine function in the left caudate of depressed patients with affective flattening and psychomotor retardation.*Am J Psychiatry.* 2001;158:314–16.

103. Haroon E, Fleischer CC, Felger JC, et al. Conceptual convergence: increased inflammation is associated with increased basal ganglia glutamate in patients with major depression. *Mol Psychiatry.* 2016;21:1351–7.

104. Segrin C. Social skills deficits associated with depression. *Clinical Psychology Review*. 2000;20:379–403.

105. Heinrich LM, Gullone E. The clinical significance of loneliness: a literature review. *Clin Psychol Rev*. 2006;26 (6):695–718.

106. Eisenberger NI, Inagaki TK, Mashal NM, Irwin MR. Inflammation and social experience: an inflammatory challenge induces feelings of social disconnection in addition to depressed mood. *Brain Behav Immun*. 2010b;24: 558–63.

107. Eisenberger NI, Inagaki TK, Rameson LT, Mashal NM, Irwin MR. An fMRI study of cytokine-induced depressed mood and social pain: the role of sex differences. *Neuroimage*. 2009;47:881–90.

108. Moieni M, Irwin MR, Jevtic I, Breen EC, Eisenberger NI. Inflammation impairs social cognitive processing: a randomized controlled trial of endotoxin. *Brain Behav Immun*. 2015a;48:132–8.

109. Cyranowski JM, Frank E, Young E, Shear MK. Adolescent onset of the gender difference in lifetime rates of major depression: a theoretical model. *Arch Gen Psychiatry*. 2000;57:21–7.

110. Dantzer R. Can immunopsychiatry help in understanding the basis of sex differences in major depressive disorder? *Biol Psychiatry Cogn Neurosci Neuroimaging*. 2019;4(7): 606–7.

111. Moieni M, Irwin MR, Jevtic I, et al. Sex differences in depressive and socioemotional responses to an inflammatory challenge: implications for sex differences in depression. *Neuropsychopharmacology*. 2015b;40:1709–16.

112. Frith CD, Frith U. Mechanisms of social cognition. *Annu Rev Psychol*. 2012;63:287–313.

113. Seminowicz DA, Mayberg HS, McIntosh AR, et al. Limbic-frontal circuitry in major depression: a path modeling meta-analysis. *Neuroimage*. 2004;22:409–18.

114. Mayberg HS, Liotti M, Brannan SK, et al. Reciprocal limbic-cortical function and negative mood: converging PET findings in depression and normal sadness. *Am J Psychiatry*. 1999;156:675–82.

115. Mayberg HS, Brannan SK, Tekell JL, et al. Regional metabolic effects of fluoxetine in major depression: serial changes and relationship to clinical response. *Biol Psychiatry*. 2000;48:830–43.

116. Mayberg HS, Lozano AM, Voon V, et al. Deep brain stimulation for treatment-resistant depression. *Neuron*. 2005;45:651–60.

117. Sheline YI, Barch DM, Donnelly JM, et al. Increased amygdala response to masked emotion faces in depressed subjects resolves with antidepressant treatment: an fMRI study. *Biol Psychiatry*. 2001;50:651–8.

118. Price JL, Drevets WC. Neurocircuitry of mood disorders. *Neuropsychopharmacology*. 2010;35:192–216.

119. Victor TA, Furey ML, Fromm SJ, Ohman A, Drevets WC. Relationship between amygdala responses to masked faces and mood state in major depressive disorder. *JAMA Psychiatry*. 2010;67:1128–38.

120. Siegle GJ, Carter CS, Thase ME. Use of fMRI to predict recovery from unipolar depression with cognitive behaviour therapy. *Am J Psychiatry*. 2006;163:735–8.

121. Labrenz F, Wrede K, Forsting M, et al. Alterations in functional connectivity of resting state networks during experimental endotoxemia – an exploratory study in healthy men. *Brain Behav Immun*. 2016;54:17–26.

122. Mehta ND, Haroon E, Xu X, et al. Inflammation negatively correlates with amygdala-ventromedial prefrontal functional connectivity in association with anxiety in patients with depression: preliminary results. *Brain Behav Immun*. 2018;73:725–30.

123. Dew MA, Hoch CC, Buysse DJ, et al. Healthy older adults' sleep predicts all-cause mortality at 4 to 19 years of

follow-up. *Psychosom Med.* 2003;65:63–73.

124. Cohen S, Doyle WJ, Alper CM, Janicki-Deverts D, Turner RB. Sleep habits and susceptibility to the common cold. *Arch Intern Med.* 2009;169:62–7.

125. Sharpley AL, Cooper CM, Williams C, Godlewska BR, Cowen PJ. Effects of typhoid vaccine on inflammation and sleep in healthy participants: a double-blind, placebo- controlled, crossover study. *Psychopharmacology (Berl).* 2016;233:3429–35.

126. Zielinski MR, Dunbrasky DL, Taishi P, Souza G, Krueger JM. Vagotomy attenuates brain cytokines and sleep induced by peripherally administered tumor necrosis factor-alpha and lipopolysaccharide in mice. *Sleep.* 2013;36:1227–38,38A.

127. Weaver JD, Huang MH, Albert M, et al. Interleukin-6 and risk of cognitive decline: MacArthur studies of successful aging. *Neurology.* 2002;59:371–8.

128. Iwashyna TJ, Ely EW, Smith DM, Langa KM. Long-term cognitive impairment and functional disability among survivors of severe sepsis. *JAMA.* 2010;304:1787–94.

129. Montagne A, Barnes SR, Sweeney MD, et al. Blood brain barrier breakdown in the aging human hippocampus. *Neuron.* 2015;85:296–302.

130. Ericsson A, Liu C, Hart RP, Sawchenko PE. Type 1 interleukin-1 receptor in the rat brain: distribution, regulation, and relationship to sites of IL-1-induced cellular activation. *J Comp Neurol.* 1995;361:681–98.

131. Hawrylycz MJ, Lein ES, Guillozet-Bongaarts AL, et al. An anatomically comprehensive atlas of the adult human brain transcriptome. *Nature.* 2012;489:391–9.

132. Suzuki WA, Amaral DG. Perirhinal and parahippocampal cortices of the macaque monkey: cortical afferents. *J Comp Neurol.* 1994;350:497–533.

133. Ban E, Haour F, Lenstra R. Brain interleukin 1 gene expression induced by peripheral lipopolysaccharide administration. *Cytokine.* 1992;4:48–54.

134. Barrientos RM, Higgins EA, Sprunger DB, et al. Memory for context is impaired by a post context exposure injection of interleukin-1 beta into dorsal hippocampus. *Behav Brain Res.* 2002;134:291–8.

135. Oitzl MS, van Oers H, Schobitz B, de Kloet ER. Interleukin-1 beta, but not interleukin-6, impairs spatial navigation learning. *Brain Res.* 1993;613:160–3.

136. Chesnokova V, Pechnick RN, Wawrowsky K. Chronic peripheral inflammation, hippocampal neurogenesis, and behavior. *Brain Behav Immun.* 2016;58:1–8. doi:10.1016/j.bbi.2016.01.017

137. Frodl T, Carballedo A, Hughes M, et al. Reduced expression of glucocorticoid-inducible genes GILZ and SGK-1: high IL-6 levels are associated with reduced hippocampal volumes in major depressive disorder. *Transl Psychiatry.* 2012;2:e88.

138. Schmaal L, Veltman D, van Erp T, et al. Subcortical brain alterations in major depressive disorder: findings from the ENIGMA Major Depressive Disorder working group. *Mol Psychiatry* 2016;21:806–12.

139. Airaksinen E, Larsson M, Lundberg I, Forsell Y. Cognitive functions in depressive disorders: evidence from a population-based study. *Psychol Med.* 2004;34:83–91.

140. Sweeney JA, Kmiec JA, Kupfer DJ. Neuropsychologic impairments in bipolar and unipolar mood disorders on the CANTAB neurocognitive battery. *Biol Psychiatry.* 2000;48:674–84.

141. Dowlati Y, Herrmann N, Swardfager W, et al. A meta-analysis of cytokines in major depression. *Biol Psychiatry.* 2010;67 (5):446–57.

142. Goldsmith DR, Rapaport MH, Miller BJ. A meta-analysis of blood cytokine network alterations in psychiatric

patients: comparisons between schizophrenia, bipolar disorder and depression. *Mol Psychiatry*. 2016b;21 (12):1696–1709.

143. Haapakoski R, Mathieu J, Ebmeier KP, Alenius H, Kivimaki M. Cumulative meta-analysis of interleukins 6 and 1beta, tumour necrosis factor alpha and C-reactive protein in patients with major depressive disorder. *Brain Behav Immun*. 2015;49:206–15.

144. Howren MB, Lamkin DM, Suls J. Associations of depression with C-reactive protein, IL-1, and IL-6: a meta-analysis. *Psychosom Med*. 2009;71 (2):171–86.

145. Osimo EF, Baxter LJ, Lewis G, Jones PB, Khandaker GM. Prevalence of low-grade inflammation in depression: a systematic review and meta-analysis of CRP levels. *Psychol Med*. 2019;49(12):1958–70.

146. Osimo EF, Pillinger T, Rodriguez IM, et al. Inflammatory markers in depression: a meta-analysis of mean differences and variability in 5,166 patients and 5,083 controls. *Brain Behav Immun*. 2020a;87:901–9.

147. Lamers F, Milaneschi Y, Smit JH, et al. Longitudinal association between depression and inflammatory markers: results from the Netherlands study of depression and anxiety. *Biol Psychiatry*. 2019;85(10):829–37.

148. Zalli A, Jovanova O, Hoogendijk WJ, Tiemeier H, Carvalho LA. Low-grade inflammation predicts persistence of depressive symptoms. *Psychopharmacology (Berl)*. 2016;233 (9):1669–78.

149. Au B, Smith KJ, Gariepy G, Schmitz N. The longitudinal associations between C-reactive protein and depressive symptoms: evidence from the English Longitudinal Study of Ageing (ELSA). *Int J Geriatr Psychiatry*. 2015;30 (9):976–84.

150. Khandaker GM, Stochl J, Zammit S, et al. Childhood inflammatory markers and intelligence as predictors of subsequent persistent depressive symptoms:

a longitudinal cohort study. *Psychol Med*. 2018b;48(9):1514–22.

151. Osimo EF, Stochl J, Zammit S, et al. Longitudinal population subgroups of CRP and risk of depression in the ALSPAC birth cohort. *Compr Psychiatry*. 2020b;96:152143.

152. Burgess S, Timpson NJ, Ebrahim S, Davey Smith G. Mendelian randomization: where are we now and where are we going? *Int J Epidemiol*. 2015;44(2):379–88.

153. Davey Smith G, Ebrahim S. 'Mendelian randomization': can genetic epidemiology contribute to understanding environmental determinants of disease? *Int J Epidemiol*. 2003;32(1):1–22.

155. Ferreira RC, Freitag DF, Cutler AJ, et al. Functional IL6R 358Ala allele impairs classical IL-6 receptor signaling and influences risk of diverse inflammatory diseases. *PLoS Genet*. 2013;9(4):e1003444.

154. Khandaker GM, Zammit S, Burgess S, Lewis G, Jones PB. Association between a functional interleukin 6 receptor genetic variant and risk of depression and psychosis in a population-based birth cohort. *Brain Behav Immun*. 2018c;69:264–72.

156. Khandaker GM, Zuber V, Rees JMB, et al. Shared mechanisms between coronary heart disease and depression: findings from a large UK general population-based cohort. *Mol Psychiatry*. 2020;25 (7):1477–86.

157. Kohler O, Benros ME, Nordentoft M, et al. Effect of anti-inflammatory treatment on depression, depressive symptoms, and adverse effects: a systematic review and meta-analysis of randomized clinical trials. *JAMA Psychiatry*. 2014;71(12):1381–91.

158. Kohler-Forsberg O, Lydholm CN, Hjorthoj C, et al. Efficacy of anti-inflammatory treatment on major depressive disorder or depressive symptoms: meta-analysis of clinical trials. *Acta Psychiatr Scand*. 2019;139(5):404–19.

159. Wittenberg GM, Stylianou A, Zhang Y, et al. Effects of immunomodulatory drugs on depressive symptoms: a mega-analysis

of randomized, placebo-controlled clinical trials in inflammatory disorders. *Mol Psychiatry.* 2020;25(6):1275–85.

160. McIntyre RS, Subramaniapillai M, Lee Y, et al. Efficacy of adjunctive infliximab vs placebo in the treatment of adults with bipolar I/II depression: a randomized clinical trial. *JAMA Psychiatry.* 2019;76 (8):783–90.

161. Raison CL, Rutherford RE, Woolwine BJ, et al. A randomized controlled trial of the tumor necrosis factor antagonist infliximab for treatment-resistant depression: the role of baseline inflammatory biomarkers. *JAMA Psychiatry.* 2013;70(1):31–41.

162. Khandaker GM, Oltean BP, Kaser M, et al. Protocol for the insight study: a randomised controlled trial of single-dose tocilizumab in patients with depression and low-grade inflammation. *BMJ Open.* 2018a;8(9):e025333.

163. Jokela M, Virtanen M, Batty GD, Kivimaki M. Inflammation and specific symptoms of depression. *JAMA Psychiatry.* 2016;73(1):87–8.

164. Kohler-Forsberg O, Buttenschon HN, Tansey KE, et al. Association between C-reactive protein (CRP) with depression symptom severity and specific depressive symptoms in major depression. *Brain Behav Immun* 2017;62:344–50.

165. Chu AL, Stochl J, Lewis G, et al. Longitudinal association between inflammatory markers and specific symptoms of depression in a prospective birth cohort. *Brain Behav Immun.* 2019;76:74–81.

166. Milaneschi Y, Lamers F, Peyrot WJ, et al. Genetic association of major depression with atypical features and obesity-related immunometabolic dysregulations. *JAMA Psychiatry.* 2017;74(12):1214–25.

167. Perry BI, Oltean BP, Jones PB, Khandaker GM. Cardiometabolic risk in young adults with depression and evidence of inflammation: a birth cohort study. *Psychoneuroendocriniology.* 2020;116:104682.

168. Stellwagen D, Malenka RC. Synaptic scaling mediated by glial TNF-α. *Nature.* 2006;440:1054–9.

169. Myint AM, Kim YK. Cytokine–serotonin interaction through IDO: a neurodegeneration hypothesis of depression. *Med Hypotheses.* 2003;61 (5–6):519–25.

170. Campbell BM, Charych E, Lee AW, Moller T. Kynurenines in CNS disease: regulation by inflammatory cytokines. *Front Neurosci.* 2014;8:12.

171. Capuron L, Neurauter G, Musselman DL, et al. Interferon-alpha-induced changes in trypto-phan metabolism. Relationship to depression and paroxetine treatment. *Biol. Psychiatry.* 2003b;54:906–14.

172. Bonaccorso S, Marino V, Puzella A, et al. Increased depressive ratings in patients with hepatitis C receiving interferon-alpha-based immunotherapy are related to interferon-alpha-induced changes in the serotonergic system. *J Clin Psychopharmacol.* 2002;22:86–90.

173. Erhardt S, Lim CK, Linderholm KR, et al. Connecting inflammation with glutamate agonism in suicidality. *Neuropsychopharmacology.* 2013;38:743–52.

174. Steiner J, Walter M, Gos T, et al. Severe depression is associated with increased microglial quinolinic acid in subregions of the anterior cingulate gyrus: evidence for an immune- modulated glutamatergic neurotransmission? *J Neuroinflammation.* 2011;8:94.

175. Miller A. Conceptual confluence: the kynurenine pathway as a common target for ketamine and the convergence of the inflammation and glutamate hypotheses of depression. *Neuropsychopharmacol.* 2013;38:1607–8.

176. Kitagami T, Yamada K, Miura H, et al. Mechanism of systemically injected interferon-alpha impeding monoamine biosynthesis in rats: role of nitric oxide as a signal crossing the blood-brain barrier. *Brain Res.* 2003;978:104–14.

177. Felger JC, Miller AH. Cytokine effects on the basal ganglia and dopamine function:

the subcortical source of inflammatory malaise. *Front Neuroendocrinol.* 2012;33:315–27.

178. Kazumori H, Ishihara S, Rumi MA, et al. Transforming growth factor-alpha directly augments histidine decarboxylase and vesicular monoamine transporter 2 production in rat enterochromaffin-like cells. *Am. J Physiol Gastrointest Liver Physiol.* 2004;286:G508–14.

179. Jha MK, Minhajuddin A, Gadad BS, et al. Can C-reactive protein inform antidepressant medication selection in depressed outpatients? Findings from the CO-MED trial. *Psychoneuroendocrinology.* 2017;78:105–13.

180. Jacobs B, van Praag H, Gage F. Adult brain neurogenesis and psychiatry: a novel theory of depression. *Mol Psychiatry.* 2000;5:262–9.

181. Pariante CM. Why are depressed patients inflamed? A reflection on 20 years of research on depression, glucocorticoid resistance and inflammation. *Eur Neuropsychopharmacol.* 2017;27:554–9.

182. Pariante CM, Lightman SL. The HPA axis in major depression: classical theories and new developments. *Trends Neurosci.* 2008;31(9):464–8.

183. Ekdahl CT, Kokaia Z, Lindvall O. Brain inflammation and adult neurogenesis: The dual role of microglia. *Neuroscience.* 2009;158(3):1021–9.

184. Wu CW, Chen YC, Yu L, et al. Treadmill exercise counteracts the suppressive effects of peripheral lipopolysaccharide on hippocampal neurogenesis and learning and memory. *J Neurochem.* 2007;103:2471–81.

185. Koo JW, Duman RS. IL-1beta is an essential mediator of the antineurogenic and anhedonic effects of stress *Proc Natl Acad Sci.* 2008;105:751–6.

186. Goshen I, Kreisel T, Ben-Menachem-Zidon O, et al. Brain interleukin-1 mediates chronic stress-induced depression in mice via adrenocortical activation and hippocampal neurogenesis suppression. *Mol Psychiatry.* 2008;13:717–28.

187. Capuron L, Raison CL, Musselman DL, et al. Association of exaggerated HPA axis response to the initial injection of interferon-alpha with development of depression during interferon-alpha therapy. *Am J Psychol.* 2003a;160: 1342–5.

188. Baumeister D, Akhtar R, Ciufolini S, et al. Childhood trauma and adulthood inflammation: a meta-analysis of peripheral C-reactive protein, interleukin-6 and tumour necrosis factor-α. *Mol Psychiatry.* 2016;21:642–9.

189. Harrison NA, Brydon L, Walker C, et al. Inflammation causes mood change through alterations in subgenual cingulate activity and mesolimbic connectivity. Biol Psychiatry. 2009;66:407–14.

Immunotherapies for Depression

Nils Kappelmann, Edward Bullmore and
Golam Khandaker

8.1 Introduction

In relation to inflammation, the real world of people living with depressive symptoms is diagnostically divided in two. On one side of the line is the large group of patients who have depressive and other mental health symptoms associated with physical health disorders, like rheumatoid arthritis, inflammatory bowel disease or psoriasis (1; 2 ; 3). These are typically categorized as cases of 'comorbid' depression, induced by the demoralizing effects of physical illness and its treatment, and the patient's mental reflection on the implications of their physical disease. They cannot be formally diagnosed as cases of major depressive disorder (MDD) because the standard DSM criteria for MDD explicitly exclude cases associated with a medical disorder. On the other side of this diagnostic fault line is another large group of patients with depressive symptoms that are *not* associated with a major medical disorder and are therefore eligible for a diagnosis of MDD (4). One of the interesting aspects of an immune strategy for new antidepressant interventions is that it cuts across this categorical distinction between comorbid depression and MDD: It offers a potentially interesting way forward for depression caused by inflammation – 'inflamed depression' – whether there is an obvious medical disorder with potentially very high levels of innate immune system activation in comorbid depression, or low-grade inflammation detectable only by a biomarker or blood test in a subset of patients with MDD.

With symptoms such as low mood, anhedonia, fatigue, concentration difficulties and changes in appetite, MDD is also not that dissimilar from symptoms accompanying an acute infection, that is, so-called sickness behaviour (5). This may not be a coincidence. It is now increasingly being recognized that MDD is linked with activation of the innate immune system. Meta-analyses of cross-sectional studies confirm that levels of pro-inflammatory cytokines are generally higher in cases of acute MDD compared to healthy controls (6; 7; 8; 9; 10). According to a recent meta-analysis, about a quarter of MDD cases have evidence of low-grade inflammation as defined by serum C-reactive protein (CRP) levels of >3mg/L (11).

Population-based longitudinal cohort and genetic Mendelian randomization (MR) studies provide evidence that the association between low-grade inflammation and MDD could be causal (see Figure 8.1), and is not fully attributable to reverse causality (e.g., depression itself causing inflammation, for instance, through psychological stress, unhealthy lifestyle and diet) or residual confounding (e.g., lifestyle factors not accounted for in cross-sectional studies underlie the association between inflammation and depression). Using longitudinal data from approximately 5,000 people born in early 1990s in Bristol and south-west England included in the ALSPAC birth cohort, a study suggests that

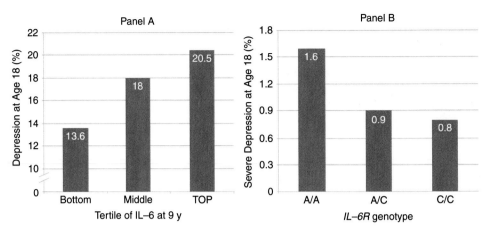

Figure 8.1 Evidence for potential role for IL-6/IL-6 R pathway in depression from the ALSPAC birth cohort. Figure 8.1a shows increased risk of depression at age 18 years for individuals with higher IL-6 levels in childhood at age 9 years. Figure 8.1b minor allele of the *IL-6 R* genetic variant Asp358Ala is associated with impaired *IL-6 R* signalling and decreased inflammation as reflected by reduced serum CRP levels. Figure 8.1b shows that carriers of this 'anti-inflammatory' minor allele have reduced risk of severe depression. Figures reproduced with permission from Khandaker et al. (17) and describe data from Khandaker et al. (12) and Khandaker et al. (18).

higher levels of IL-6 in childhood at age 9 years are associated with increased risk of depression at age 18 years in a linear dose-response fashion (12). Similarly, high levels of IL-6 and CRP have been reported to be associated with subsequent incidence or persistence of depressive symptoms in the ALSPAC, Generation R and Whitehall II cohorts (13; 14; 15). These findings convergently indicate that inflammation precedes the onset of depressive symptoms. Similarly, pharmacological treatment of the hepatitis C virus with interferon therapy, a potent inducer of innate immune response, precedes incidence of MDD in 21–58% (16).

MR analyses of ALSPAC and UK Biobank cohorts provide further evidence for potential causal associations of IL-6 and CRP with depression (18; 19). MR analyses make use of Mendel's law of inheritance, which states that genetic variants are inherited randomly from parents to offspring. This provides a 'natural Randomized Controlled Trial (RCT)' (see Figure 8.2), so that genetic variants associated with an exposure (here, inflammation) can be used as proxy variables to assess a causal association between exposure and outcome (20; 21; 22). Importantly, genetic variants are fixed at conception, so are not influenced by or related to socioeconomic or other confounders (23). Using MR analysis, data from ALSPAC and UK Biobank cohorts suggest that genetic variants in *IL6R* and *CRP* genes, known to be associated with circulating IL-6 and CRP levels, respectively, are also associated with depression (18; 19). Together, these population-based longitudinal cohort and genetic MR studies provide strong evidence that inflammation could be a causal risk factor for depression.

Taken together with the large literature of animal experiments, demonstrating expression of depressive behavioural phenotypes as a consequence of peripheral (body) and central (brain) inflammation (see 5; 24), these findings in clinical studies indicate that inflammation can be a causal mechanism of depressive symptoms in humans. If inflammation is causal, then it follows that anti-inflammatory interventions could be therapeutic.

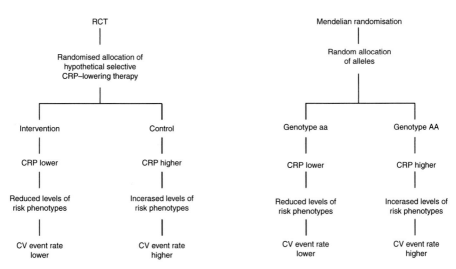

Figure 8.2 Comparison between RCT and MR analysis.
This shows the comparison and equivalent concept of RCTs and MR studies of a hypothetical CRP-lowering drug and CRP-lowering genotype, respectively. The outcome of this example is cardiovascular (CV) event rate. Figure reproduced with permission from Hingorani and Humphries (20).

Currently there is a great deal of interest in exploring whether immunotherapies may offer a potential new treatment option for patients with inflamed depression (i.e., depression *plus* evidence of inflammation such as elevated circulating CRP levels).

This chapter reviews the current evidence base regarding potential clinical relevance of inflammation in depression. Particularly, we discuss: (i) association between inflammation and current treatments for depression; (ii) evidence for effectiveness of different types of anti-inflammatory drugs in depression; (iii) potential adverse effects of immunotherapies; and (iv) potential MDD patients who may benefit from immunotherapy. We also discuss key gaps in current knowledge and offer testable questions for future research.

Throughout this chapter, we rely on evidence from systematic reviews, meta-analyses and key original studies. Wherever possible, we report effect sizes as standardized mean difference (SMD) to quantify immunotherapy effectiveness along with 95% confidence intervals (CIs). For reference, effect sizes (SMDs or Cohen's d) are typically considered as small (SMD = 0.2), medium (SMD = 0.5), and large (SMD = 0.8).

8.2 Association between Inflammation and Current Treatments for Depression

MDD is commonly treated with monoaminergic antidepressant medication such as selective serotonin reuptake inhibitors (SSRIs), selective norepinephrine reuptake inhibitors (SNRIs), monoamine oxidase (MAO) inhibitors, or tricyclics as well as with psychological therapies such as cognitive behavioural therapy (CBT). Several studies have highlighted that antidepressants affect blood levels of inflammatory markers. A recent meta-analysis of these studies has reported that levels of inflammatory markers such as IL-6, IL-10, tumour necrosis factor TNF-α, and C-C Motif Ligand 2 Chemokine CCL-2 are reduced following antidepressant treatment (25). Similarly, there is preliminary evidence that CBT may have anti-inflammatory properties, although this is based on a relatively small number of studies (26).

Studies also suggest that inflammation is associated with poor antidepressant treatment response and recovery. Specifically, patients presenting with low-grade inflammation prior to treatment initiation are less likely to respond to antidepressant medication (25; 27). Such patients have also been reported to have a greater number of unsuccessful treatment trials (28), and have a higher likelihood of symptom recurrence over a five-year period (14). In line with these studies, preliminary evidence indicates a similar pattern for psychotherapy. MDD patients with evidence of low-grade inflammation, compared to those without, have worse treatment outcomes (26).

Preliminary evidence indicates that inflammation could be related to response to specific antidepressant drugs. Results from the Genome-Based Therapeutic Drugs for Depression (GENDEP) trial, comparing an SSRI (escitalopram) with an SNRI (nortriptyline), suggest that patients with evidence of inflammation (CRP $\geq$1mg/L) responded better with nortriptyline, while those without evidence of inflammation responded better with escitalopram (29). Another study reported that patients with evidence of inflammation (CRP $\geq$1mg/L) benefitted from antidepressant augmentation with bupropion, while monotherapy was more effective for those without evidence of inflammation (30).

Evidence from these studies supports the idea that assessment of inflammatory markers could help to guide treatment choice and to identify patients who are less likely to benefit from current treatments. More research is now needed to understand how inflammatory markers can be used for prediction of treatment response in conjunction with other clinical and biochemical markers. An important consideration in this regard will be to clarify the causes of low-grade inflammation that are also linked with depression. For example, several clinically recognized risk factors for depressive disorder, such as obesity and childhood adversity, are also recognized as risk factors for low-grade peripheral inflammation. The causal relationships between psychosocial stress, inflammation and depression would be a particularly useful research focus for future studies, with the potential to identify 'upstream' therapeutic targets that reduce the inflammatory drive by mitigating the causes of inflammation, rather than blocking the effects of inflammation, which is the prevalent therapeutic strategy today.

Evidence of association between inflammation and poor response to current treatment has also raised the possibility that immunotherapies may provide an alternative treatment choice, at least for some MDD patients. In the next section we discuss evidence for the effectiveness of different types of anti-inflammatory drugs, specifically, non-steroidal anti-inflammatory drugs (NSAIDs), anti-cytokine drugs (including monoclonal antibodies (mAbs) and cytokine inhibitors), and other anti-inflammatory interventions.

8.3 Antidepressant Effects of Non-Steroidal Anti-Inflammatory Drugs

NSAIDs comprise a group of small-molecule, anti-inflammatory drugs that target the enzyme cyclooxygenase (COX) implicated in biosynthesis of prostaglandins (31). COX has two isoforms, COX-1 and COX-2. COX-1 is mainly involved in platelet aggregation and is responsible for cytoprotective effects in the stomach, while COX-2 is specifically upregulated in an inflammatory state, so provides a more specific target for anti-inflammatory treatment (31). Traditional NSAIDs such as aspirin are less specific for COX-2, which explains their potential adverse gastrointestinal side effects. On the other hand, newer NSAIDs such as the 'coxibs' show greater specificity for COX-2, which favours their anti-inflammatory potential over traditional NSAIDs (31).

A number of RCTs have tested the effectiveness of NSAIDs as add-on to antidepressant therapy in patients with depression. One of the earliest double-blind, placebo-controlled randomized trials was conducted by Müller et al. (32), which tested whether celecoxib was an effective add-on treatment to the SNRI reboxetine in a relatively small sample of 40 MDD patients treated over a period of six weeks. Addition of celecoxib resulted in significantly greater improvement in depressive symptoms over the course of six-week treatment.

A number of other RCTs have also tested antidepressant effects of NSAID add-on treatment or monotherapy in patients with MDD (33; 34; 35), and in patients with comorbid depression associated with osteoarthritis (36), brucellosis (37), fibromyalgia (38) and colorectal cancer (39). Meta-analyses of these RCTs (40; 41) suggest that adding NSAIDs along with antidepressants could offer an additional benefit for depressive symptoms over antidepressant treatment alone. The pooled effect size for the antidepressant effect of add-on NSAIDs treatment was 0.82 (95% CI: 0.46–1.17) and 0.29 (95% CI: 0.06–0.51) for NSAID monotherapy.

Thus, NSAIDs show promise as add-on treatment along with antidepressants and particularly for patients with comorbid inflammatory physical illness. It is worth noting that RCTs of NSAIDs in MDD patients without physical illness are relatively rare; combined sample size from existing RCTs is 132 patients (32; 33; 34; 35). In future, further RCTs with larger samples are required to determine whether NSAIDs could be useful for MDD patients without an inflammatory physical illness.

8.4 Antidepressant Effects of Anti-Cytokine Drugs

Anti-cytokine monoclonal antibodies (mAbs), like the anti-TNF-α antibody adalimumab, are large biological molecules engineered to target a specific inflammatory cytokine. Treatment using these agents has had major therapeutic impact in many areas of medicine because of the high specificity of target engagement and resulting low prevalence of off-target effects. These drugs are now routinely used for the treatment of psoriasis, rheumatoid arthritis, inflammatory bowel disease and other inflammatory physical illnesses (42). An advantage of mAbs is that they are administered as injection/infusion typically monthly and confer prolonged passive immunity against their target molecule over weeks or months. This means patients do not need to take a medication daily, which also ensures treatment adherence.

A number of clinical trials have investigated effects of anti-cytokine drugs on comorbid depressive symptoms in patients treated for an inflammatory physical illness such as psoriasis, Crohn's disease, atopic dermatitis, rheumatoid arthritis and multicentric Castleman's disease (a lymphoproliferative disorder associated with high levels of IL-6). Mental health or depression were not the primary clinical outcome or study endpoint in any of these studies; however, in all of them, some simple questions about mood and energy were completed as secondary or exploratory endpoints. We have conducted a meta-analysis of the antidepressant effect of anti-cytokine drugs based on such trials (43). These studies include placebo-controlled RCTs of (i) the anti-TNF-α antagonists etanercept (44; 45) and adalimumab (46; 47); (ii) the IL-12 and IL-23 inhibitor ustekinumab (48); (iii) the IL-4 R-α antagonist dupilumab (49; 50); (iv) the IL-17a inhibitor ixekizumab (51); and (v) the IL-6 inhibitors sirukumab and siltuximab (52). Based on meta-analysis of seven double-blind RCTs, our results suggest robust antidepressant effect of anti-cytokine drugs, with a medium effect size of 0.40 (95% CI: 0.22–0.59; see Figure 8.3) (43). Trials without a placebo arm showed a larger effect size of 0.51 (95% CI: 0.34–0.67) when comparing baseline and follow-up depressive symptoms, which is to be expected considering the non-adjustment for potential placebo effects. With regards to specific type of treatment, most RCTs have been conducted for anti-TNF-α drugs and two non-randomized studies evaluated the IL-6R inhibitor tocilizumab. Based on our analyses of all available clinical trial data (43), the effect size for anti-TNF-α treatment compared to placebo was 0.33 (95% CI: 0.06–0.60) and the effect size from baseline to follow-up in non-randomized clinical trials of anti-IL-6R treatment was 0.31 (95% CI: 0.20–0.42).

Other meta-analyses have reported similar findings. For instance, anti-cytokine treatment showed favourable antidepressant effect size, compared to placebo, of 0.56 (95% CI: 0.19–0.93) (41) and 0.29 (95% CI: 0.12–0.45) (53). With regards to specific drug targets, the results by Wittenberg and colleagues (53) further suggest most promising effects for anti-TNF-α (SMD = 0.30, 95% CI: -0.08–0.67), anti-IL-12/23 (SMD = 0.48, 95% CI: 0.26–0.70), anti-IL-6 (SMD = 0.80, 95% CI: 0.20–1.41), anti-CD20 (SMD = 0.32, 95% CI: -0.03–0.68), and anti-B-lymphocyte stimulator (BLγS) monoclonal antibodies (SMD = 0.34, 95% CI: -0.07–0.76).

Together, these meta-analyses provide evidence that anti-cytokine drugs have antidepressant effects, consistent with previous studies suggesting inflammation as a potential causal mechanism for depression. Indeed, since monoclonal antibodies administered by intravenous infusion are generally too large to pass through the blood-brain barrier (BBB) and do not achieve significant tissue concentrations in the brain, their apparent antidepressant efficacy is consistent more specifically with peripheral (bodily) inflammation as a cause of depression.

However, an important question regarding interpretation of these results is whether the observed antidepressant effects are secondary to improvement in physical illness. Two meta-analyses have addressed this issue. Kappelmann et al. (43) used meta-regression analyses of clinical trial data from anti-cytokine drugs to investigate whether the antidepressant effect sizes for anti-cytokine treatment (compared to a placebo) were related to the effect sizes for improvements in physical illness, i.e., the primary endpoint for respective trial (see Figure 8.4a). For the six trials included in this meta-regression analysis, there was no significant association of improvements in depressive and primary physical illness symptoms. These findings indicate that anti-inflammatory drugs improve mood independently of improving physical illness. However, this analysis was based on a relatively small number of RCTs and it did not look at individual patient-level data, which could be more powerful in disentangling these effects.

Another, more recent meta-analysis (53) has overcome this issue by combining individual patient-level data on depressive and primary disease symptoms across 18 clinical trials of anti-inflammatory drugs conducted by the pharmaceutical companies Janssen Research & Development and GlaxoSmithKline. When the estimation of antidepressant treatment effect size was restricted to individuals who did *not* respond to treatment on the primary endpoint (see Figure 8.4b), results still suggested a significant antidepressant effect of anti-cytokine antibodies (SMD = 0.38, 95% CI: 0.21–0.55), which was most pronounced for mAbs targeting IL-6 (SMD = 0.88, 95% CI: 0.16–1.59). Further

(a) RCTs of anti-cytokine drug vs. placebo

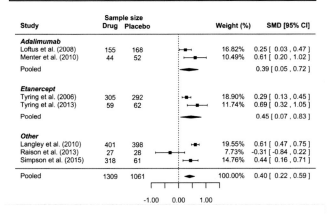

Study	Sample size Drug	Placebo		Weight (%)	SMD [95% CI]
Adalimumab					
Loftus et al. (2008)	155	168		16.82%	0.25 [0.03 , 0.47]
Menter et al. (2010)	44	52		10.49%	0.61 [0.20 , 1.02]
Pooled					0.39 [0.05 , 0.72]
Etanercept					
Tyring et al. (2006)	305	292		18.90%	0.29 [0.13 , 0.45]
Tyring et al. (2013)	59	62		11.74%	0.69 [0.32 , 1.05]
Pooled					0.45 [0.07 , 0.83]
Other					
Langley et al. (2010)	401	398		19.55%	0.61 [0.47 , 0.75]
Raison et al. (2013)	27	28		7.73%	-0.31 [-0.84 , 0.22]
Simpson et al. (2015)	318	61		14.76%	0.44 [0.16 , 0.71]
Pooled	1309	1061		100.00%	0.40 [0.22 , 0.59]

-1.00   0.00   1.00

(b) RCTs of anti-cytokine drug plus DMARD vs. DMARD

Study	Sample size Treatment	Control		Weight (%)	SMD [95% CI]
Etanercept					
Kekow et al. (2010)	265	263		54.31%	0.10 [-0.07 , 0.27]
Machado et al. (2014)	279	142		45.69%	0.29 [0.09 , 0.49]
Pooled	544	405		100.00%	0.19 [0.00 , 0.37]

-1.00   0.00   1.00

Standardised Mean Difference (SMD)

(c) Other trials (non-randomised and/or non-placebo)

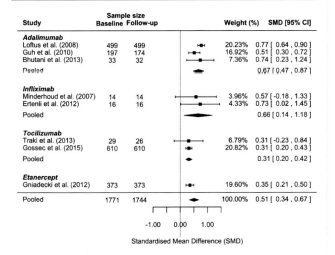

Study	Sample size Baseline	Follow-up		Weight (%)	SMD [95% CI]
Adalimumab					
Loftus et al. (2008)	499	499		20.23%	0.77 [0.64 , 0.90]
Guh et al. (2010)	197	174		16.92%	0.51 [0.30 , 0.72]
Bhutani et al. (2013)	33	32		7.36%	0.74 [0.23 , 1.24]
Pooled					0.67 [0.47 , 0.87]
Infliximab					
Minderhoud et al. (2007)	14	14		3.96%	0.57 [-0.18 , 1.33]
Ertenli et al. (2012)	16	16		4.33%	0.73 [0.02 , 1.45]
Pooled					0.66 [0.14 , 1.18]
Tocilizumab					
Traki et al. (2013)	29	26		6.79%	0.31 [-0.23 , 0.84]
Gossec et al. (2015)	610	610		20.82%	0.31 [0.20 , 0.43]
Pooled					0.31 [0.20 , 0.42]
Etanercept					
Gniadecki et al. (2012)	373	373		19.60%	0.35 [0.21 , 0.50]
Pooled	1771	1744		100.00%	0.51 [0.34 , 0.67]

-1.00   0.00   1.00

Standardised Mean Difference (SMD)

Figure 8.3 Antidepressant effect of anti-cytokine drugs.
These forest plots from Kappelmann et al. (43) show evidence for antidepressant effect of anti-cytokine drugs (positive values favour anti-cytokine treatment) with separate pooled effect estimates for different drugs. Figure 8.3a and 8.3b show evidence for anti-cytokine treatment versus placebo from RCTs without and with concomitant disease-modifying antirheumatic drugs (DMARDs), respectively. Figure 8.3c shows evidence from non-randomized and/or non-placebo trials, so effect sizes compare baseline versus follow-up symptoms. Figure 8.3 has been reproduced with permission from Kappelmann et al. (43).

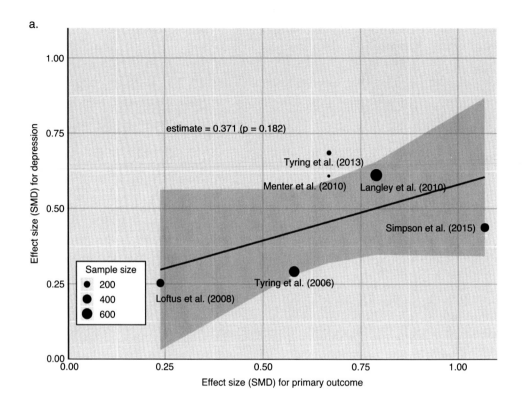

Figure 8.4 Anti-cytokine drugs improve depressive symptoms independently of improvements in physical illness. Figure 8.4a shows meta-regression analysis from Kappelmann et al. (43) showing no evidence for an association between effect size for primary physical illness and that for depression. Figure 8.4b from Wittenberg et al. (53) shows antidepressant effect size of anti-cytokine drugs in patients who did not show any improvement in physical illness for which the drug was trialled. Figure 8.4 reproduced with permission from Kappelmann et al. (43) and Wittenberg et al. (53).

analyses were performed by statistically controlling antidepressant effect sizes for improvements in primary illness symptoms. Averaging across trials and anti-inflammatory drug classes, results suggested that antidepressant effect sizes decreased slightly following such statistical correction for primary illness symptoms, but still remained statistically significant overall with a small effect size (unadjusted SMD = 0.29, 95% CI: 0.12–0.45; adjusted SMD = 0.20, 95% CI: 0.06–0.35), confirming our previous finding that anti-cytokine drugs improve depressive symptoms independently of improvements in physical illness.

In summary, evidence from secondary analysis of existing clinical trials in inflammatory physical illness suggests that anti-cytokine drugs have antidepressant properties and this may indeed be independent from improvements in primary physical disease. These findings have two important implications. First, they provide further support for the idea that inflammation could be a causal risk factor for depression. Second, they support therapeutic targeting of the immune system in MDD patients and especially those with evidence of inflammation. This calls for further RCTs of anti-cytokine drugs in patients with comorbid depression designed to measure treatment-related changes in mood as the primary outcome carefully and repeatedly over time starting within a few days of intravenous infusion of anti-cytokine antibody or placebo.

The existing database of RCTs of anti-cytokine antibodies for comorbid depression is much larger than the relatively few (currently, three) studies that have been designed specifically to test antidepressant efficacy in patients with MDD or bipolar depression without any major physical comorbidity (54; 55; clinical trial ID: NCT02473289). Raison and colleagues (54) tested the effect of the anti-TNF-α mAb infliximab in 60 patients with treatment-resistant depression. Patients with evidence for treatment resistance and at least a moderately severe depressive episode were recruited and randomized to three infusions of 50mg/kg infliximab or placebo at baseline, 2 weeks, and 6 weeks, with depressive symptoms measured at 12 weeks using a standard clinical questionnaire. Results did not show a significant placebo-controlled effect of infliximab on the primary outcome of depression symptoms. The second study tested the effect of the same drug (infliximab), same dosing regimen (5mg/kg at weeks 0, 2, & 6), and same study duration (12 weeks) in patients with bipolar depression (55). Again, results did not show a significant placebo-controlled effect of infliximab on depressive symptoms at 12 weeks, although infliximab led to faster symptom improvement visible at 2 weeks post-infusion.

One explanation for these negative findings could be strategies for patient recruitment, since both studies mainly used the clinical criteria of treatment-resistant depression as the basis for recruiting patients. Treatment-resistant depression has indeed been associated with low-grade inflammation, as indexed by CRP levels (56). However, secondary analyses of data from the Raison et. al. (54) study suggest increased peripheral inflammation at baseline, indexed by serum CRP levels, was associated with greater improvements in depressive symptoms following infliximab treatment, while lower levels of CRP at baseline were associated with greater benefit from the placebo. As such, biomarker evidence for innate immune system activation may be a more specific and useful inflammation-related inclusion criterion as compared to treatment resistance.

Raison et al. (54) did not use any biomarker inclusion criteria and McIntyre et al. (55) used inclusion criteria relatively unspecific for inflammation, e.g., high BMI, daily cigarette smoking, etc. Lastly, the McIntyre trial reported some evidence of antidepressant effect for participants with a history of childhood trauma (55). Similar to treatment-resistant depression, there is evidence of associations between childhood trauma and inflammatory markers (57), so childhood trauma may also capture some of the variance of inflammation-related depression. It is also important to note that both trials had low power to detect the small-to-moderate effect sizes of anti-cytokine drugs reported in meta-analyses (including data from patients suffering from chronic inflammatory conditions).

Recently, Janssen Pharmaceuticals tested a novel anti-IL-6 mAb, sirukumab, using an RCT where 193 patients with unipolar depression and serum CRP levels >3 mg/L were enrolled, of which 169 patients completed the trial (clinical trial ID: NCT02473289). This was the first clinical trial of an anti-inflammatory intervention for depression to use an inflammatory biomarker prospectively as an eligibility criterion designed to enrich the sample for inflamed depression. Although main results reported on clinicaltrials.gov suggest no significant benefit of sirukumab over placebo on depressive symptoms, those with higher baseline CRP levels (>8mg/L) had greater improvements in depression after sirukumab treatment compared with the placebo. In addition, the drug appeared to decrease anhedonia, a key symptom of depression, specifically (from presentation at the Lancet Conference 2018, Barcelona). Together, findings from these three RCTs highlight that, in addition to large sample size, careful inclusion of patients who are likely to benefit from immunotherapy, selected based on biomarker evidence of inflammation and/or other criteria, is likely to be crucial for the success of future RCTs in this field (see Section 8.7 below).

8.5 Antidepressant Effects of Other Anti-Inflammatory Drugs

A number of drugs with anti-inflammatory properties such as statins, omega-3 fatty acids, minocycline and glucocorticoids have been tested in clinical trials and observational studies of depression, which have been subject to systematic reviews and meta-analyses.

8.5.1 Statins

Statins are typically used for their lipid lowering properties to prevent cardiovascular disease and stroke (58). They have anti-inflammatory properties, for example, statins have been reported to reduce inflammation induced by a high-fat diet in mice (59). A meta-analysis of epidemiological cohort, case-control and cross-sectional studies has suggested that statin users develop depression less frequently compared with non-users (60), although more recent large register-based analysis of 193,977 Danish individuals has contradicted this finding (61).

In terms of acute effects of statin treatment on depressive symptoms, several RCTs of statin monotherapy (62; 63; 64; 65) or add-on treatment (66; 67; 68) have been conducted. Of note, three of these trials have looked at effects of statins on depressive symptoms in patients with a history of acute myocardial infarction or hospitalisation for unstable angina pectoris (63), hypercholesterolemia (64) and multiple sclerosis (65), so not specific to MDD. Meta-analysis pooling all of these monotherapy and add-on trials shows a small antidepressant effect size of 0.26 (95% CI: 0.04–0.48) for statins compared with a placebo (41).

8.5.2 Minocycline

Minocycline is a tetracycline antibiotic that has a range of different effects on pathways implicated in depression aetiology, such as oxidative stress, apoptosis, modulation of glutamatergic and monoaminergic systems, and inflammation (69). To date, three RCTs have investigated minocycline as a treatment for MDD (70; 71) or comorbid depression in HIV patients (72). Meta-analyses of these studies have indicated overall large effect sizes of 0.87 (95% CI: 0.29–1.45) in MDD and of 0.78 (0.24–1.33) in comorbid MDD in HIV patients. However, this is based on relatively small pooled sample sizes of 151 and 158 patients, respectively (41; 73). Thus, further studies with larger samples are required. We are aware of a larger RCT of add-on minocycline in treatment-resistant depression currently underway (clinical trial ID: NCT02456948), which will add to the evidence base.

8.5.3 Glucocorticoids

Glucocorticoids have long been used as anti-inflammatory agents due to their well-known anti-inflammatory effects on innate immune system activity. Endogenously, glucocorticoid release from the Hypothalamus-Pituitary-Adrenal (HPA) axis is upregulated following inflammation in response to infection or tissue damage, which in turn reduces the transcription of pro-inflammatory genes (74). However, patients with depression tend to show chronic low-grade inflammation in the presence of hypercortisolemia, which has been attributed to glucocorticoid insensitivity or resistance (75). Two RCTs have tested the antidepressant effects of glucocorticoids by evaluating the effects of: (i) single intravenous administration of hydrocortisone and ovine corticotropin-releasing hormone (CRH) versus a placebo (76); and (ii) dexamethasone versus a placebo for four days (77). These two RCTs show a rather large pooled effect size of 0.90 (95% CI: 0.36–1.44), but this evidence is based on a very small sample of 59 patients (two trials combined) who were treated for a very short duration of time. In future, larger RCTs with longer follow-up and repeated treatment are needed, including careful assessment of known side effects of corticosteroids, particularly mood disturbance and psychotic symptoms (78), to assess potential usefulness of corticosteroids in MDD.

8.5.4 Omega-3 Fatty Acids

Omega-3 fatty acids are abundant in fish and the Mediterranean diet and have been suggested to downregulate inflammation (79). The body usually maintains a physiologic balance between omega-3 and omega-6 fatty acids. Omega-6 fatty acids increase pro-inflammatory eicosanoid metabolites, and it is thought that the modern diet/lifestyle has shifted this balance towards more omega-6 compared to prehistoric times (79). While a recent meta-analysis of 15 clinical trials involving a total of 916 participants confirmed an antidepressant effect of fish oil supplement, on closer examination the composition of supplement seemed crucial (80). Specifically, the relative balance of eicosapentaenoic acid (EPA) and docosahexaenoic acid (DHA) determined the efficacy of supplement versus placebo. Studies with a supplement containing EPA/DHA ratio ≥60% showed antidepressant effects with a moderate effect size of 0.56 (95% CI: 0.28–0.84), while no antidepressant benefit was observed if EPA/DHA ratio was <60% (SMD = -0.03; 95% CI: -0.20–0.15). While these findings require careful evaluation due to likely publication bias, they offer preliminary evidence for a potential role of dietary supplementation with omega-3 fatty acids for treatment of depression.

In summary, similar to NSAIDs and anti-cytokine drugs, there is some evidence that other drugs with anti-inflammatory properties show promise as treatments of depression.

However, unlike NSAIDs and anti-cytokine drugs the number of RCTs for these interventions is small. Due to the broad ranging effects of these drugs, it also remains unclear whether anti-inflammatory mechanisms are solely responsible for their putative antidepressant effect.

Lastly, it is worth noting that many other non-pharmacological interventions may also improve mood by modulating inflammation. For example, yoga and mindfulness training have been proposed to have both antidepressant and anti-inflammatory properties (81). Mindfulness-based cognitive therapy (MBCT) is an evidence-based treatment for depression relapse prevention (82), and mindfulness training has been reported to improve mental well-being and decrease circulating inflammatory maker levels in university students (83; 84). As these non-pharmacological interventions are likely to be acceptable by many, and even be preferred over pharmacological treatment especially for those with relatively mild depressive symptoms, potential usefulness of these interventions merits further investigation.

8.6 Potential Adverse Effects of Immunotherapies for Depression

When considering immunotherapies for patients with depression, it will be important to balance their potential clinical utility against possible side effects. Side effects of NSAIDs predominantly involve the gastrointestinal system, but they can also increase risk for cardiovascular disease. As mentioned previously, NSAIDs differ in their balance of COX-1/COX-2 inhibition with newer drugs showing greater specificity for COX-2. Due to the physiological role of COX-1 in gastrointestinal function, unspecific COX inhibitors such as aspirin can cause pronounced gastrointestinal side effects (e.g., dyspepsia and ulcers), potentially limiting their long-term use. COX-2 specific drugs (i.e., coxibs) also have gastrointestinal side effects especially in older patients, albeit less frequently compared with COX-1 inhibitors (85). COX-2 drugs can also increase the risk of cardiovascular disease (86; 87). Considering that depression is itself associated with increased risk of cardiovascular disease (88), long-term use of these NSAIDs could be problematic for some patients and would require careful monitoring of cardiovascular risk.

While anti-cytokine drugs are usually well-tolerated due to their high target specificity, side effects can range from general, target-independent effects such as rare autoimmunity (e.g., acute anaphylaxis or serum sickness) to target-specific side effects, so patients on these drugs require careful monitoring (89). Clinically, liver function is routinely assessed due to increases in liver enzymes by some cytokine inhibitors (90). Regarding the target-specific effects of anti-cytokine drugs, a meta-analysis of RCTs testing anti-TNF-α mAbs adalimumab and infliximab for rheumatoid arthritis (91), has reported a dose-dependent increase in the risks for serious infections and malignancies. Here, low dosage (infliximab: <3mg/kg every four weeks; adalimumab: 20mg/week) significantly increased the risk of serious infection (OR = 1.8, 95% CI: 1.1–3.1) and high dosage (infliximab: ≥6mg/kg every eight weeks; adalimumab: 40mg every other week) increased the risk of both serious infection (OR = 2.3, 95% CI: 1.5–3.6) and malignancy (OR = 4.3, 95% CI: 1.6–11.8). However, the increased risk of malignancies was contradicted recently, and has been attributed to publication bias (92). Anti-TNF-α drugs can also lead to reactivation of latent tuberculosis infection, which is usually maintained by TNF-α (93). For other monoclonal antibodies, side effects can be diverse including infections, cancer, autoimmune disease, platelet and thrombotic disorders and cardiotoxicity depending on the drug target (89).

Regarding other anti-inflammatory drugs, a recent systematic review and meta-analysis of RCTs investigating minocycline in depression, bipolar disorder and schizophrenia found minocycline prevented headaches and there were no significant differences in other adverse events compared to a placebo (94). However, minocycline treatment for other disease indications was reported to be associated with dizziness, vertigo, skin rash, gastrointestinal disturbance, ringing ears and teratogenicity (95; 96; 97).

Glucocorticoids can have a range of side effects depending on type and duration of treatment. Side effects range from increased risk of infections, cardiovascular effects such as hypertension, and gastrointestinal effects like peptic ulcers or gastrointestinal bleeding (98). When taken over prolonged periods of time, glucocorticoids also promote glucocorticoid receptor resistance (74), which is itself implicated in MDD pathogenesis (99; 75).

A recent meta-analysis of antidepressant effects of anti-inflammatory drugs also synthesized evidence on side effects (41). Out of all categories of side effects (gastrointestinal symptoms, pain, muscle ache, infections and cardiovascular events), anti-inflammatory treatment was reported to be associated only with risk of infection (OR = 1.14, 95% CI: 0.99–1.31). However, reporting of side effects in 36 trials included in this meta-analysis was inconsistent with only 19 trials reporting any side effects. Not all studies recorded all side effects. For example, cardiovascular events were recorded in 3 trials and gastrointestinal symptoms in 13 trials. This highlights the need for better side-effect reporting in future trials including those of depressed patients without chronic inflammatory condition. Immunotherapy, at least in theory, could lead to more pronounced side effects in these patients as they have less severe immune dysfunction compared to patients with autoimmune/other chronic inflammatory physical illness. In sum, there are a number of side effects of immunotherapies, which need to be considered carefully before prescribing these medications. As ever, balancing potential risk-benefit by taking into account individual patient history, risk factors, need and preference would be key as well as appropriate monitoring during ongoing treatment.

8.7 Which Patients May Benefit from Immunotherapy?

Which patients may benefit from immunotherapy is now a key question for the field. Several lines of evidence point towards the idea that immunotherapy may be specifically helpful for patients who show evidence of inflammation. First, many of the trials demonstrating treatment effectiveness include patients with chronic inflammatory conditions. As these patients present with an abnormally functioning immune system by definition, they may etiologically be more likely to suffer from an 'inflamed depression'. Consistent with this idea, the infliximab trial by Raison et al. (55) reported that higher levels of CRP at baseline were associated with greater improvement in mood symptoms after treatment with infliximab. There is also similar evidence from a trial of omega-3 fatty acid supplementation (100).

Considering the prevalence of low-grade inflammation (CRP levels >3mg/L) in patients with depression is about 27% (11), it may be necessary to first stratify patients suffering from MDD into those with probable low-grade inflammation versus those without inflammation. Immunotherapy could have a role for 'inflamed' patients, while in 'non-inflamed' patients it may be more appropriate to consider treatment with SSRIs (cf., 29; 30) or psychotherapy (e.g., CBT). This approach would avoid unnecessary risk of immunotherapy side effects.

A number of ongoing immunotherapy clinical trials are currently using CRP and other measures of inflammation as part of the inclusion criteria (Table 8.1). For instance, the Insight study, a double-blind RCT of single-dose, intravenous tocilizumab (anti-IL-6 receptor mAb) infusion for patients with depression, is using persistent inflammation (CRP ≥3mg/L on two occasions) and inflammation-related symptoms along with other criteria for patient selection (17). Refining selection criteria to ensure inclusion of patients most likely to benefit from anti-inflammatory treatment is an important ongoing endeavour for the field, which would be vital for the success of future RCTs.

Detailed immuno-profiling may prove a useful tool in this regard. For example, a recent study by Lynall et al. (101) conducted in-depth immunophenotyping analysis of depressed patients and healthy controls, which identified subgroups of individuals with distinct immunological profiles. Depressed patients with evidence of inflammation ('inflamed') were characterized by both increased myeloid and lymphoid cell counts as well as increased serum CRP and IL-6 levels compared to healthy controls. The study also highlighted further heterogeneity within the 'inflamed' group reflected in the balance of myeloid and lymphoid cell counts.

Clinically, another promising avenue for patient stratification may be the depressive symptom profile. It is well known that there is a great deal of heterogeneity in the symptom profile of patients with depression. Emerging evidence suggests specific associations of individual depressive symptoms with certain risk factors (102). For instance, elevated levels of circulating inflammatory markers, such as CRP and IL-6, are mostly associated with somatic symptoms of depression, including fatigue and sleep disturbances, rather than psychological symptoms, such as hopelessness or excessive/inappropriate guilt (103; 104; 105; 106; 107). Symptoms of so-called 'atypical depression' such as an increased weight/appetite are associated with immuno-metabolic alterations including high BMI, waist circumference, and levels of CRP and TNF-α (104). There is also discussion on covarying anxiety symptoms in interferon-induced depression (108), which needs to be explored in future studies. If individual symptoms or symptom dimensions continue to show reliable specificity for inflamed depression, symptoms could offer an easy and quick means of identifying patients potentially benefiting from immunotherapy. Potential usefulness of this strategy is currently being assessed in the Insight study (17).

Genetic testing could also be helpful depending on mechanism of effect of the anti-inflammatory drug under investigation. For example, an ongoing RCT (clinical trial IDs: NCT04116606/ISRCTN44411633) is testing a novel anti-inflammatory drug JNJ-54175446 that acts as an antagonist to the P2X7 receptor, which is located on microglia, and down-regulates pro-inflammatory IL-1β stimulation via the NLRP3 inflammasome. In this trial, patients are selected based on genetic polymorphisms of P2X7 receptors associated with the activity of this pathway. Other clinical and biochemical measures could also be useful for selecting patients in future RCTs of anti-inflammatory treatment. As described in Section 8.4, a recent RCT reported that history of childhood maltreatment was associated with improvement in mood after treatment with infliximab in patients with bipolar depression (55). There is a rich literature linking childhood maltreatment and chronic low-grade inflammation characterized by elevated levels of circulating inflammatory markers (109).

Neuroimaging positron emission tomography (PET) studies provide evidence for microglia activation, a marker of neuroinflammation, in patients with depression (110). This could also

Table 8.1 Ongoing/unpublished clinical trials of anti-inflammatory drugs for depression

Trial Identifier	Published Protocol	Drug	Key immune/related inclusion criteria	Status at Apr 2020
NCT02362529	-	Minocycline, Celecoxib	TSPO VT ≥10.5 (HAB) or ≥8.5 (MAB) in any of the primary regions of interest (prefrontal cortex, anterior cingulate cortex or insula)	Completed
NCT02473289	-	Sirukumab	Serum/plasma hsCRP level ≥3mg/L	Completed
ISRCTN16942542	17	Tocilizumab	Serum hsCRP level ≥3mg/L; somatic symptoms	Recruiting
NCT02660528	-	Tocilizumab	-	Recruiting
NCT02456948	-	Minocycline	-	Active, not recruiting
NCT04116606/ ISRCTN44411633	-	P2X7 receptor blocker JNJ-54175446	Venous hsCRP blood level ≤1 mg/L; no loss of function allele at one or both of two SNPs on the P2RX7 gene: rs3751143 (1487 A >C) and rs1653624 (1703 T >A)	Recruiting

be a useful measure for patient selection, though perhaps limited to centres with appropriate facilities. An ongoing RCT comparing minocycline, celecoxib and placebo is currently testing whether evidence of microglia activation measured by PET imaging could be useful for patient selection (clinical trial ID: NCT02362529). In general, however, further developments in PET radiochemistry and other methods of measuring inflammation in the central nervous system (not just in blood samples) is likely to be crucial to the optimal stratification of patients with MDD and other neuropsychiatric disorders for anti-inflammatory drug treatment.

8.8 Conclusions and Future Outlook

The idea of immunotherapies for depression is revolutionary because it not only offers new mechanistic insights into the causes of this illness, but it also flies in the face of Cartesian dualistic views about the mind and body as separate entities. Pathophysiologic explanations and drug therapy for depression is largely predicated on monoamine neurotransmitters, such as serotonin, but heterogeneity in clinical presentation and treatment response suggests that other mechanisms are involved. Inflammation could be one such mechanism relevant for some patients with depression. Traditionally, the brain has been considered as an 'immune privileged' site shielded by the BBB, but research over the last few decades now confirms that there is a great deal of interaction between the immune system and the brain, challenging the divide between mind and body.

As we have highlighted in this chapter, research on immunotherapy for depression is an exciting and active area within psychiatry today. Current empirical work emphasizes that a significant minority of depressed patients display evidence of low-grade inflammation. Importantly, these patients do not do too well on antidepressant treatments such as SSRIs or psychotherapy currently used. This highlights two key points.

First, inflammatory markers may serve as decision tools for determining which depressed patients are likely to respond to currently available treatments. Preliminary evidence indicates the potential usefulness of this approach, for instance, using peripheral blood levels of CRP and other inflammatory markers. This could be game changing for psychiatry, as there is no reliable test to predict antidepressant treatment response as of yet. Thus, immunopsychiatry holds promise of identifying accessible biomarkers to guide clinical decision making.

Informed by existing evidence, clinicians today could test for evidence of inflammation/infection (e.g., full blood count and CRP) along with careful history taking and physical examination as part of the initial assessment of patients with depression, which is already being done in some specialist services. This could identify inflammatory physical illness in need of appropriate treatment. It could also identify inflammation-related factors, such as obesity, physical inactivity, smoking and alcohol abuse, which could be managed accordingly using both pharmacological and lifestyle interventions, and would lead to better long-term outcomes for patients.

Second, immunotherapy could offer effective alternative treatment options for some patients with depression. As we have discussed, there is evidence that NSAIDs could be useful as an add-on treatment to antidepressants, so clinicians could consider these relatively low-risk options for suitable patients. There is evidence that novel anti-cytokine anti-inflammatory drugs improve depressive symptoms independently of chronic inflammatory physical illness. More RCTs, especially those based on patients without comorbid inflammatory physical illness, are required to test conclusively whether these drugs could have a place in psychiatric clinics. More studies are also needed to establish long-term efficacy and safety.

Which patients would benefit from immunotherapy is an important question, and is subject to ongoing research. Emerging evidence indicates that low-grade inflammation, as measured by circulating CRP levels, may be a useful approach for identifying such patients. However, more work is needed to refine patient selection criteria in future RCTs. It is clear that inflammation is unlikely to be relevant for all patients with depression, so a one-size-fits-all approach to immunotherapy is unlikely to be successful. Recent examples of refined patient selection include the Insight trial (17), which is recruiting depressed patients based on evidence of inflammation and inflammation-related symptoms along with other criteria. We have also discussed other examples of stratified patient selection such as detailed immunophenotyping, neuroimaging and genetic tests. More research, especially clinical trials, is needed to determine how useful these approaches are and to further refine selection criteria.

In this regard, RCTs of immunotherapies are clear examples of precision medicine in psychiatry, which could inform more personalized care in the future. It is possible that in future we will test patients at first presentation for suitability for different treatment options including suitable and effective immunotherapies, which would avoid years of unsuccessful treatment largely guided by trial and error. Research underway now will determine to what extent this vision lives up to these expectations in the face of rigorous scientific tests.

8.9 Competing Interests

Mr Kappelmann has no financial or other competing interests to declare.

Professor Bullmore is a member of the scientific advisory board of Sosei Heptares; until May 2019 he was employed half-time by GlaxoSmithKline and he currently leads the Wellcome Trust-funded consortium for Neuroimmunology of Mood Disorders and Alzheimer's disease (NIMA) with matching funds from Janssen, GSK, Lundbeck and Alzheimer's Research UK.

Dr Khandaker has no financial interests to declare. Dr Khandaker is Head of the Inflammation and Psychiatry Research Group at the University of Cambridge. The group investigates novel immunological mechanisms and treatment options for major psychiatric disorders including depression. He is chief investigator for the Insight trial (ISRCTN16942542).

8.10 Funding

Mr Kappelmann is funded by the Max Planck Institute of Psychiatry and the International Max Planck Research School for Translational Psychiatry (IMPRS-TP) in Munich, Germany. Dr Khandaker acknowledges funding support from the Wellcome Trust (Intermediate Clinical Fellowship; grant code: 201486/Z/16/Z), BMA Foundation (J Moulton grant 2019), the MQ: Transforming Mental Health (Data Science Award; grant code: MQDS17/40), and the Medical Research Council (MICA: Mental Health Data Pathfinder; grant code: MC_PC_17213 and Therapeutic Target Validation in Mental Health; grant code: MR/S037675/1). Professor Bullmore is an NIHR Senior Investigator and Chief Investigator of the NIMA consortium.

References

1. Bruce TO. 2008. Comorbid Depression in Rheumatoid Arthritis: Pathophysiology and Clinical Implications. *Current Psychiatry Reports*. 10(3):258–64. https://doi.org/10.1007/s11920-008-0042-1

2. Takeshita J, Sungat Grewal S, Langan SM, et al. 2017. Psoriasis and Comorbid Diseases. *Journal of the American Academy of Dermatology*. 76(3):377–90. https://doi.org/10.1016/j.jaad.2016.07.064

3. Graff LA, Walker JR, Bernstein CN. 2009. Depression and Anxiety in Inflammatory Bowel Disease: A Review of Comorbidity and Management. *Inflammatory Bowel Diseases*. 15(7):1105–18. https://doi.org/10.1002/ibd.20873

4. Otte C, Gold SM, Penninx BWJH, et al. 2016. Major Depressive Disorder. *Nat Rev Dis Primers*. 2(1):16065. https://doi.org/10.1038/nrdp.2016.65

5. Dantzer R, O'Connor JC, Freund GG, Johnson RW, Kelley KW. 2008. From Inflammation to Sickness and Depression: When the Immune System Subjugates the Brain. *Nature Reviews Neuroscience*. 9(1):46–56. https://doi.org/10.1038/nrn2297

6. Dowlati, Y, Herrmann, N, Swardfager, W, et al. 2010. A Meta-Analysis of Cytokines in Major Depression. *Biological Psychiatry*. 67(5):446–57. https://doi.org/10.1016/j.biopsych.2009.09.033

7. Howren MB, Lamkin DM, Suls J. 2009. Associations of Depression with C-Reactive Protein, IL-1, and IL-6: A Meta-Analysis. *Psychosomatic Medicine*. 71(2):171–86. https://doi.org/10.1097/PSY.0b013e3181907c1b

8. Goldsmith DR, Rapaport MH, Miller BJ. 2016. A Meta-Analysis of Blood Cytokine Network Alterations in Psychiatric Patients: Comparisons between Schizophrenia, Bipolar Disorder and Depression. *Molecular Psychiatry*. 21:1696–709. https://doi.org/10.1038/mp.2016.3

9. Haapakoski R, Mathieu J, Ebmeier KP, Alenius H, Kivimäki M. 2015. Cumulative Meta-Analysis of Interleukins 6 and 1β, Tumour Necrosis Factor α and C-Reactive Protein in Patients with Major Depressive Disorder. *Brain, Behavior, and Immunity*. 49:206–15. https://doi.org/10.1016/j.bbi.2015.06.001

10. Köhler CA, Freitas TH, Maes M, et al. 2017. Peripheral Cytokine and Chemokine Alterations in Depression: A Meta-Analysis of 82 Studies. *Acta Psychiatrica Scandinavica*. 135(5):373–87. https://doi.org/10.1111/acps.12698

11. Osimo EF, Baxter LJ, Lewis G, Jones PB, Khandaker GM. 2019. Prevalence of Low-Grade Inflammation in Depression: A Systematic Review and Meta-Analysis of CRP Levels. *Psychological Medicine*. 49(12):1958–70. https://doi.org/10.1017/S0033291719001454

12. Khandaker GM, Pearson RM, Zammit S, Lewis G, Jones PB. 2014. Association of Serum Interleukin 6 and C-Reactive Protein in Childhood with Depression and Psychosis in Young Adult Life: A Population-Based Longitudinal Study. *JAMA Psychiatry*. 71(10):1121–8. https://doi.org/10.1001/jamapsychiatry.2014.1332

13. Gimeno, D, Kivimaki, M, Brunner, EJ, et al. 2009. Associations of C-Reactive Protein and Interleukin-6 with Cognitive Symptoms of Depression: 12-Year Follow-up of the Whitehall II Study. *Psychological Medicine*. 39(3):413–23. https://doi.org/10.1017/S0033291708003723

14. Zalli A, Jovanova O, Hoogendijk WJG, Tiemeier H, Carvalho LA. 2016. Low-Grade Inflammation Predicts Persistence of Depressive Symptoms. *Psychopharmacology*. 233:1669–78. https://doi.org/10.1007/s00213-015-3919-9

15. Khandaker GM, Stochl J, Zammit S, et al. 2018a. Childhood Inflammatory Markers and Intelligence as Predictors of Subsequent Persistent Depressive Symptoms: A Longitudinal Cohort Study. *Psychological Medicine*. 48(9):1514–22. https://doi.org/10.1017/S0033291717003038

16. Raison CL, Demetrashvili M, Capuron L, Miller AH. 2005. Neuropsychiatric Adverse Effects of Interferon-α. *CNS Drugs*. 19(2):105–23. https://doi.org/10.2165/00023210-200519020-00002

17. Khandaker GM, Oltean BP, Kaser M, et al. 2018b. Protocol for the Insight Study: A Randomised Controlled Trial of Single-Dose Tocilizumab in Patients with Depression and Low-Grade Inflammation. *BMJ Open.* 8:e025333. https://doi.org/10.1136/bmjopen-2018-025333

18. Khandaker GM, Zammit S, Burgess S, Lewis G, Jones PB. 2018c. Association between a Functional Interleukin 6 Receptor Genetic Variant and Risk of Depression and Psychosis in a Population-Based Birth Cohort. *Brain, Behavior, and Immunity.* 69 (March):264–72. https://doi.org/10.1016/j.bbi.2017.11.020

19. Khandaker GM, Zuber V, Rees, JMB, et al. 2019. Shared Mechanisms between Coronary Heart Disease and Depression: Findings from a Large UK General Population-Based Cohort. *Molecular Psychiatry.* March:533828. https://doi.org/10.1038/s41380-019-0395-3

20. Hingorani A, Humphries S. 2005. Nature's Randomised Trials. *The Lancet.* 366 (9501):1906–8. doi.org/10.1016/S0140-6736(05)67767-7

21. Davey Smith G, Ebrahim S. 2003. 'Mendelian Randomization': Can Genetic Epidemiology Contribute to Understanding Environmental Determinants of Disease?* *International Journal of Epidemiology.* 32(1): 1–22. https://doi.org/10.1093/ije/dyg070

22. Davey Smith G, Ebrahim S. 2005. What Can Mendelian Randomisation Tell Us about Modifiable Behavioural and Environmental Exposures? *BMJ.* 330 (7499):1076–79. https://doi.org/10.1136/bmj.330.7499.1076

23. Lawlor DA, Harbord RM, Sterne JAC, et al. 2008. Mendelian Randomization: Using Genes as Instruments for Making Causal Inferences in Epidemiology. *Statistics in Medicine.* 27(8):1133–63. https://doi.org/10.1002/sim.3034

24. Ma Li, Demin KA, Kolesnikova,TO, et al. 2017. Animal Inflammation-Based Models of Depression and Their Application to Drug Discovery. *Expert Opinion on Drug Discovery.* 12(10):995–1009. https://doi.org/10.1080/17460441.2017.1362385

25. Köhler CA, Freitas TH, Stubbs B, et al. 2017. Peripheral Alterations in Cytokine and Chemokine Levels After Antidepressant Drug Treatment for Major Depressive Disorder: Systematic Review and Meta-Analysis. *Molecular Neurobiology.* 16(June):4195–206. https://doi.org/10.1007/s12035-017-0632-1

26. Lopresti AL. 2017. Cognitive Behaviour Therapy and Inflammation: A Systematic Review of Its Relationship and the Potential Implications for the Treatment of Depression. *Australian & New Zealand Journal of Psychiatry.* 51(6):565–82. https://doi.org/10.1177/0004867417701996

27. Strawbridge R, Arnone D, Danese A, et al. 2015. Inflammation and Clinical Response to Treatment in Depression: A Meta-Analysis. *European Neuropsychopharmacology.* 25:1532–43. https://doi.org/10.1016/j.euroneuro.2015.06.007

28. Haroon E, Daguanno AW, Woolwine BJ, et al. 2018. Antidepressant Treatment Resistance Is Associated with Increased Inflammatory Markers in Patients with Major Depressive Disorder. *Psychoneuroendocrinology.* 95:43–9. https://doi.org/10.1016/j.psyneuen.2018.05.026

29. Uher R, Tansey KE, Dew T, et al. 2014. An Inflammatory Biomarker as a Differential Predictor of Outcome of Depression Treatment With Escitalopram and Nortriptyline. *American Journal of Psychiatry.* 171(12):1278–86. https://doi.org/10.1176/appi.ajp.2014.14010094

30. Jha MK, Minhajuddin A, Gadad BS, et al. 2017. Can C-Reactive Protein Inform Antidepressant Medication Selection in Depressed Outpatients? Findings from the CO-MED Trial. *Psychoneuroendocrinology.* 78(April):105–13. https://doi.org/10.1016/j.psyneuen.2017.01.023

31. Vane JR, Botting RM. 1998. Mechanism of Action of Nonsteroidal Anti-Inflammatory Drugs. *The American Journal of Medicine.* 104(3):2S–8S. https://doi.org/10.1016/S0002-9343(97)00203-9

32. Müller N, Schwarz MJ, Dehning S, et al. 2006. The Cyclooxygenase-2 Inhibitor Celecoxib Has Therapeutic Effects in Major Depression: Results of a Double-Blind, Randomized, Placebo Controlled, Add-on Pilot Study to Reboxetine. *Molecular Psychiatry*. 11(7):680–4. https://doi.org/10.1038/sj.mp.4001805

33. Akhondzadeh S, Jafari S, Raisi F, et al. 2009. Clinical Trial of Adjunctive Celecoxib Treatment in Patients with Major Depression: A Double Blind and Placebo Controlled Trial. *Depression and Anxiety*. 26(7):607–11. https://doi.org/10.1002/da.20589

34. Abbasi S-H, Hosseini F, Modabbernia A, Ashrafi M, Akhondzadeh S. 2012. Effect of Celecoxib Add-On Treatment on Symptoms and Serum IL-6 Concentrations in Patients with Major Depressive Disorder: Randomized Double-Blind Placebo-Controlled Study. *Journal of Affective Disorders*. 141(2–3):308–14. https://doi.org/10.1016/j.jad.2012.03.033

35. Majd M, Hashemian F, Hosseini SM, Shariatpanahi MV Sharifi A. 2015. A Randomized, Double-Blind, Placebo-Controlled Trial of Celecoxib Augmentation of Sertraline in Treatment of Drug-Naive Depressed Women: A Pilot Study. *Iranian Journal of Pharmaceutical Research : IJPR*. 14(3):891–9. https://c7ljem051wudj6bdbogn0sefchly.amc-literatuur.amc.nl/pmc/articles/PMC4518118/pdf/ijpr-14-891.pdf

36. Iyengar RL, Gandhi S, Aneja A, et al. 2013. NSAIDs Are Associated with Lower Depression Scores in Patients with Osteoarthritis. *The American Journal of Medicine*. 126(11):1017.e11–1017.e18. https://doi.org/10.1016/j.amjmed.2013.02.037

37. Jafari S, Ashrafizadeh S-G, Zeinoddini A, et al. 2015. Celecoxib for the Treatment of Mild-to-Moderate Depression Due to Acute Brucellosis: A Double-Blind, Placebo-Controlled, Randomized Trial. *Journal of Clinical Pharmacy and Therapeutics*. 40(4):441–6. https://doi.org/10.1111/jcpt.12287

38. Mahagna H, Amital D, Amital H. 2016. A Randomised, Double-blinded Study

Comparing Giving Etoricoxib vs. Placebo to Female Patients with Fibromyalgia. *International Journal of Clinical Practice*. 70 (2):163–70. https://doi.org/10.1111/ijcp.12760

39. Alamdarsaravi M, Ghajar A, NoorbalaA-A, et al. 2017. Efficacy and Safety of Celecoxib Monotherapy for Mild to Moderate Depression in Patients with Colorectal Cancer: A Randomized Double-Blind, Placebo Controlled Trial. *Psychiatry Research*. 255 (June 2016):59–65. https://doi.org/10.1016/j.psychres.2017.05.029

40. Köhler O, Benros ME, Nordentoft M, et al. 2014. Effect of Anti-Inflammatory Treatment on Depression, Depressive Symptoms, and Adverse Effects: A Systematic Review and Meta-Analysis of Randomized Clinical Trials. *JAMA Psychiatry*. 71(12):1381–91. https://doi.org/10.1001/jamapsychiatry.2014.1611

41. Köhler-Forsberg O, Lydholm CN, Hjorthøj C, et al. 2019. Efficacy of Anti-Inflammatory Treatment on Major Depressive Disorder or Depressive Symptoms: Meta-Analysis of Clinical Trials. *Acta Psychiatrica Scandinavica*. March:0–2. https://doi.org/10.1111/acps.13016

42. Taylor PC, Feldmann M. 2009. Anti-TNF Biologic Agents: Still the Therapy of Choice for Rheumatoid Arthritis. *Nature Reviews Rheumatology*. 5(10):578–82. https://doi.org/10.1038/nrrheum.2009.181

43. Kappelmann N, Lewis G, Dantzer R, Jones PB, Khandaker GM. 2018. Antidepressant Activity of Anti-Cytokine Treatment: A Systematic Review and Meta-Analysis of Clinical Trials of Chronic Inflammatory Conditions. *Molecular Psychiatry*. 23(2):335–43. https://doi.org/10.1038/mp.2016.167

44. Tyring S, Gottlieb A, Papp K, et al. 2006. Etanercept and Clinical Outcomes, Fatigue, and Depression in Psoriasis: Double-Blind Placebo-Controlled Randomised Phase III Trial. *The Lancet*. 367(9504):29–35. https://doi.org/10.1016/S0140-6736(05)67763-X

45. Tyring S, Bagel J, Lynde C, et al. 2013. Patient-Reported Outcomes in

Moderate-to-Severe Plaque Psoriasis with Scalp Involvement: Results from a Randomized, Double-Blind, Placebo-Controlled Study of Etanercept. *Journal of the European Academy of Dermatology and Venereology.* 27 (1):125–28. https://doi.org/10.1111/j.1468-3083.2011.04394.x

46. Loftus EV, Feagan BG, Colombel JF, et al. 2008. Effects of Adalimumab Maintenance Therapy on Health-Related Quality of Life of Patients with Crohn's Disease: Patient-Reported Outcomes of the CHARM Trial. *The American Journal of Gastroenterology.* 103(12):3132–41. https://doi.org/10.1111/j.1572-0241.2008.02175.x

47. Menter A, Augustin M, Signorovitch J, et al. 2010. The Effect of Adalimumab on Reducing Depression Symptoms in Patients with Moderate to Severe Psoriasis: A Randomized Clinical Trial. *Journal of the American Academy of Dermatology.* 62 (5):812–18. https://doi.org/10.1016/j.jaad.2009.07.022

48. Langley RG, Feldman SR, Han C, et al. 2010. Ustekinumab Significantly Improves Symptoms of Anxiety, Depression, and Skin-Related Quality of Life in Patients with Moderate-to-Severe Psoriasis: Results from a Randomized, Double-Blind, Placebo-Controlled Phase III Trial. *Journal of the American Academy of Dermatology.* 63(3):457–65. https://doi.org/10.1016/j.jaad.2009.09.014

49. Simpson EL, Gadkari A, Worm M, et al. 2016. Dupilumab Therapy Provides Clinically Meaningful Improvement in Patient-Reported Outcomes (PROs): A Phase IIb, Randomized, Placebo-Controlled, Clinical Trial in Adult Patients with Moderate to Severe Atopic Dermatitis (AD). *Journal of the American Academy of Dermatology.* 75(3):506–15. https://doi.org/10.1016/j.jaad.2016.04.054

50. Cork MJ, Eckert L, Simpson EL, et al. 2019. Dupilumab Improves Patient-Reported Symptoms of Atopic Dermatitis, Symptoms of Anxiety and Depression, and Health-Related Quality of Life in Moderate-to-Severe Atopic Dermatitis:

Analysis of Pooled Data from the Randomized Trials SOLO 1 and SOLO 2. *Journal of Dermatological Treatment.* 31 (6):606–14. https://doi.org/10.1080/09546634.2019.1612836

51. Griffiths CEM, Fava M, Miller AH, et al. 2017. Impact of Ixekizumab Treatment on Depressive Symptoms and Systemic Inflammation in Patients with Moderate-to-Severe Psoriasis: An Integrated Analysis of Three Phase 3 Clinical Studies. *Psychotherapy and Psychosomatics.* 86(5):260–67. https://doi.org/10.1159/000479163

52. Sun Y, Wang D, Salvadore G, et al. 2017. The Effects of Interleukin-6 Neutralizing Antibodies on Symptoms of Depressed Mood and Anhedonia in Patients with Rheumatoid Arthritis and Multicentric Castleman's Disease. *Brain, Behavior, and Immunity* 66:156–64. https://doi.org/10.1016/j.bbi.2017.06.014

53. Wittenberg GM, Stylianou A, Zhang Y, et al. 2020. Effects of Immunomodulatory Drugs on Depressive Symptoms: A Mega-Analysis of Randomized, Placebo-Controlled Clinical Trials in Inflammatory Disorders. *Molecular Psychiatry.* 25(6):1275–85. https://doi.org/10.1038/s41380-019-0471-8

54. Raison CL, Rutherford RE, Woolwine BJ, et al. 2013. A Randomized Controlled Trial of the Tumor Necrosis Factor Antagonist Infliximab for Treatment-Resistant Depression: The Role of Baseline Inflammatory Biomarkers. *JAMA Psychiatry.* 70(1):31–41. https://doi.org/10.1001/2013.jamapsychiatry.4

55. McIntyre RS, Subramaniapillai M, Lee Y, et al. 2019. Efficacy of Adjunctive Infliximab vs Placebo in the Treatment of Adults With Bipolar I/II Depression. *JAMA Psychiatry.* 76(8):783–90. https://doi.org/10.1001/jamapsychiatry.2019.0779

56. Chamberlain SR, Cavanagh J, de Boer P, et al. 2019. Treatment-Resistant Depression and Peripheral C-Reactive Protein. *British Journal of Psychiatry.* 214 (1):11–19. https://doi.org/10.1192/bjp.2018.66

57. Baumeister D, Akhtar R, Ciufolini S, Pariante CM, Mondelli.V 2016. Childhood Trauma and Adulthood Inflammation: A Meta-Analysis of Peripheral C-Reactive Protein, Interleukin-6 and Tumour Necrosis Factor-α. *Molecular Psychiatry.* 21 (5):642–49. https://doi.org/10.1038/mp.2015.67

58. Fracassi A, Marangoni M, Rosso P, et al. 2018. Statins and the Brain: More than Lipid Lowering Agents? *Current Neuropharmacology.* 17(1):59–83. https://doi.org/10.2174/1570159X15666170703101816

59. Wu H, Lv W, Pan Q, et al. 2019. Simvastatin Therapy in Adolescent Mice Attenuates HFD-Induced Depression-like Behavior by Reducing Hippocampal Neuroinflammation. *Journal of Affective Disorders.* 243(January):83–95. https://doi.org/10.1016/j.jad.2018.09.022

60. Parsaik AK, Singh BM, Hassan M, et al. 2014. "Statins Use and Risk of Depression: A Systematic Review and Meta-Analysis." *Journal of Affective Disorders* 160 (May):62–7. https://doi.org/10.1016/j.jad.2013.11.026

61. Köhler-Forsberg O, Gasse C, Petersen L, et al. 2019. Statin Treatment and the Risk of Depression. *Journal of Affective Disorders.* 246(March):706–15. https://doi.org/10.1016/j.jad.2018.12.110

62. Santanello NC, Barber BL, Applegate WB, et al. 1997. Effect of Pharmacologic Lipid Lowering on Health-Related Quality of Life in Older Persons: Results from the Cholesterol Reduction in Seniors Program (CRISP) Pilot Study. *Journal of the American Geriatrics Society.* 45(1):8–14. https://doi.org/10.1111/j.1532–5415.1997.tb00971.x

63. Stewart RA. 2000. Long-Term Assessment of Psychological Well-Being in a Randomized Placebo-Controlled Trial of Cholesterol Reduction With Pravastatin. *Archives of Internal Medicine.* 160 (20):3144. https://doi.org/10.1001/archinte.160.20.3144

64. Carlsson CM, Papcke-Benson K, Carnes M, et al. 2002. Health-Related Quality of Life and Long-Term Therapy with Pravastatin and Tocopherol (Vitamin E) in Older Adults. *Drugs & Aging.* 19 (10):793–805. https://doi.org/10.2165/00002512–200219100-00008

65. Chan D, Binks S, Nicholas JM, et al. 2017. Effect of High-Dose Simvastatin on Cognitive, Neuropsychiatric, and Health-Related Quality-of-Life Measures in Secondary Progressive Multiple Sclerosis: Secondary Analyses from the MS-STAT Randomised, Placebo-Controlled Trial. *The Lancet Neurology.* 16(8):591–600. https://doi.org/10.1016/S1474-4422(17)30113–8

66. Ghanizadeh A, Hedayati A. 2013. Augmentation of Fluoxetine with Lovastatin for Treating Major Depressive Disorder, a Randomized Double-Blind Placebo Controlled-Clinical Trial. *Depression and Anxiety.* 30(11):1084–88. https://doi.org/10.1002/da.22195

67. Haghighi M, Khodakarami S, Jahangard L, et al. 2014. In a Randomized, Double-Blind Clinical Trial, Adjuvant Atorvastatin Improved Symptoms of Depression and Blood Lipid Values in Patients Suffering from Severe Major Depressive Disorder. *Journal of Psychiatric Research.* 58 (2014):109–14. https://doi.org/10.1016/j.jpsychires.2014.07.018

68. Gougol A, Zareh-Mohammadi N, Raheb S, et al. 2015. Simvastatin as an Adjuvant Therapy to Fluoxetine in Patients with Moderate to Severe Major Depression: A Double-Blind Placebo-Controlled Trial. Edited by David J Nutt and Pierre Blier. *Journal of Psychopharmacology.* 29 (5):575–81. https://doi.org/10.1177/0269881115578160

69. Soczynska JK, Mansur RB, Brietzke E, et al. 2012. Novel Therapeutic Targets in Depression: Minocycline as a Candidate Treatment. *Behavioural Brain Research.* 235(2).302–17. https://doi.org/10.1016/j.bbr.2012.07.026

70. Husain MI, Chaudhry IB, Husain N, et al. 2017. Minocycline as an Adjunct for Treatment-Resistant Depressive Symptoms: A Pilot Randomised Placebo-Controlled Trial. *Journal of Psychopharmacology.* 31(9):1166–75.

https://doi.org/10.1177
/0269881117724352

71. Dean OM, Kanchanatawan B, Ashton M, et al. 2017. Adjunctive Minocycline Treatment for Major Depressive Disorder: A Proof of Concept Trial. *Australian & New Zealand Journal of Psychiatry*. 51 (8):829–40. https://doi.org/10.1177 /0004867417709357

72. Emadi-Kouchak H, Mohammadinejad P, Asadollahi-Amin A, et al. 2016. Therapeutic Effects of Minocycline on Mild-to-Moderate Depression in HIV Patients. *International Clinical Psychopharmacology*. 31(1):20–26. https://doi.org/10.1097/YIC .0000000000000098

73. Rosenblat JD, McIntyre RS. 2018. Efficacy and Tolerability of Minocycline for Depression: A Systematic Review and Meta-Analysis of Clinical Trials. *Journal of Affective Disorders*. 227 (September 2017):219–25. https://doi.org/ 10.1016/j.jad.2017.10.042

74. Ronchetti S, Migliorati G, Bruscoli S, Riccardi C. 2018. Defining the Role of Glucocorticoids in Inflammation. *Clinical Science*. 132(14):1529–43. https://doi.org/1 0.1042/CS20171505

75. Zunszain PA, Anacker C, Cattaneo A, Carvalho LA, Pariante CM. 2011. Glucocorticoids, Cytokines and Brain Abnormalities in Depression. *Progress in Neuro-Psychopharmacology and Biological Psychiatry*. 35(3):722–9. https://doi.org/10 .1016/j.pnpbp.2010.04.011

76. DeBattista C, Posener JA, Kalehzan BM, Schatzberg AF. 2000. Acute Antidepressant Effects of Intravenous Hydrocortisone and CRH in Depressed Patients: A Double-Blind, Placebo-Controlled Study. *American Journal of Psychiatry*. 157 (8):1334–37. https://doi.org/10.1176/appi .ajp.157.8.1334

77. Arana GW, Roberts JM, Santos AB, et al. 1995. Dexamethasone for the Treatment of Depression: A Randomized, Placebo-Controlled, Double-Blind Trial. *American Journal of Psychiatry*. 152 (2):265–67. https://doi.org/10.1176/ajp .152.2.265

78. Brown ES, Khan DA, Nejtek VA .1999. The Psychiatric Side Effects of Corticosteroids. *Annals of Allergy, Asthma & Immunology*. 83(6):495–504. https://doi.org/10.1016/S1 081-1206(10)62858-X

79. Grosso G, Galvano F, Marventano S, et al. 2014. Omega-3 Fatty Acids and Depression: Scientific Evidence and Biological Mechanisms. *Oxidative Medicine and Cellular Longevity*. 313570. https://doi.org/10.1155/2014/313570

80. Sublette ME, Ellis SP, Geant AL, Mann JJ. 2011. Meta-Analysis of the Effects of Eicosapentaenoic Acid (EPA) in Clinical Trials in Depression. *The Journal of Clinical Psychiatry*. 72(12):1577–84. https://doi.org /10.4088/JCP.10m06634

81. Bower JE, Irwin MR. Mind–Body Therapies and Control of Inflammatory Biology: A Descriptive Review. *Brain, Behavior, and Immunity*. 2016 Jan;51:1–11. https://doi.org/http://dx.doi.org/10.1016/j .bbi.2015.06.012

82. Kuyken W, Warren FC, Taylor RS, et al. 2016. Efficacy of Mindfulness-Based Cognitive Therapy in Prevention of Depressive Relapse: An Individual Patient Data Meta-Analysis From Randomized Trials. *JAMA Psychiatry*. 73(6):565–74. https://doi.org/10.1001/jamapsychiatry .2016.0076

83. Galante J, Dufour G, Vainre M, et al. 2018. A Mindfulness-Based Intervention to Increase Resilience to Stress in University Students (the Mindful Student Study): A Pragmatic Randomised Controlled Trial. *The Lancet Public Health*. 3(2):e72–81. https://doi.org/10.1016/S2468- 2667(17)30231-1

84. Turner L, Galante J, Vainre M, et al. 2020. Immune Dysregulation among Students Exposed to Exam Stress and Its Mitigation by Mindfulness Training: Findings from an Exploratory Randomised Trial. *Scientific Reports*. 10(1):5812. https://doi.org/10 .1038/s41598-020-62274-7

85. Sostres C, Gargallo CJ, Arroyo MT, Lanas A. 2010. Adverse Effects of Non-Steroidal Anti-Inflammatory Drugs (NSAIDs, Aspirin and Coxibs) on Upper Gastrointestinal Tract. *Best Practice &*

Research Clinical Gastroenterology. 24 (2):121–32. https://doi.org/10.1016/j .bpg.2009.11.005

86. Trelle S, Reichenbach S, Wandel S, et al. 2011. Cardiovascular Safety of Non-Steroidal Anti-Inflammatory Drugs: Network Meta-Analysis. *BMJ.* 342 (Jan11 1):c7086. https://doi.org/10.1136/b mj.c7086

87. Ray WA, Stein CM, Hall K, Daugherty JR, Griffin MR. 2002. Non-Steroidal Anti-Inflammatory Drugs and Risk of Serious Coronary Heart Disease: An Observational Cohort Study. *The Lancet.* 359(9301):118–23. https://doi.org/10.1016 /S0140-6736(02)07370-1

88. Van der Kooy K, van Hout H, Marwijk H, et al. 2007. Depression and the Risk for Cardiovascular Diseases: Systematic Review and Meta Analysis. *International Journal of Geriatric Psychiatry.* 22 (7):613–26. https://doi.org/10.1002/gps .1723

89. Hansel TT, Kropshofer H, Singer T, Mitchell JA, George AJT. 2010. The Safety and Side Effects of Monoclonal Antibodies. *Nature Reviews Drug Discovery.* 9 (4):325–38. https://doi.org/10.1038 /nrd3003

90. Sokolove J, Strand V, Greenberg JD, et al. 2010. Risk of Elevated Liver Enzymes Associated with TNF Inhibitor Utilisation in Patients with Rheumatoid Arthritis. *Annals of the Rheumatic Diseases.* 69 (9):1612–17. https://doi.org/10.1136/ard .2009.112136

91. Bongartz T, Sutton AJ, Sweeting MJ, et al. 2006. Anti-TNF Antibody Therapy in Rheumatoid Arthritis and the Risk of Serious Infections and Malignancies. *JAMA.* 295(19):2275. https://doi.org/10 .1001/jama.295.19.2275

92. Bonovas S, Minozzi S, Lytras T, et al. 2016. Risk of Malignancies Using Anti-TNF Agents in Rheumatoid Arthritis, Psoriatic Arthritis, and Ankylosing Spondylitis: A Systematic Review and Meta-Analysis. *Expert Opinion on Drug Safety.* 15 (sup1):35–54. https://doi.org/10.1080/147 40338.2016.1238458

93. Keane J. 2005. TNF-Blocking Agents and Tuberculosis: New Drugs Illuminate an Old Topic. *Rheumatology.* 44(6):714–20. https://doi.org/10.1093/rheumatology/ keh567

94. Zheng W, Zhu X-M, Zhang Q-E, et al. 2019. Adjunctive Minocycline for Major Mental Disorders: A Systematic Review. *Journal of Psychopharmacology.* 33 (10):1215–26. https://doi.org/10.1177/ 0269881119858286

95. Brogden RN, Speight TM, Avery GS. 1975. Minocycline. *Drugs.* 9(4):251–91. https://doi.org/10.2165/00003495- 197509040-00005

96. Garner SE, Eady A, Bennett C, et al. 2012. Minocycline for Acne Vulgaris: Efficacy and Safety. *Cochrane Database of Systematic Reviews.* 2012(8):CD002086. https://doi.org/10.1002/14651858 .CD002086.pub2

97. Knothe H, Dette GA. 1986. Antibiotics in Pregnancy: Toxicity and Teratogenicity. *Obstetrical & Gynecological Survey.* 41 (1):31–2.

98. Schäcke H, Döcke W-D, Asadullah K. 2002. "Mechanisms Involved in the Side Effects of Glucocorticoids." *Pharmacology & Therapeutics* 96(1):23–43. https://doi .org/10.1016/S0163-7258(02)00297-8

99. Pariante CM, Miller AH. 2001. Glucocorticoid Receptors in Major Depression: Relevance to Pathophysiology and Treatment. *Biological Psychiatry.* 49 (5):391–404. https://doi.org/10.1016/S0006- 3223(00)01088-X

100. Rapaport MH, Nierenberg AA, Schettler PJ, et al. 2016. Inflammation as a Predictive Biomarker for Response to Omega-3 Fatty Acids in Major Depressive Disorder: A Proof-of-Concept Study. *Molecular Psychiatry.* 21(1):71–9. https:// doi.org/10.1038/mp.2015.22

101. Lynall M-E, Turner L, Bhatti J, et al. 2020. Peripheral Blood Cell-Stratified Subgroups of Inflamed Depression. *Biological Psychiatry.* 88(2):185–96. https://doi.org/10.1016/j .biopsych.2019.11.017

102. Fried EI, Nesse RM. 2015. Depression Sum-Scores Don't Add up: Why Analyzing Specific Depression Symptoms Is Essential. *BMC Medicine*. 13(1):72. https://doi.org/10.1186/s12916-015-0325-4

103. Jokela M, Virtanen M, Batty G, Kivimäki M. 2016. Inflammation and Specific Symptoms of Depression. *JAMA Psychiatry*. 73(1):87–8. https://doi.org/10.1001/jamapsychiatry.2015.1977

104. Lamers F, Milaneschi Y, de Jonge P, Giltay EJ, Penninx BWJH. 2018. Metabolic and Inflammatory Markers: Associations with Individual Depressive Symptoms. *Psychological Medicine*. 48(7):1102–10. https://doi.org/10.1017/S0033291717002483

105. Köhler-Forsberg O, Buttenschøn HN, Tansey KE, et al. 2017. Association between C-Reactive Protein (CRP) with Depression Symptom Severity and Specific Depressive Symptoms in Major Depression. *Brain, Behavior, and Immunity*. 62(May):344–50. https://doi.org/10.1016/j.bbi.2017.02.020

106. Chu AL, Stochl J, Lewis G, et al. 2019. Longitudinal Association Between Inflammatory Markers and Specific Symptoms of Depression in a Prospective Birth Cohort. *Brain, Behavior, and Immunity*. 76(November):74–81. https://doi.org/10.1016/j.bbi.2018.11.007

107. Fried EI, von Stockert S, Haslbeck JMB, et al. 2019. Using Network Analysis to Examine Links between Individual Depressive Symptoms, Inflammatory Markers, and Covariates. *Psychological Medicine*. October:1–9. https://doi.org/10.1017/S0033291719002770

108. Whale R, Fialho R, Field AP, et al. 2019. Factor Analyses Differentiate Clinical Phenotypes of Idiopathic and Interferon-Alpha-Induced Depression. *Brain, Behavior, and Immunity*. 80(August):519–24. https://doi.org/10.1016/j.bbi.2019.04.035

109. Coelho R, Viola TW, Walss-Bass C, Brietzke E, Grassi-Oliveira R. 2014. Childhood Maltreatment and Inflammatory Markers: A Systematic Review. *Acta Psychiatrica Scandinavica*. 129(3):180–92. https://doi.org/10.1111/acps.12217

110. Mondelli V, Vernon AC, Turkheimer F, Dazzan P, Pariante CM. 2017. Brain Microglia in Psychiatric Disorders. *The Lancet Psychiatry*. 4(7):563–72. https://doi.org/10.1016/S2215-0366(17)30101-3

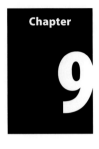

The Effect of Systemic Inflammation on Cognitive Function and Neurodegenerative Disease

Colm Cunningham and Donal T. Skelly

9.1 Introduction

Chronic neurodegenerative diseases represent a major challenge for health systems worldwide. The most common diseases are Alzheimer's disease (AD), Parkinson's disease (PD), Lewy body dementia, frontotemporal dementia, amyotrophic lateral sclerosis (ALS), Huntington's disease (HD) and prion diseases. Multiple sclerosis (MS) is classically considered to be an autoimmune disease but increasingly, it is viewed as a degenerative disease (1).

Despite meaningful advances in understanding of protein aggregation, metabolic dysfunction, neuroinflammation and neuronal and synaptic loss (2) no treatment has been shown to ameliorate the major neurodegenerative processes. In the absence of disease-modifying treatments, an ability to mitigate the effects of factors that exacerbate disease progression would be of considerable value at an individual and societal level. It is now apparent that systemic inflammation, caused by infection, tissue trauma or inflammatory disease, has negative consequences for the brain, particularly when there is an underlying vulnerability, such as neurodegenerative disease.

This chapter will explore the clinical evidence that circulating systemic inflammation outside the central nervous system (CNS) can produce acute brain dysfunction and exacerbate and accelerate neurodegenerative disease. It will then examine experimental work that can help understand the underlying pathophysiological mechanisms. Given current evidence, we will focus predominantly on the role of innate immune system cells, microglia and circulating monocytes.

9.2 Clinical Evidence for the Effects of Systemic Inflammation on Neurodegenerative Disease

9.2.1 Cognitive Decline and Peripheral Inflammation

Systemic inflammation is associated with cognitive impairment and progression of neurodegenerative disease. A meta-analysis of 40 studies and 1,500 participants reported significantly elevated circulating pro-inflammatory mediators in the blood of AD participants in comparison with control participants (3). A prospective study of 300 community-based patients with AD found that both acute and chronic systemic inflammation was associated with an accelerated rate of cognitive decline (4). Acute systemic inflammatory events, associated with the pro-inflammatory cytokine TNF-α, led to a two-fold increase in the rate of cognitive decline, while baseline elevation of TNF-α was associated with a four-fold increase in the rate of cognitive decline. Patients with prodromal AD and dementia with Lewy bodies (DLB), but not those with more advanced disease, have significantly elevated inflammatory makers, suggesting that peripheral inflammation may have a role early in these neurodegenerative processes (5).

While there is no consistent evidence for one specific infective pathogen in the aetiology of neurodegenerative disease, peripheral infections seem to have a role in initiating or accelerating cognitive dysfunction and systemic infection demonstrably produces acute injury to the brain (6). In the very elderly, the occurrence of acute infection increases the risk of dementia diagnosis (7), while previous infection burden is associated with chronic cognitive impairment (8). Severe sepsis due to infection can cause chronic cognitive impairment and functional disability, especially in the elderly (9) and it is clear from post-mortem studies that sepsis activates microglia and the perivascular macrophages of the brain (10). Evidence also suggests that amyloid beta (Aβ) is an anti-microbial peptide that is induced by bacterial (11) and viral (12) infection, implying that a broad range of infections might drive amyloid pathology directly, but non-infectious sources of peripheral inflammation such as surgery are also associated with post-operative cognitive dysfunction (13). This ill-defined impairment, especially common in the elderly and those with dementia, appears to be related to inflammatory burden, as opposed to reduced blood flow or anaesthesia (14).

Chronic inflammatory conditions also confer an increased risk of cognitive decline and dementia (120). A meta-analysis found a significantly increased risk of dementia in those with rheumatoid arthritis (15). Chronic periodontitis is associated with an increased risk of AD and PD (16,17). In AD it is associated with circulating pro-inflammatory mediators, and linked with a six-fold increased rate of cognitive decline over six months (18). Metabolic syndrome is also associated with cognitive decline but this relationship occurs only in those with high inflammation (19). Indeed, inflammaging, the chronic low-grade inflammation that accompanies the age-related decline in adaptive immunity has been linked with frailty and vulnerability to acute stressors (20) and may contribute to progression of neurodegenerative disease.

9.2.2 Peripheral Inflammation and Acute CNS Dysfunction

A clear, common and obvious consequence of acute systemic inflammation in aged people, especially those with neurodegenerative disease, is delirium (21–23). Studies have reported significant differences in systemic inflammation between delirious and non-delirious cohorts and specific inflammatory markers have been associated with delirium (24). Systemic infections (24,26) and sterile systemic inflammation, from trauma, such as hip fracture (27), burns or surgery, especially cardiac surgery (28), can induce delirium. Relatively benign inflammatory events appear to precipitate delirium in those with dementia (29). Urinary tract infections are often (30) thought to be drivers of delirium in elderly or demented patients but this is not universally accepted (31).

The greater the burden of neurodegenerative disease a person has the higher their risk of developing delirium. Severity of existing cognitive impairment, as measured by the Mini Mental State Examination (MMSE), correlates with the risk of developing delirium

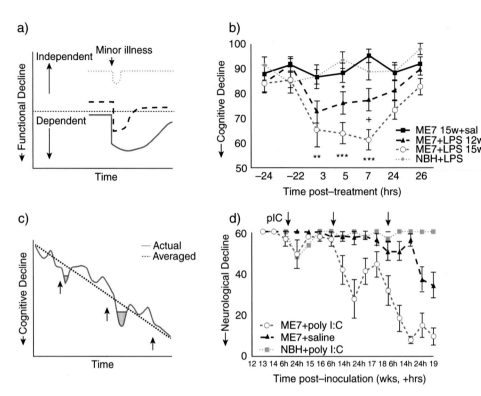

Figure 9.1 Transient and lasting effects of systemic inflammation on the diseased brain. **a)** Conceptual depiction of the differential impact of stressors in the context of prior frailty/functional ability. Adapted (with permission from © Elsevier; Clegg et al., 2013 *The Lancet*, (21)) to show that relatively minor illness can produce progressively more severe deficits on a background of progressively reduced reserve. This adapted scheme is supported by: **b)** Experimental mouse model work showing that underlying neurodegenerative disease progression increases the incidence, severity and duration of acute exacerbations of cognitive dysfunction induced by standardized systemic inflammation (LPS). Working memory performance assessed with T-maze alteration task. Adapted with permission from *Journal of Neuroscience*, © Society for Neuroscience. See (141) for experimental detail. **c)** Schematic diagram illustrating that cognition, in an individual with dementia declines over time but does not typically follow the linear progression represented by the population when averaged. Rather rate changes and fluctuations occur, some of which may meet criteria for delirium (shaded areas). We propose that these fluctuations are triggered by episodic systemic inflammation or other stressors (arrows). Adapted with permission from Perry et al. 2007 *Nature Reviews Immunology* (71), © Nature Research. This proposal is also supported by experimental mouse model work: **d)** Repeated acute systemic inflammatory challenges, with the viral mimetic poly(I:C), induce episodic acute neurological impairment followed by partial recovery on a test of motor coordination, but also accelerates disease progression. See (84) for experimental detail. Adapted with permission from *Brain, Behaviour & Immunity* © Elsevier.

(32, Figure 9.1). The syndrome is associated with loss of independence, early institutionalisation, persistent functional and cognitive decline, and death (33,34). A large prospective cohort study demonstrated that delirium accelerates the trajectory of cognitive decline in AD (35). Delirium also increases the likelihood of subsequently developing dementia: up to eight-fold in the 'oldest-old' (≥85 years of age) (36). A recent study using 900 autopsied brains, with population-based sampling, demonstrated that delirium, in the presence of the features of neurodegenerative pathology, hastens cognitive decline beyond that which would be expected for dementia alone (37) and appears to do so independent of an increase in classical neuropathological features of dementia. This suggests that delirium triggers an interrelated but distinct pathologic pathway to effect cognitive decline.

There are other recognized acute consequences of systemic inflammation in neurodegenerative disease. In AD, neuropsychiatric symptoms, termed behavioural and psychological symptoms of dementia (BPSD), are poorly understood and under-investigated but peripheral infection and inflammation have been implicated as causes (38). Motor deterioration due to systemic inflammation in PD is well recognized, and also often includes delirium, but these phenomena are poorly understood (39). In MS, acute relapses, focal symptoms persisting for more than 24 hours, are a characteristic part of the disease and intra-current infections are implicated in about 25% of cases (40). A prospective study following 73 patients for over 6,400 patient weeks demonstrated that infections can induce prolonged relapses and neurologic deterioration (41). Pseudoflares are a short-lasting stereotyped recapitulation of previously experienced symptoms, classically provoked by fever, infection, hot temperatures or menstruation. Nerve-conduction block due to pyrexia is commonly understood to be the underlying mechanism (42) but there are data that implicate inflammatory mediators in these flares: aspirin prophylaxis reduces luteal phase-associated MS pseudoflares, without altering body temperature (43). The idea that inflammatory mediators can drive acute deterioration of symptoms in human disease is further supported by data on the first infusion of alemtuzumab, an anti-CD52 humanized monoclonal antibody in patients with MS, which resulted in acute but short-lived recapitulation of previous symptoms in 12 of 14 MS patients (44). The symptoms were correlated with elevated systemic cytokines but not pyrexia. Monoclonal antibody-induced cytokine-release syndrome is now well recognized (45) and this CNS manifestation supports our hypothesis that acute systemic inflammation drives acute dysfunction in neurodegenerative disease. Therefore the evidence that systemic inflammation may episodically drive acute impairments and accelerate decline is mounting in humans and, as discussed in Section 9.3.6, this is supported by demonstrations in experimental models (see Figure 9.1).

9.3 Experimental Evidence

9.3.1 Routes to the Brain and Induction of Sickness Behaviour

Understanding of how the peripheral immune system signals to the CNS has been largely garnered from animal studies. Communication can be via fast neural or slower humoral routes (46). Afferent cranial nerves, the vagus and trigeminus, activated by locally synthesized cytokines, can signal from visceral organs to the brainstem, to elicit hypothalamic and limbic activation (47,48). The cells of the CNS vasculature, perivascular macrophages and endothelial cells, can be activated by circulating pathogen-associated molecular patterns (PAMPs) such as lipopolysaccharide (LPS) – a component of the outer membrane of some Gram-negative bacteria – and by pro-inflammatory mediators such as IL-1β, TNF-α and prostaglandins (49–52). Circulating mediators can also directly signal into the parenchyma at circumventricular organs (CVOs), where there is an absence of the usual endothelial tight junctions that are characteristic of the blood-brain-barrier (BBB) (53). Cytokines can, to some extent, be transported across the BBB by saturable receptors (54,55). Evidence suggests that inflammation can damage the BBB, while in ageing and dementia there is evidence of BBB dysfunction (56,57). Recently, extracellular vesicles (EV), containing miRNAs and other modulatory molecules, were shown to be released by the epithelial

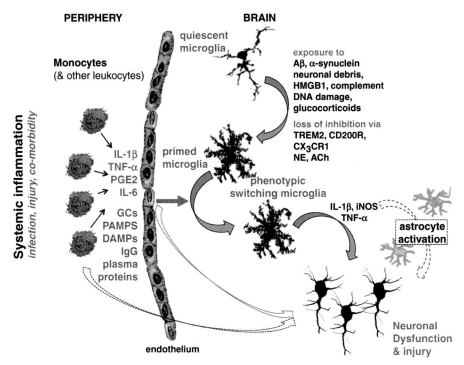

Figure 9.2 Systemic inflammation induces neuronal dysfunction and damage via inflammatory phenotypic switching of microglia and other cell types. Systemic inflammation may be induced by peripheral infection, surgery or injury-induced trauma and these, as well as chronic co-morbidities, induce a range of inflammatory mediators (red) that circulate in the blood or activate leukocytes to secrete such mediators at or close to the brain endothelium. These mediators and both pathogen-associated and damage-associated molecular patterns robustly activate the brain endothelium to transduce an inflammatory signal into the brain. BBB permeability is also affected in neurodegenerative states and further affected by DAMPs/PAMPs and cytokines. Therefore, some plasma proteins and leukocytes may also penetrate the brain parenchyma, while molecules such as prostanoids and glucocorticoids (GCs) can readily cross the BBB. The nature of microglial activation occurring upon systemic inflammatory insult to the brain is highly dependent on the microglial activation status prior to systemic stimulation. During neurodegenerative disease microglia are 'primed' by a number of damage-associated factors to show exaggerated responses to LPS and other stimuli. The priming factors are many, including *exposure to Aβ, α-synuclein, HMGB1, activated complement C3, neurodegenerative debris, glucocorticoids,* or *the loss of normal inhibitory influences* on microglia such as CX3CR1-CX3CL1, CD200-CD200R binding interactions, loss of tonic inhibition by neurotransmitters such as noradrenaline and acetylcholine. Systemic inflammatory stimulation can induce phenotypic switching of primed microglia leading to more robust microglial activation and synthesis of IL-1β and iNOS specifically in areas of prior pathology. These molecules have known neuronal disrupting actions and have been shown to mediate systemic inflammation-induced neuronal death and dysfunction. Microglial secretory products also activate astrocytes, which can also be primed by prior disease, to produce a range of secretory products that may disrupt and/or damage neurons, although astrocytes may also be activated directly by secretory products of the endothelium. Similarly, although monocytes and other leukocytes interact with the brain endothelium there is also evidence for their infiltration of the brain parenchyma to disrupt neuronal function. Neither the list of microglial priming factors, nor the list of circulating mediators capable of endothelial activation, is exhaustive and cell types are not drawn to scale. Abbreviations: SIE, systemic inflammatory event; LPS, lipopolysaccharide; DAMPs/PAMPs, damage/pathogen-associated molecular patterns; IL-1β, interleukin 1β; TNF-α, tumor necrosis factor-α; IgG, immunoglobulins; PGs, prostaglandins; BBB, blood brain barrier; iNOS, inducible nitric oxide synthase. (A black and white version of this figure will appear in some formats. For the colour version, please refer to the plate section.)

cells of the choroid plexus, in response to systemic inflammation, and to enter the brain parenchyma (58). Some of these basic mechanisms are shown in Figure 9.2.

The interplay between the peripheral milieu and CNS immune function is further complicated by the composition of the gut microbiota. Germ-free mice and mice with limited microbiota complexity demonstrate dysfunctional central immune responses (59,60). Microglia bear receptors for short chain fatty acids and tryptophan (aryl hydrocarbons) derived from the microbiota and these receptors are important in modulating central neuroinflammatory responses to systemic inflammation (59,60).

9.3.2 The Degenerating Brain Is Primed to Produce Exaggerated Responses to Systemic Inflammation

It is normal and adaptive that the presence of systemic inflammation is signalled to the healthy brain so that the individual can implement behavioural and metabolic strategies, effectively reorganizing physiological priorities in order to effect a return to homeostasis as soon as possible (see Chapter 7). However, given that much of the mechanism underpinning sickness behaviour consists of signalling by inflammatory mediators, it seems intuitive that the brain, already inflamed by neurodegeneration might show a more robust response to these inflammatory signals arising in the periphery.

Microglia have been known to be a consistent feature of neurodegenerative processes for three decades (61) but have become a more mainstream interest of late due to a series of genome-wide association studies in AD that have implicated genetic loci pertinent to immune signalling in cells of myeloid origin, including microglia. These include Triggering Receptor Expressed on *Myeloid* cells 2 (*TREM2*), *CD33*, *CR1*, *MS4Q*, *ABCA7* and *EPHA1* (62–65). In particular, rare heterozygous variants in the *TREM2* gene confer an increased risk of late-onset AD equivalent to apolipoprotein E ε4 allele (66,67). The field investigating the general role of microglia in neurodegenerative disease is a complex and rapidly expanding one that cannot be covered in detail here but what is important to stress is that neurodegenerative disease leaves these cells susceptible to further stimulation during comorbid systemic infection, disease or trauma.

The first demonstration that the diseased brain was more susceptible to the effects of systemic inflammation was in animals with the ME7 strain of prion disease that were challenged with bacterial endotoxin (LPS; lipopolysaccharide), a widely used, potent activator of an inflammatory response. LPS induced hypothermia and robust activity suppression in normal animals but these changes were significantly exaggerated in animals with neurodegeneration (68) and these animals also showed significantly larger hippocampal and hypothalamic elevation of IL-1β, which we demonstrated to be microglial (69,70). These experiments demonstrated that the brain, and specifically the microglia, is primed by prior pathology to respond disproportionately to subsequent inflammatory stimulation. Importantly, the systemic inflammatory response to peripheral immune challenge is equivalent in diseased and normal animals (71). Hence, it is specifically the CNS response that is amplified (see Figure 9.2). The same phenomenon was subsequently shown in aged rodents (72,73). The terminology of priming alludes to the similar phenomenon of macrophage priming described in the 1980s, whereby macrophages primed with IFN-γ showed more robust IL-1 and inducible nitric oxide synthase (iNOS) synthesis upon exposure to LPS (74). IFN-γ was undetectable in the ME7 model but the outputs (IL-1, iNOS) of the restimulated primed microglial cell matched that of the primed macrophage (75). Thus, we used the term 'primed' based on a functional definition.

As the expression profile of microglia during neurodegenerative disease is revealed in ever more detail there are constant additions to the nomenclature but these are highly overlapping and it would seem prudent to rationalize and reconcile much of this terminology (76–79). Although there are novel data suggesting different stages of activation during evolving neurodegenerative disease, such as 'disease-associated microglia' ((DAM) – stage 1 and 2; (80)) and 'early response' and 'late response' populations (77), broadly speaking microglia show a phagocytic, lysosomal, antigen-presenting and lipid-metabolising phenotype. This can be observed by histological or functional means, or with novel single-cell transcriptomic and weighted co-expression analysis in sorted populations or unsorted homogenates (76,78,81). The 'primed' signature, as described by Holtman et al., (76) is largely concordant with signatures of primed microglia in our own hands, with upregulation of *Clec7a* (Dectin 1), *Lgals3* (Galectin 3) and *Itgax* (Cd11c) and also with several features of the 'DAM' profile (80) and it is likely the DAMs are also primed microglia. It is clear that microglia tightly regulate expression of cytokines and that these transcriptomic profiles are distinct from the strong NFκB-inducing, classical pro-inflammatory 'M1-type' microglial cell, produced by LPS (76,82). However, when subjected to a secondary stimulus, these microglia acutely synthesize substantial levels of IL-1β. This tendency to be hyperreactive to secondary stimuli has been confirmed in multiple animal models following our initial demonstrations in prion disease (69,83): AD (84–86), PD (87), Wallerian degeneration (88), ageing (72).

9.3.3 What Primes Microglia?

Microglia detect parenchymal disruption via recognition of products of damaged tissue: the ever-growing collection of damage-associated molecular patterns (DAMPs), which stimulate pattern recognition receptors (PRRs) on immune cells. Many of these receptors recognize both microbial products and endogenous molecules released during injury. For example, TLR4 is the receptor for LPS and high mobility box group 1 (HMGB1). The emerging consensus (76,80,89) is that microglial priming/DAM is broadly similar across several chronic neurodegenerative diseases and we propose that microglia may be exposed to multiple different DAMPs during any given neurodegenerative disease (see Figure 9.2). Here we briefly detail a number of DAMPs/PRRs that may be relevant to priming but a more detailed overview is available elsewhere (90,91).

Aggregated proteins constitute one major class of DAMP. Although there is no consensus on the main receptor for Aβ, it clearly acts as a DAMP: microglia adjacent to amyloid plaques have the classical primed transcriptional signature and generate exaggerated levels of IL-1 in response to LPS stimulation (84,85). Likewise, extracellular α-synuclein, injected directly into the substantia nigra, provokes a robust pro-inflammatory response and animals challenged 18 hours later with systemic LPS produced exaggerated levels of pro-inflammatory mediators LPS (91).

Multiple indicators of cellular damage, such as ATP and HMGB1, or indeed neuronal and synaptic loss also activate microglia. HMGB1, a DAMP implicated in sterile inflammation and infection (92), has been implicated as a key mediator of neuroinflammation in traumatic brain injury (TBI), epilepsy and ischaemia (93) and contributes to microglial priming in ageing and stress (94,95). Microglia become primed in aged rats upon *E. coli* infection (96). HMGB1 is modestly increased in the CSF of these rats and intra-cisterna magna injection of an antagonist (Box-A) is sufficient to block exaggerated IL-1 responses, sickness behaviour and cognitive impairment (94).

Activation of the complement system via C1q and activated C3 is proposed as a major mechanism of synaptic removal (97) and may contribute to priming: deletion of the C3 convertase regulator complement receptor 1-related protein γ (Crry) activates C3 and leads to microglial priming, which is abrogated in Crry/C3 double knockout animals, implicating C3 as a key factor (98). In mice with deficient DNA repair, due to expression of a mutant endonuclease (Ercc1$^{\Delta/-}$), microglia are hypertrophic and synthesize exaggerated IL-1β levels upon systemic LPS challenge (99). It is neuronal DNA damage that drives the microglial priming although precise mechanisms are unclear. In the ME7 prion disease model, a number of Fcγ receptors have been shown to be elevated in microglia and the ability to synthesize CNS IL-1β in response to systemic LPS was significantly impaired in Fcγ chain knockout mice (100), indicating that the Fcγ chain and recognition of IgGs in the brain may be important in phenotypic switching.

Among major genetic risk factors for AD, *TREM2* and the *APoE ε4* allele also appear to predispose to exaggerated responses to inflammatory stimulation. TREM2 has emerged as a likely PRR binding lipoproteins – like APOE, LDL and clusterin/APoJ-, phosphatidyl serine exposed on the surface of apoptotic cells, sphingolipids released from damaged myelin (101,102) and Aβ with nanomolar affinity (103). Some caution is required however: although TREM2 may drive a DAM/primed phenotype in mice, recent studies in human brain suggest that TREM2 is selectively expressed on recruited monocytes, rather than microglia (104). The inflammatory response to innate immune challenge is also reportedly elevated in ε4 carriers. In APoE ε4 transgenic animals, LPS causes an exaggerated inflammatory response in both microglia and macrophages when compared to *APoE ε3* mice (105). In human, inflammatory responses triggered by innate immune agonists are highest in *APoE ε4* carriers (106).

There are a number of ligand-receptor interactions between microglia and surrounding neurons that help to maintain a quiescent microglial state (107). These include CD200 R and CX3CR1 on microglia and their corresponding ligands CD200 (108) and CX3CL1 (109). Transcript expression for these receptors, along with other 'homeostatic' genes such as *P2ry12*, *Cd33* and *Tmem119*, is reduced in the first stage of the proposed DAM phenotypic transition (78). This is consistent with earlier ideas that down-regulation of these molecules constitutes a sort of 'removal of the brakes', facilitating exaggerated responses to subsequent inflammatory stimuli. In a similar vein, loss of the 'don't eat me' neuronal signalling protein CD47 or its microglial receptor SIRPα results in excessive microglial phagocytosis of synapses and loss of preferential protection of active inputs (110).

Loss of normal neurotransmitter tone also affects microglial reactivity to secondary stimulation. The neurotransmitter noradrenaline (NA) exerts anti-inflammatory effects on microglia, via the β2 adrenergic receptor (111). Removal of its influence, via lesioning, exacerbates Aβ pathology, while microglial pro-inflammatory cytokine responses to Aβ are suppressed by NA administration (112,192). Acetylcholine (ACh) may also exert suppression of microglial pro-inflammatory actions, as it does on macrophages in the viscera, via the nicotinic α7 receptor (113).

Even psychological stress in vivo primes microglia, via glucocorticoid signalling, for an exaggerated response to LPS ex vivo. Adrenalectomy and GC receptor inhibition with the antagonist RU486 abrogate this effect (114). Thus, although the microglial glucocorticoid receptor may limit microglial activation in degenerative states per se (115), it may leave microglia vulnerable to subsequent phenotypic switching upon systemic inflammation (116).

Finally, priming can occur due to a persistently heightened, albeit low grade, systemic inflammatory states. Immune ageing and chronic conditions such as, diabetes, atherosclerosis and arthritis have a systemic inflammatory component (19) and there is evidence that these conditions can drive central inflammatory changes (117). There are also now studies examining the impact of chronic peripheral inflammatory conditions on amyloid pathology (86,117) and other features of age-related cognitive decline (119) but this is beyond the scope of the current chapter.

9.3.4 Primed for Exaggerated Responses: Duration, Turnover and Memory

Thus far, we have discussed microglia primed by evolving neurodegenerative pathology but discrete acute brain or nerve injury and axon degeneration events also prime local microglia for extended periods. These microglia undergo phenotypic switching when subsequently challenged with LPS or other stimuli (88,120). Indeed there is evidence for persistence of features of microglial activation long after brain injury, in one report up to 18 years after a single episode of TBI (121). Like 'innate immune memory' in peripheral monocytes (122) there is evidence that microglia retain relatively long-term memory of prior systemic inflammatory events. Systemic infection with *Salmonella typhimurium* leads to an exaggerated central inflammatory response to intra-cerebral LPS challenge four weeks later (123) and a similar exaggerated responsiveness could be achieved with three consecutive systemic LPS challenges despite diminishing peripheral cytokine responses (peripheral immune tolerance). A 2018 paper showed that systemic inflammation can produce epigenetically-mediated long-lasting (up to six months) microglial memory of prior activation that may confer exaggerated (primed) or suppressed (tolerant) responses to subsequent inflammatory stimuli (124). These differential microglial states are highly dependent on the number, timing and dose of LPS treatments and other studies showed highly damaging microglial phenotypes upon similar sequential LPS regimes (125). The real-life relevance of these 'repeated challenge' regimes require study since long-term microglial memory has important implications. Although traditionally thought of as long-lived, estimations for the renewal of the population vary from 95 days to 15 months (126,127). This implies that if microglia persist in a primed state these primed microglia must either be especially long-lived or daughter cells from recent divisions must rapidly assume the primed phenotype from the milieu or retain a 'memory' for the phenotype of its lineage, via epigenetic modifications, such as those described above.

9.3.5 Does Microglial Priming Occur in Humans?

A meta-analysis of 113 AD post-mortem studies showed that, in the majority of cases, MHC-II and CD68 were elevated in AD versus controls (128). The increase in these markers appears to reflect the phagocytic and antigen presentation phenotype typical of primed microglia and in another post-mortem study with 299 samples, CD-68 and MSR-A were positively correlated with cognitive decline, while IBA-1 was negatively associated (129).

While some post-mortem studies have reported evidence of M1 activation around amyloid plaques in AD (130,131), sepsis clearly activates microglia in humans (132) and therefore systemic inflammation associated with a terminal illness may alter microglial protein expression.

Studies of isolated human microglia have begun to emerge. It is clear that the brain environment heavily influences the microglial signature and length of time in culture dramatically alters the phenotype (133). The microglia express a transcriptomic signature that appears to overlap with mouse microglia and with risk genes for neurodegenerative disease. In one recent study of the microglia transcriptome, using autopsy samples of healthy-brain aged patients, marked divergence from that of the mouse was reported, with many immune-related genes activated uniquely in humans (134). Comparisons were, however, between healthy aged mice from specific pathogen-free environments and humans who had recently died, so it is plausible that preceding ill health impacted upon microglial phenotype. Plaque-associated microglia from post-mortem tissue from patients with early- and late-onset AD exhibit many of the hallmarks of microglial priming identified in mouse studies (*Clec7a*, *Axl*, *Itgax* and *Trem2*; (84,85) at significantly higher levels than non-plaque microglia. However, an exaggerated IL-1 response to subsequent inflammatory stimulation is yet to be demonstrated in humans.

9.3.6 Mechanisms Underlying Acute and Long-term Impairments after Systemic Inflammation

Since systemic inflammation has disproportionate acute and long-term consequences in those with neurodegenerative disease and microglia are well placed to mediate some or all of these changes, here we examine recent evidence that inflammatory changes, triggered by acute systemic inflammation, contribute to acute exacerbations of function and altered trajectory of disease in animal models of disease. The key output in describing microglial priming, was an exaggerated acute production of IL-1β which, when superimposed on existing degeneration in the vulnerable brain, may have deleterious effects on brain function and integrity. However, inflammation-induced effects on brain integrity may occur via direct effects on microglia, astrocytes, neurons and indeed the brain vasculature. There is some evidence for each of these possibilities and below we provide some exemplar studies. This section is constrained by available space and is by no means exhaustive.

There are well-established data that IL-1 impairs memory consolidation (using the contextual fear-conditioning test; CFC) and inhibits long-term potentiation (the best known molecular paradigm for explaining memory) via direct interaction with IL-1RI on hippocampal neurons (135–137). This mechanism has been implicated in memory deficits in models of LPS-induced sepsis (135), *E. coli* infection (138) and trauma (139). In examining those and other studies it is important to differentiate between acute and reversible effects of IL-1 (or other mediators) on cognitive function and effects of IL-1 that may cause lasting brain injury and cognitive decline. Our own work also supports a role for IL-1 in acute brain dysfunction in a model of delirium during dementia. Notably, in those studies systemic IL-1 mediated acute LPS-induced cognitive dysfunction, but neuropathological and in vitro slice experiments suggested that CNS IL-1β produced selective deleterious effects on neuronal integrity (140,141, Figure 9.2). This suggests that acute dysfunction and acute brain injury are dissociable. Studies with viral mimetics also support the idea of repeated challenges producing dissociable acute deficits and long-term decrements, with the latter accumulating, upon repeated challenge, to accelerate decline (84, Figure 9.1d). If true in humans, it would be of considerable significance that acute disruption, like delirium, may be dissociable from the long-term decline that is associated with such episodes.

Systemic inflammation can also worsen AD and PD pathology in animal models. Using repeated LPS dosing schedules that produce significant peripheral tolerance to LPS and complex responses in microglia (124,125). This has meant that mechanistic interpretations are complicated. Repeated LPS drives increased lysosomal and complement activation with deleterious consequences (125) but its impact on microglial phagocytosis of amyloid may depend on when the systemic inflammation occurs with respect to the onset or stage of amyloidosis (124). Indeed, although LPS (0.5 mg/Kg) weekly for 12 weeks was reported to increase amyloid precursor protein processing and amyloid deposition (118), LPS once a week for 13 weeks at the same dose was recently shown to reduce amyloid load (142). With respect to tau pathology, one study used a single high dose of LPS (10 mg/Kg) in mice and showed significantly increased tau hyperphosphorylation that was IL-1 dependent and neuronal p38 MAP kinase-mediated (143). Other studies support the idea that systemic LPS drives new central IL-1β and that this contributes to new brain pathology. Two PD models report that peripheral inflammation leads to increased death of substantia nigra neurons and IL-1 and nitric oxide, the very hallmarks of phenotypic switching of primed microglia (see Figure 9.2), are causative in this nigral degeneration (87,144). That same IL-1β and iNOS profile was shared by microglia in two models of axonal injury in which peripheral LPS challenge-induced new axonal injury and phagocytosis: optic nerve crush-induced Wallerian degeneration (88) and experimental autoimmune encephalomyelitis (EAE) (145).

However, although we and others have shown that IL-1β and TNF-α in the brain originate largely from microglia and that these cytokines have direct effects on neuronal function, they also act on astrocytes to trigger significant chemokine production (85,119). Astrocytes are abundant in the CNS, particularly at the interface between the peripheral and central environments, and are universally activated during neurodegeneration (147). We have now shown that these cells too are primed and show exaggerated chemokine production in response to local IL-1 (85,119) or TNF-α stimulation (85). When cytokines like IL-1β or TNF-α are generated, either outside or inside the brain, they can also impact on the integrity of the BBB. IL-1β, for example impacts on connexin 43-containing gap junctions, on sonic hedgehog, on platelet activation at the vasculature and on claudin expression and patency of the BBB (147–149).

Both increases in chemotactic signals for peripheral inflammatory cells and loosening of the barriers that impede their infiltration to the brain are likely to contribute to the occurrence of increased inflammatory cell infiltrates and these may have significant consequences for neuronal integrity. D'Mello and colleagues showed that microglia drive recruitment of monocytes in response to peripheral inflammation (150). Subsequent studies in post-operative cognitive dysfunction (POCD), sepsis and viral encephalitis demonstrate that infiltrating immune cells contribute directly to cognitive dysfunction and loss of integrity (151–153). Using poly(I:C), it was demonstrated that peripheral and central TNF-α, dependent on CX3CR1-positive circulating monocytes, causes synaptic and motor learning deficits, independently of microglia (154). Furthermore, in a model of stroke, systemic inflammation induced by LPS lead to an IL-1-dependent secretion of peripheral chemokines, which, in turn, mobilized neutrophils, driving an exacerbation of ischaemia-induced neuronal damage (155).

In addition to the chemotactic roles of chemokines, they also have direct neuromodulatory actions that may contribute to cognitive and functional deficits. Endothelial and epithelial IFN-induced CXCL10-CXCR3 signalling contributes to cognitive and behavioural effects of systemically administered RNA viruses and IFN-β (156). CCL2 produced in the hypothalamus drives LPS-induced cachexia, via direct effects on peptide hormone-containing neurons (157) and CCL3 has direct impacts on synaptic transmission and memory (158). Finally, astrocyte-derived CCL11 has been reported to contribute to hippocampal neuronal damage and cognitive impairment in response to systemic immune activation (159), while circulating CCL11 has been reported to penetrate the brain and impair neurogenesis and cognition (160).

In summary, IL-1 and TNF-α may have dissociable roles in acute cognitive impairments and lasting brain injury and may act independently on multiple brain cell types, with a wide range of demonstrated deleterious effects in animal models (Figure 9.2).

9.4 Future Perspectives for Clinical Interrogation of Systemic Inflammation Effects on the Degenerating Brain

As discussed, there are converging strands of evidence implicating systemic inflammation and heightened innate immune activation in neurodegenerative processes. Continuing rapid development in understanding of neuroimmune interactions and microglial biology will likely generate clinically relevant findings and testable hypotheses. This knowledge will have to be coupled with powerful new techniques to overcome some of the obstacles presented by the relatively inaccessible brain. However, there is scope to use already available techniques to interrogate dysregulated immune function in neurology and psychiatry.

9.4.1 Neuroimaging

Position emission tomography (PET) ligands targeting microglia have been developed to quantify neuroinflammation in vivo in CNS disease. Translocator protein (TPSO) is highly expressed on phagocytic immune cells and there is evidence that microglia express higher levels in disease and during systemic inflammation (161,162). TPSO is, by a distance, the most widely used target in studies of microglial changes in neurodegenerative disease but it has limitations. Increased signal does not necessarily equate to increased microglial activation and human microglial TPSO expression has been reported to be reduced following immune challenge, in contrast to the rodent microglial response (163). Moreover, both astrocytes and endothelial cells have been reported to bind TPSO tracers (164). However, additional ligands, most notably P2X7 and CSF1 R, are being studied to be used in tandem with, or in place of, TPSO (165,166). PET also remains expensive but despite its limitations, it retains powerful potential as a biomarker of neuroinflammation, capable of observing in vivo spatial and temporal alterations in the phenotype of microglia during neurodegeneration, and in response to systemic inflammation or putative treatments. Functional magnetic resonance imaging (167) and quantification magnetization transfer (168) have also been used to illustrate that experimentally applied inflammatory stimuli can produce regionally specific changes in brain metabolism/activation and these approaches, most commonly associated with assessing neuronal activation/neurovascular coupling, could be pursued more avidly.

9.4.2 Cerebrospinal Fluid (CSF)

The CSF represents an important fluid interface between the periphery and brain that allows researchers to identify mediators and biomarkers of brain inflammation, injury and neurodegeneration. However, its collection is a relatively skilled and time-consuming undertaking and not all patients are keen to undergo the procedure.

The theoretical underpinnings of immunopsychiatry hold that neuroimmune processes mediate a variety of CNS diseases. In the context of neurodegenerative disease there is a need for detailed analysis of human CSF soluble inflammatory mediators and infiltrating immune cells in response to systemic inflammatory events or peripheral inflammatory comorbidities. A series of mass spectrometry studies have mapped the CSF proteome, both in health and disease (169,170) aiding selection of proteins for targeted quantification assays and comparisons with animal studies. To date, most studies of acute inflammatory events with CNS sequelae remain relatively small but studies of the central response to peripheral inflammation resulting from hip fracture show association between cytokines (IL-1β and IL-8) and incidence of delirium (171,172). Modern multiplex protein assays are capable of parallel and sensitive detection of many soluble CSF inflammatory mediators. In ALS, this method has been used to establish that follistatin, IL-1α and kallikrein-5 are significantly reduced in comparison to controls (173). Similarly, studies have examined the CNS cytokine response to bacterial meningitis (174) showing the ability of relatively few infiltrating cells to generate high levels of pro-inflammatory cytokines and differences in the inflammatory profiles triggered by common bacterial pathogens that cause meningitis.

In a healthy-brain state, there is minimal influx of peripheral innate or adaptive immune cells. In CNS disease, however, circulating immune cells can infiltrate the brain, most evident in MS and ischaemia (175). It remains to be seen whether these changes are important in the pathogenesis of other neurodegenerative diseases. Using immunophenotyping approaches one can characterize the phenotypic features of peripheral immune cells that infiltrate the CSF. Antibodies against cell surface markers (usually functional membrane proteins) are used to identify specific cell populations but given that, in some cases, different cell types can express the same protein, the co-expression of multiple markers is required to characterize and differentiate cell types.

Immunophenotyping has been utilized in clinical laboratory tests by medical specialties such as haematology and oncology for decades. Flow cytometry, traditionally the most widely utilized method, uses fluorochromes conjugated to antibodies against proteins. Utilizing this approach it has been shown that IL-17-producing CD4+ cells are increased in CNS vasculitis from secondary angiitis and giant cell arteritis (176) (see Bielekova and Pranzatelli for a comprehensive review of CSF immunophenotyping (177)). However, the number of cell proteins that can be simultaneously measured with flow cytometry is limited to less than 20 by spectral overlap of the fluorescent antibodies. In contrast, a new approach, mass cytometry, has seen an increase in the number of potential cell surface protein targets to 40, by using heavy metal ion antibody conjugates in place of fluorescent dyes. This technique also benefits from high signal-to-noise ratio and the ability to target intracellular proteins. It has been used to demonstrate the characteristics of DAMs in animal models of AD, HD and EAE and infiltrating macrophages in EAE (178). Techniques for characterization of cellular protein expression are progressing rapidly and even newer approaches, such as CITE-seq and REAP-seq, offer the possibility of accurate large-scale simultaneous measurement of gene and protein expression at a single-cell level (179).

9.4.3 Blood

Collection of blood for analysis of biomarkers is obviously more practical than CSF (180) and development of peripheral biomarkers of neurodegeneration is ongoing. Neurofilament light chain protein, in particular, is a promising, non-specific marker of neurodegenerative events (181). However, identification of reliable plasma markers of CNS changes is fraught with difficulty. The small fraction of CNS proteins that reaches the plasma is greatly diluted in the matrix of abundant albumin and immunoglobulins. Moreover, variations in liver metabolism and renal clearance bring further complexity to measurement.

Approximating central inflammation by measuring peripheral markers of inflammation is also problematic. The relationship between the peripheral and central inflammatory milieux, in both health and neurodegeneration, is not adequately characterized. Felger and colleagues (182) examined the strength of CRP as a marker of peripheral and central inflammation in context of depression. Multiple peripheral cytokines, including soluble TNF receptor 2 (sTNFR2), TNF-α, IL-1RA and IL-6, and central CRP were correlated with elevated systemic CRP. In turn, central CRP correlated with central IL-6 soluble receptor and TNF-α. Thus, a clinically available inflammatory marker appears to reflect some degree of central inflammation, at least in depression. However, in a study of 221 neurology patients, immunophenotyping of CSF and peripheral leukocytes showed a poor correlation between the peripheral and central compartments in disease states (183). They demonstrated that peripheral and central inflammatory biomarkers only correlated in patients without neuroinflammation. This study suggests that the CNS environment shapes the phenotype of infiltrating cells and ultimately that peripheral measures of inflammation alone are probably insufficient to make reliable inferences about CNS inflammation. Once central inflammation is established, the authors showed, the correlation between the periphery and CNS environment diminishes significantly as there is selective recruitment, expansion and retention of certain cell types intrathecally. As with CSF, immunophenotyping of peripheral immune cells offers great potential insights. In a similar vein to peripheral soluble inflammatory mediators, the relationship between the phenotype of circulating peripheral immune cells and central disease processes is unclear. One obvious possibility is that the upregulation of innate inflammatory responses that accompanies the decline in adaptive immunity in inflammaging (184) contributes to worsening of cognitive decline and merits detailed immunophenotyping. Indeed, peripheral signatures may offer information about vulnerability of the CNS to disease occurrence, exacerbation or progression: HD patients show peripheral immune activation 16 years before onset of clinical symptoms and monocytes from these patients are also hyperreactive to stimulation (185).

9.5 Summary

Our aim here has been to convey to psychiatrists, allied health professionals and researchers that peripheral inflammation has clinical consequences in neurodegenerative disease and that the mechanisms underpinning this interplay are becoming clearer. Understanding that common inflammatory events contribute to and worsen

Table 9.1 Selected methodological approaches for future progress

Area	Current Knowledge	Future directions
Neuroimaging: PET/MRI	PET ligands for neuroinflammation developed (mainly targeting TPSO) but questions of reliability, biological interpretation and cost remain	Development of reliable, specific, robust and affordable non-invasive techniques to elucidate neuroinflammatory responses in vivo in humans
CSF markers of neuroinflammation	Analysis of CSF proteins and biochemistry is available as standard in clinical practice	Increasingly detailed characterization of the soluble mediator components of the central inflammatory response with multiplex assays and 'omics' platforms
Immunophenotyping of infiltrating cells in the CNS	At homeostasis, peripheral innate or adaptive cells show limited migration into the CNS compartment, but these cells can be analyzed	New powerful approaches will allow characterization of any infiltrating peripheral populations identified in the CSF of those with CNS disease, with and without the imposition of peripheral inflammatory insults
Peripheral immunophenotyping	Established in both clinical practice and research for disciplines like haematology. Limited numbers of studies showing immunophenotyping of peripheral cells in those with neurodegenerative diseases and in those with acute exacerbations of disease	Establishing whether those who have evidence of exacerbation of neurological dysfunction have unique cellular and molecular signatures in peripheral inflammation. Establishing whether inflammaging contributes to differential responses or trajectories for neurodegenerative disease

neurodegenerative conditions offers new avenues for prevention and treatment of these challenging, deleterious conditions. In addition to the effect of innate immunity, it is clear from studies on MS and autoimmune encephalitis that adaptive immunity will also likely be important in mediating the relationship between inflammatory events and neurodegeneration.

A generation ago it was noted in cohort studies that NSAIDs usage was associated with lower dementia incidence (186). Since then, the vast majority of the information we have on systemic inflammation and neurodegeneration has been garnered from observational studies. Ongoing well-designed current cohort studies such as DELPHIC and SAGES will bring further insights into the impact of acute illness or surgery on trajectories of cognitive and functional decline (187–189).

A key aim of the nascent immunopsychiatry field must be to generate treatments that affect intractable diseases. This can only come from design and implementation of clinical trials that test hypotheses generated from the field. IL-1 and TNF-α are prime candidates for thorough clinical investigation. Immunosuppressive biologics are commonplace in medical practice. Anti-TNF-α treatments are well-established in rheumatological and inflammatory bowel conditions. Indeed, a phase II clinical trial showed that subcutaneous anti-TNF-α was well tolerated in an AD (190). Anti-IL-1 treatments are not as widely used but, like anti-TNF-αs, have acceptable safety profiles. Thus, there are readily available anti-IL-1 and TNF-α strategies that merit testing in new clinical settings (191). Understandably, this will be complex given the central role of IL-1 and TNF-α in regulating innate and adaptive immune responses. There are clear potential benefits to examining their impact in acute-on-chronic settings. However, before such work we could consider trials testing well-known, cheap, broadly targeted anti-inflammatory treatments such as NSAIDs, steroids or colchicine in vulnerable populations since these anti-inflammatory drugs clearly are effective in suppressing cytokine and/or prostaglandin synthesis and in treating fever and other manifestations of cytokine response syndromes (45). Altering the peripheral immune response using these drugs may plausibly alter the acute dysfunction and/or long-term sequelae of acute inflammation's effects on neurodegenerative disease. Such studies may be highly informative on functional domains and neuroanatomical areas that are most vulnerable to effects of peripheral inflammation and perhaps bring us closer to novel treatments for intractable conditions.

References

1. Trapp BD, Nave K-A. Multiple sclerosis: an immune or neurodegenerative disorder? *Annu Rev Neurosci.* 2008 Jun 17; 31(1):247–69.

2. Redmann M, Darley-Usmar V, Zhang J. The role of autophagy, mitophagy and lysosomal functions in modulating bioenergetics and survival in the context of redox and proteotoxic damage: implications for neurodegenerative diseases. *Aging Dis.* 2016 Mar 15;7(2):150.

3. Swardfager W, Lanctt K, Rothenburg L, et al. A meta-analysis of cytokines in Alzheimer's disease. *Biol Psychiatry.* 2010;68(10):930–41.

4. Holmes C, Cunningham C, Zotova E, et al. Systemic inflammation and disease progression in alzheimer disease. *Neurology,* 2009;73(10); 768–74.

5. King E, Tiernan O'Brien J, Donaghy P, et al. Peripheral inflammation in prodromal Alzheimer's and Lewy body dementias. *Journal of Neurology, Neurosurgery and Psychiatry.* 2018;89:339–45.

6. McManus RM, Heneka MT. Role of neuroinflammation in neurodegeneration: new insights. *Alzheimers Res Ther.* 2017;9(1):14.

7. Dunn N, Mullee M, Perry VH, Holmes C. Association between dementia and infectious disease. *Alzheimer Dis Assoc Disord.* 2005;19 (2):91–4.

8. Katan M, Moon YP, Paik MC, et al. Infectious burden and cognitive function. *Neurology.* 2013 Mar 26;80(13): LP1209–15.

9. Widmann CN, Heneka MT. Long-term cerebral consequences of sepsis. *Lancet Neurol.* 2014 Jun 1;13(6):630–6.

10. Zrzavy T, Höftberger R, Berger T, et al. Pro-inflammatory activation of microglia in the brain of patients with sepsis. *Neuropathol Appl Neurobiol.* 2019 April;45 (3):278–90.

11. Kumar DKV, Choi SH, Washicosky KJ, et al. Amyloid-β peptide protects against microbial infection in mouse and worm models of Alzheimer's disease. *Sci Transl Med.* 2016 May 25;8 (340):340ra72.

12. Eimer WA, Vijaya Kumar DK, Navalpur Shanmugam NK, et al. Alzheimer's disease-associated β-amyloid is rapidly seeded by herpesviridae to protect against brain infection. *Neuron.* 2018 Jul 11;99 (1):56–63.e3.

13. Rasmussen LS. Postoperative cognitive dysfunction: Incidence and prevention. *Best Pract Res Clin Anaesthesiol.* 2006;20 (2):315–30.

14. Nadelson MR, Sanders RD, Avidan MS. Perioperative cognitive trajectory in adults. *BJA Br J Anaesth.* 2014 Mar 1;112 (3):440–51.

15. Ungprasert P, Wijarnpreecha K, Thongprayoon C. Rheumatoid arthritis and the risk of dementia: a systematic review and meta-analysis. *Neurol India.* 2016;64(1):56.

16. Chen C-K, Wu Y-T, Chang Y-C. Association between chronic periodontitis and the risk of Alzheimer's disease: a retrospective, population-based, matched-cohort study. *Alzheimers Res Ther.* 2017;9(1):56.

17. Chen C-K, Wu Y-T, Chang Y-C. Periodontal inflammatory disease is associated with the risk of Parkinson's disease: a population-based retrospective matched-cohort study. Emsley H, editor. *PeerJ.* 2017;5:e3647.

18. Ide M, Harris M, Stevens A, et al. Periodontitis and cognitive decline in Alzheimer's disease. *PLoS One.* 2016;11(3): e0151081.

19. Yaffe K, Kanaya A, Lindquist K, et al. The metabolic syndrome, inflammation, and risk of cognitive decline. *J Am Med Assoc.* 2004;292(18):2237–42.

20. Clegg A, Young J, Iliffe S, Rikkert MO, Rockwood K. Frailty in elderly people. *Lancet.* 2013;381(9868):752–62.

21. Cunningham C. Systemic inflammation and delirium: important co-factors in the progression of dementia. *Biochem Soc Trans.* 2011;39(4):945–53.

22. Cerejeira J, Firmino H, Vaz-Serra A, Mukaetova-Ladinska EB. The neuroinflammatory hypothesis of delirium. *Acta Neuropathol.* 2010;119 (6):737–54.

23. van Gool WA, van de Beek D, Eikelenboom P. Systemic infection and delirium: when cytokines and acetylcholine collide. *Lancet.* 2010;375 (9716):773–5.

24. Khan BA, Zawahiri M, Campbell NL, Boustani MA. Biomarkers for deliriuma – a review. *J Am Geriatr Soc.* 2011;59(SUPPL. 2):S256–61.

25. George J, Bleasdale S, Singleton SJ. Causes and prognosis of delirium in elderly patients admitted to a district general hospital. *Age Ageing.* 1997;26(6):423–7.

26. Chang YL, Tsai YF, Lin PJ, Chen MC, Liu CY. Prevalence and risk factors for postoperative delirium in a cardiovascular intensive care unit. *AmJCrit Care.* 2008;17 (6):567–75.

27. Kat MG, Vreeswijk R, De Jonghe JFM, et al. Long-term cognitive outcome of delirium in elderly hip surgery patients: a prospective matched controlled study over two and a half years. *Dement Geriatr Cogn Disord.* 2008;26(1):1–8.

28. Rudolph JL, Jones RN, Levkoff SE, et al. Derivation and validation of a preoperative prediction rule for delirium after cardiac surgery. *Circulation.* 2009;119(2):229–36.

29. Inouye SK, Charpentier PA. Precipitating factors for delirium in hospitalized elderly persons: predictive model and interrelationship with baseline vulnerability. *J Am Med Assoc*. 1996;275 (11):852–7.

30. Eriksson I, Gustafson Y, Fagerstrom L, Olofsson B. Urinary tract infection in very old women is associated with delirium. *Int Psychogeriatr*. 2011;23(3):496–502.

31. McKenzie R, Stewart MT, Bellantoni MF, Finucane TE. Bacteriuria in individuals who become delirious. *Am J Med*. 2014 Apr 1;127(4):255–7.

32. Davis DHJ, Skelly DT, Murray C, et al. Worsening cognitive impairment and neurodegenerative pathology progressively increase risk for delirium. *Am J Geriatr Psychiatry*. 2015;23(4):403–15.

33. Witlox J, Eurelings LSM, De Jonghe JFM, et al. Delirium in elderly patients and the risk of postdischarge mortality, institutionalization, and dementia: a meta-analysis. *JAMA*. 2010;304(4):443–51.

34. Saczynski JS, Marcantonio ER, Quach L, et al. Cognitive trajectories after postoperative delirium. *N Engl J Med*. 2012 Jul 5;367(1):30–9.

35. Fong TG, Jones RN, Shi P, et al. Delirium accelerates cognitive decline in Alzheimer disease. *Neurology*. 2009;72(18):1570–5.

36. Davis DHJ, Muniz Terrera G, Keage H, et al. Delirium is a strong risk factor for dementia in the oldest-old: a population-based cohort study. *Brain*. 2012 Sep 9;135(9):2809–16.

37. DJ D, Muniz-Terrera G, HD K, et al. Association of delirium with cognitive decline in late life: a neuropathologic study of 3 population-based cohort studies. *JAMA Psychiatry*. 2017 Mar 1;74 (3):244–51.

38. Holmes C, Butchart J. Systemic inflammation and Alzheimer's disease. *Biochem Soc Trans*. 2011 Aug 1;39(4): LP898–901.

39. Brugger F, Erro R, Balint B, et al. Why is there motor deterioration in Parkinson's disease during systemic infections – a hypothetical view. *npj Park Dis*. 2015;1 (1):15014.

40. Correale J, Fiol M, Gilmore W. The risk of relapses in multiple sclerosis during systemic infections. *Neurology*. 2006 Aug 22;67(4):LP652–9.

41. Buljevac D, Flach HZ, Hop WCJ, et al. Prospective study on the relationship between infections and multiple sclerosis exacerbations. *Brain*. 2002 May 1;125 (5):952–60.

42. Smith KJ, McDonald WI. The pathophysiology of multiple sclerosis: the mechanisms underlying the production of symptoms and the natural history of the disease. *Philos Trans R Soc London Ser B Biol Sci*. 1999 Oct 29;354(1390): LP1649–73.

43. DM W, Rodriguez M. Premenstrual multiple sclerosis pseudoexacerbations: role of body temperature and prevention with aspirin. *Arch Neurol*. 2006 Jul 1;63 (7):1005–8.

44. Moreau T, Coles A, Wing M, et al. Transient increase in symptoms associated with cytokine release in patients with multiple sclerosis. *Brain*. 1996;119 (1):225–37.

45. Shimabukuro-Vornhagen A, Gödel P, Subklewe M, et al. Cytokine release syndrome. *J Immunother Cancer*. 2018;6(1):56.

46. Dantzer R, O'Connor JC, Freund GG, Johnson RW, Kelley KW. From inflammation to sickness and depression: When the immune system subjugates the brain. *Nat Rev Neurosci*. 2008;9 (1):46–56.

47. Matsumura K, Kaihatsu S, Imai H, et al. Cyclooxygenase in the vagal afferents: is it involved in the brain prostaglandin response evoked by lipopolysaccharide? *Auton Neurosci Basic Clin*. 2000; 85(1–3):88–92.

48. Hosoi T, Okuma Y, Matsuda T, Nomura Y. Novel pathway for LPS-induced afferent vagus nerve activation: possible role of nodose ganglion. *Auton Neurosci Basic Clin*. 2005;120(1–2):104–7.

49. Chakravarty S. Toll-like receptor 4 on nonhematopoietic cells sustains CNS inflammation during endotoxemia, independent of systemic cytokines. *J Neurosci.* 2005;25(7):1788–96.

50. Gosselin D, Rivest S. MyD88 signaling in brain endothelial cells is essential for the neuronal activity and glucocorticoid release during systemic inflammation. *Mol Psychiatry.* 2008;13(5):480–97.

51. Murray CL, Skelly DT, Cunningham C. Exacerbation of CNS inflammation and neurodegeneration by systemic LPS treatment is independent of circulating IL-1β and IL-6. *J Neuroinflammation.* 2011 May 17;8:50.

52. Saper CB, Romanovsky AA, Scammell TE. Neural circuitry engaged by prostaglandins during the sickness syndrome. *Nat Neurosci.* 2012 Jul 26;15:1088.

53. Quan N, Stern EL, Whiteside MB, Herkenham M. Induction of pro-inflammatory cytokine mRNAs in the brain after peripheral injection of subseptic doses of lipopolysaccharide in the rat. *J Neuroimmunol.* 1999 Jan 1;93 (1–2):72–80.

54. Gutierrez EG, Banks WA, Kastin AJ. Murine tumor necrosis factor alpha is transported from blood to brain in the mouse. *J Neuroimmunol.* 1993;47 (2):169–76.

55. Banks WA, Kastin AJ. Blood to brain transport of interleukin links the immune and central nervous systems. *Life Sci.* 1991;48(25):PL117–21.

56. Varatharaj A, Galea I. The blood-brain barrier in systemic inflammation. *Brain Behav Immun.* 2017;60:1–12.

57. Zlokovic B. The blood-brain barrier in health and chronic neurodegenerative disorders. *Neuron.* 2008;57(2):178–201.

58. Balusu S, Van Wonterghem E, De Rycke R, et al. Identification of a novel mechanism of blood–brain communication during peripheral inflammation via choroid plexus-derived extracellular vesicles. *EMBO Mol Med.* 2016 Oct 8;10:1162–83.

59. Erny D, de Angelis ALH, Jaitin D, et al. Host microbiota constantly control maturation and function of microglia in the CNS. *Nat Neurosci.* 2015 Jul 1;18 (7):965–77.

60. Rothhammer V, Borucki DM, Tjon EC, et al. Microglial control of astrocytes in response to microbial metabolites. *Nature.* 2018;557(7707):724–8.

61. Itagaki S, McGeer PL, Akiyama H, Zhu S, Selkoe D. Relationship of microglia and astrocytes to amyloid deposits of Alzheimer disease. *J Neuroimmunol.* 1989;24(3):173–82.

62. Harold D, Abraham R, Hollingworth P, et al. Genome-wide association study identifies variants at CLU and PICALM associated with Alzheimer's disease. *Nat Genet.* 2009; 41(10):1088–93.

63. Hollingworth P, Sims R, Gerrish A, et al. ABCA7 and BIN1 are susceptibility genes for Alzheimer's disease. *Nat Genet.* 2011;43:429–35.

64. Lambert JC, Ibrahim-Verbaas CA, Harold D, et al. Meta-analysis of 74,046 individuals identifies 11 new susceptibility loci for Alzheimer's disease. *Nat Genet.* 2013;45(12):1452–8.

65. Shi H, Belbin O, Medway C, et al. Genetic variants influencing human aging from late-onset Alzheimer's disease (LOAD) genome-wide association studies (GWAS). *Neurobiol Aging.* 2012 Aug 23;33(8): 1849.e5–1849.18.

66. Jonsson T, Stefansson H, Steinberg S, et al. Variant of *TREM2* associated with the risk of Alzheimer's disease. *N Engl J Med.* 2013 Nov 14;368(2):107–16.

67. Guerreiro R, Wojtas A, Bras J, et al. *TREM2* variants in Alzheimer's disease. *N Engl J Med.* 2013 Nov 14;368(2): 117–27.

68. Combrinck MI, Perry VH, Cunningham C. Peripheral infection evokes exaggerated sickness behaviour in pre-clinical murine prion disease. Neuroscience. 2002;112 (1):7–11.

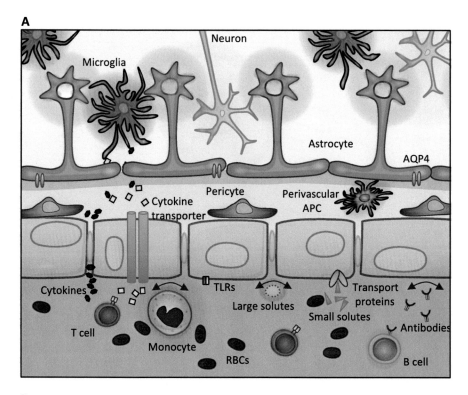

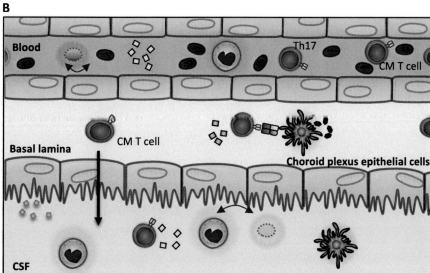

Figure 1.1 Schematic representation of the Blood Brain Barrier and the blood cerebrospinal fluid barrier (BCSFB).

A. The BBB consists of highly specialized endothelial cells joined by tight junctions. They deposit an endothelial basement membrane (yellow) in which pericytes are embedded. The parenchymal basement membrane (orange) is deposited by astrocytes and together with astrocytic endfeet forms the glia limitans perivascularis. The endothelial layer prevents the unrestricted movement of large solutes, antibodies and immune cells while allowing the passage of smaller solutes, cytokines and other proteins through dedicated transport systems.

B. The BCSFB is made up by the choroid plexus epithelial cells which similarly prevent the unrestricted passage of molecules between the blood and the CSF. Central memory T cells are the predominant immune population in the CSF, and it is thought that they may cross the BCSFB, although the molecular mechanisms behind this are still unclear.

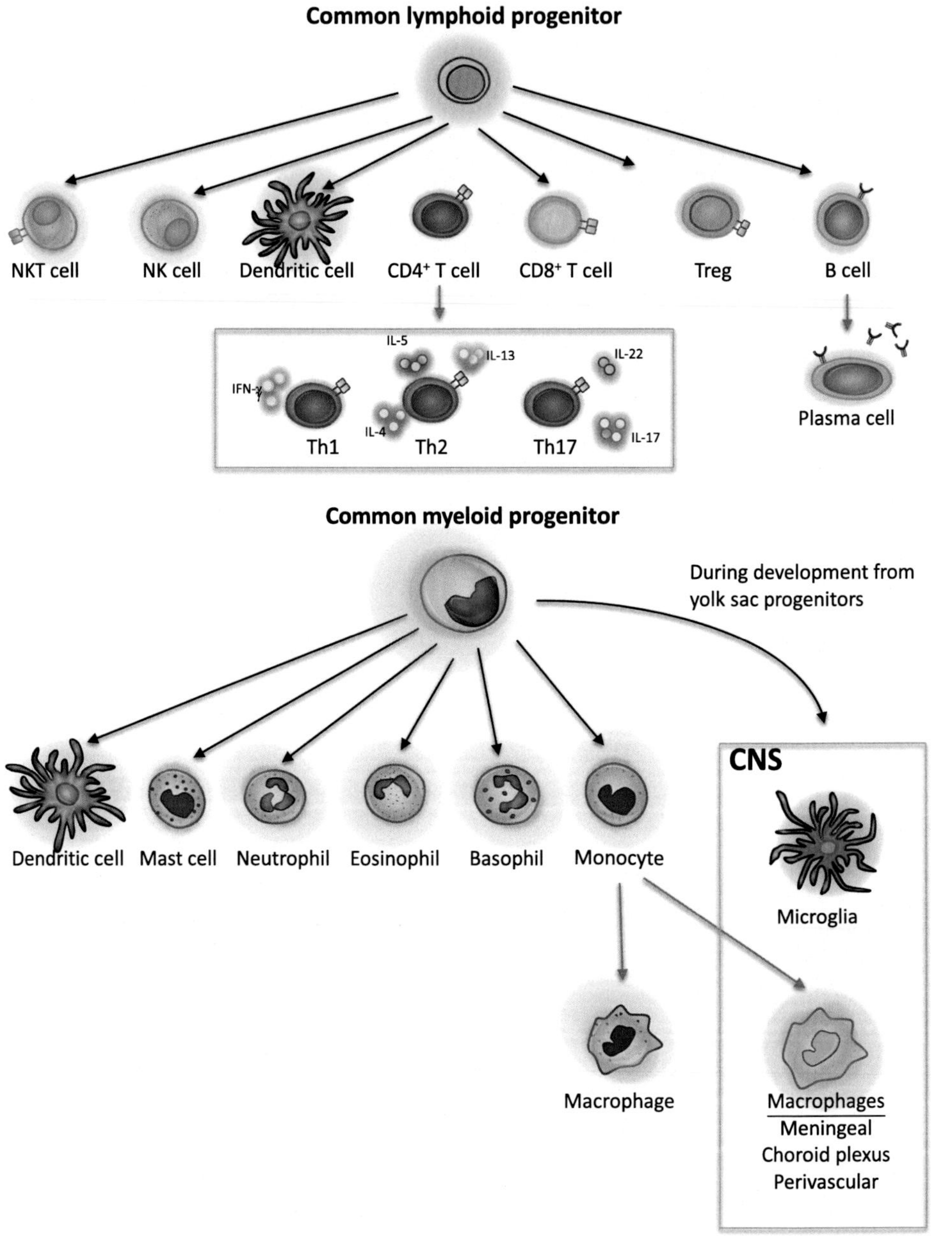

Figure 1.2 Developmental origins of immune cells.
Lymphocytes and some dendritic cells derive from the common lymphoid progenitor cell line. CD4+ T cells can differentiate into T helper cells with specific functions, defined by their cytokine profiles. Activated B cells give rise to antibody secreting plasma cells. Granulocytes (mast cells, neutrophils, eosinophils and basophils), monocytes, some dendritic cells and microglia derive from the common myeloid progenitor cell line. However, microglia are established in the brain prenatally during development from yolk sac progenitors and are transcriptionally distinct from other myeloid cells. Monocytes give rise to macrophages, some in peripheral tissues and others in the CNS.

A

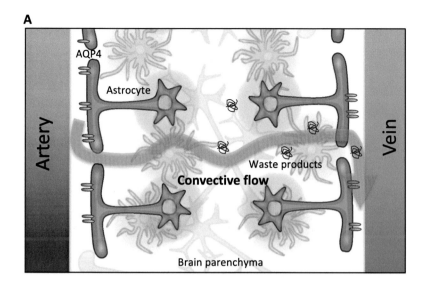

B

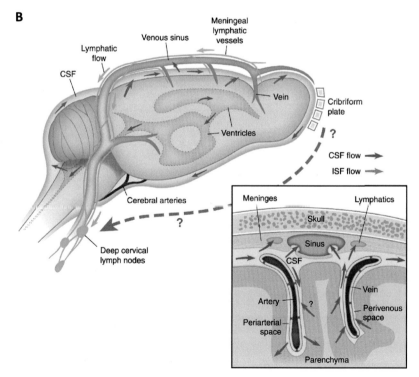

Figure 1.3 CNS lymphatic and glymphatic systems.
A. Schematic of the glymphatic system. CSF enters the brain parenchyma along paraarterial routes, exchanges with interstitial fluid and is cleared along paravenous routes. Convective flow is facilitated by AQP4 pores which are abundantly expressed on astrocytic endfeet. Clearance of solutes, proteins and waste products such as amyloid-β occur along this pathway. Draining fluid may be dispersed into the subarachnoid CSF, venous circulation or lymphatics.
B. Schematic representation of lymphatic drainage of the brain. Meningeal lymphatic vessels (green) adjacent to the venous sinuses and arteries drain molecules and meningeal immune cells in the CSF into the deep cervical lymph nodes. Adapted with permission from Louveau et al. *Neuron*. 2016; 91:957–73 (109).

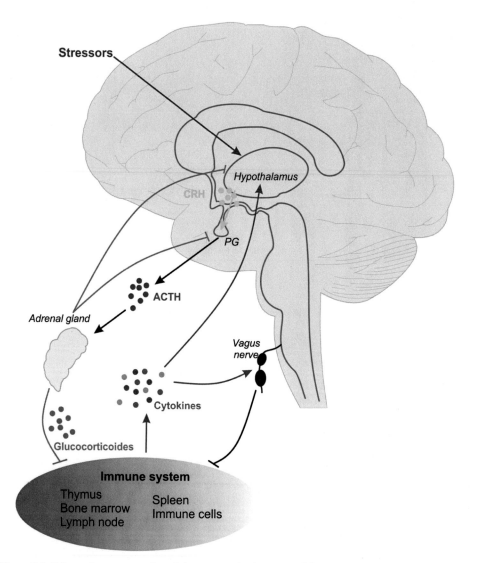

Figure 3.1 Schematic representation of the communication network between the HPA axis, the ANS and the immune system in response to stress (modified from Sternberg, Nature Reviews Immunology, 2006 (4)). Exposure to stressors like pro-inflammatory cytokines leads to the production of corticotropin-releasing hormone (CRH) from the hypothalamus into the vicinity of the pituitary gland (PG). This triggers the release of adrenocorticotropic hormone (ACTH), which promotes the production of glucocorticoids. Glucocorticoids regulate inflammation via their anti-inflammatory properties and also downregulate the HPA axis in order to maintain homeostasis. Another negative-feedback control of systemic inflammation is provided by the vagus nerve fibres following their activation by pro-inflammatory molecules.

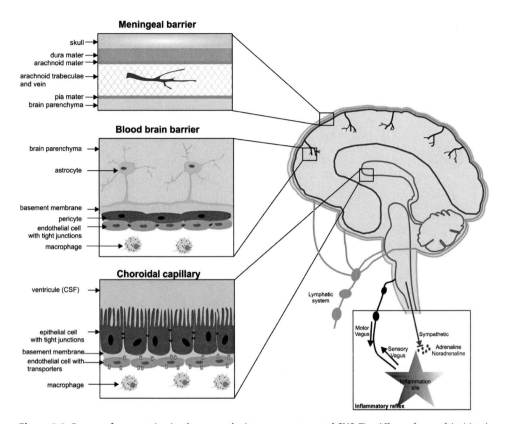

Figure 3.2 Routes of communication between the immune system and CNS. The different facets of the blood-brain interface can become leaky or break down following inflammation or physical trauma. In the meningeal barrier, the pia mater allows cerebrospinal fluid (CSF) that circulates in the subarachnoid space to enter the brain interstitial fluid. The BBB is formed by small blood capillaries that infiltrate information into the deeper structures of the brain. Any leakage from the blood into the brain is prevented by the presence of pericytes and astrocytes wrapped around the endothelial cells bearing tight junctions. The choroid plexus is formed by epithelial cells with tight junctions in order to prevent the passage of molecules from the CSF into the brain. However, the choroidal endothelial cells contain transporters that allow selective active transport of substances into and out of the CSF. The lymphatic drainage system is another tool for the organism to filter inflammatory signals as well as maintain water and solute balance, homeostasis and metabolism. Finally, the inflammatory reflex is a neural circuit that regulates the immune response to injury and infection The vagus nerve sends the inflammatory information via the nucleus tractus solitarius to the forebrain where the information is integrated, and a response is sent back via the efferent vagus branch of the inflammatory reflex to peripheral organs in order to suppress pro-inflammatory cytokine release. Sympathetic output directs adrenaline and noradrenaline to the inflammation site to attenuate the response.

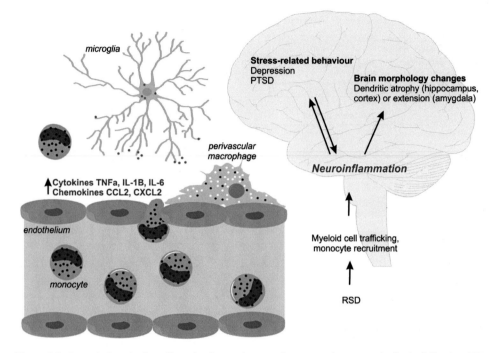

Figure 3.3 **Stress-induced microglia activation and macrophage recruitment to the brain following RSD have long-term effects on brain morphology and behaviour.** Repeated social defeat triggers inflammatory monocytes to cross the BBB and differentiate into perivascular and parenchymal macrophages. These cells and activated microglia contribute to the neuroinflammatory signalling and the enhanced production of cytokines and chemokines, which are involved in specific regional morphology changes and stress-related behaviour.

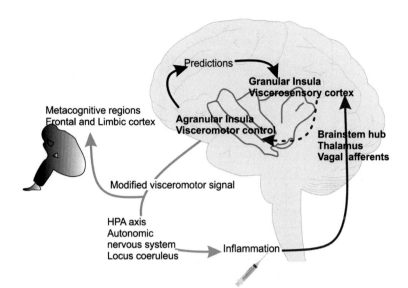

Figure 3.4 Bayesian-brain connections. Blue arrow represents visceromotor predictions (model) of the inflammatory state of the body. The red arrow represents the inflammatory stimulus that is conveyed to the brain through interoceptive/humoral pathways. The mismatch between predictions and incoming sensory signals give rise to prediction error signals (dotted red arrow), conveyed back to the VMC. This leads to activation of LC, SNS and HPA axis – that lead to allostatic/homoeostatic control. Failure of this system would lead to metacognitive appraisal of the homoeostatic/allostatic dyscontrol, manifesting as fatigue/ depressive symptoms.

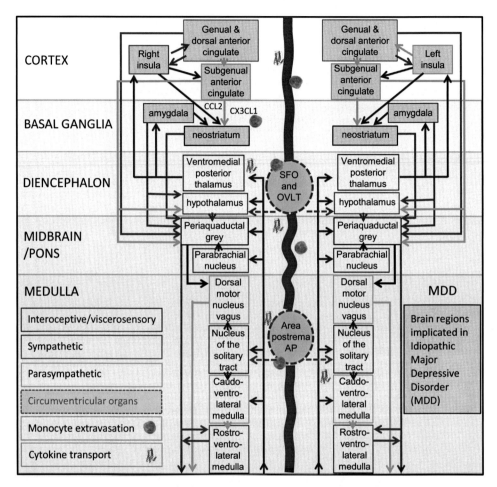

Figure 7.2 Circuit diagram illustrating visceral, humoral, and cellular interoceptive signalling pathways and the major points of interaction. AP, area postrema; CCL2, chemokine (C-C motif) ligand 2; CXCL1, chemokine (C-X3-C motif) ligand 1; OVLT, organum vasculosum laminae terminalis; SFO, subfornical organ. Shaded areas highlight brain regions implicated in the aetiology of idiopathic MDD.

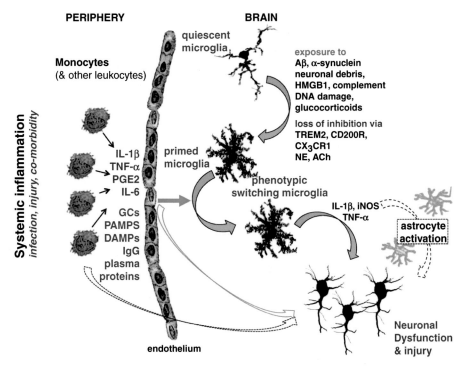

Figure 9.2 Systemic inflammation induces neuronal dysfunction and damage via inflammatory phenotypic switching of microglia and other cell types. Systemic inflammation may be induced by peripheral infection, surgery or injury-induced trauma and these, as well as chronic co-morbidities, induce a range of inflammatory mediators (red) that circulate in the blood or activate leukocytes to secrete such mediators at or close to the brain endothelium. These mediators and both pathogen-associated and damage-associated molecular patterns robustly activate the brain endothelium to transduce an inflammatory signal into the brain. BBB permeability is also affected in neurodegenerative states and further affected by DAMPs/PAMPs and cytokines. Therefore, some plasma proteins and leukocytes may also penetrate the brain parenchyma, while molecules such as prostanoids and glucocorticoids (GCs) can readily cross the BBB. The nature of microglial activation occurring upon systemic inflammatory insult to the brain is highly dependent on the microglial activation status prior to systemic stimulation. During neurodegenerative disease microglia are 'primed' by a number of damage-associated factors to show exaggerated responses to LPS and other stimuli. The priming factors are many, including *exposure to Aβ, α-synuclein, HMGB1, activated complement C3, neurodegenerative debris, glucocorticoids, or the loss of normal inhibitory influences* on microglia such as CX3CR1-CX3CL1, CD200-CD200R binding interactions, loss of tonic inhibition by neurotransmitters such as noradrenaline and acetylcholine. Systemic inflammatory stimulation can induce phenotypic switching of primed microglia leading to more robust microglial activation and synthesis of IL-1β and iNOS specifically in areas of prior pathology. These molecules have known neuronal disrupting actions and have been shown to mediate systemic inflammation-induced neuronal death and dysfunction. Microglial secretory products also activate astrocytes, which can also be primed by prior disease, to produce a range of secretory products that may disrupt and/or damage neurons, although astrocytes may also be activated directly by secretory products of the endothelium. Similarly, although monocytes and other leukocytes interact with the brain endothelium there is also evidence for their infiltration of the brain parenchyma to disrupt neuronal function. Neither the list of microglial priming factors, nor the list of circulating mediators capable of endothelial activation, is exhaustive and cell types are not drawn to scale. Abbreviations: SIE, systemic inflammatory event; LPS, lipopolysaccharide; DAMPs/PAMPs, damage/pathogen-associated molecular patterns; IL-1β, interleukin 1β; TNF-α, tumor necrosis factor-α; IgG, immunoglobulins; PGs, prostaglandins; BBB, blood brain barrier; iNOS, inducible nitric oxide synthase.

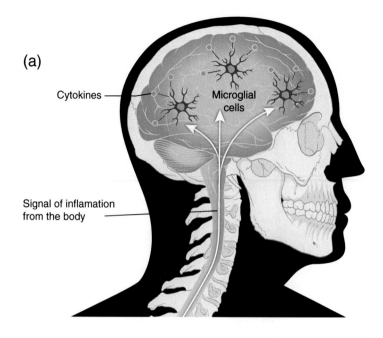

(a)

Cytokines

Microglial cells

Signal of inflamation from the body

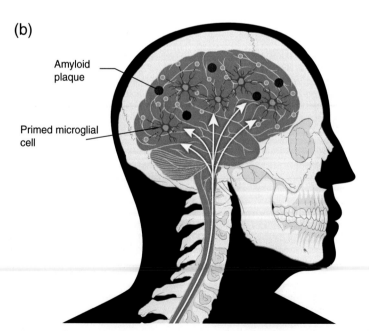

(b)

Amyloid plaque

Primed microglial cell

Figure 11.1 (a) Signals of peripheral inflammation are relayed (e.g., by the vagus nerve) to the immune cells of the brain. In turn, these cells produce cytokines that signal to different areas of the brain to bring about specific sickness behaviours (e.g., lethargy, loss of appetite, depression etc.) (b) In AD the presence of amyloid deposits 'prime' immune cells such as microglial cells causes them to respond more aggressively to the peripheral inflammatory signal with a greater cytokine response resulting in detrimental downstream changes including neuronal degeneration.

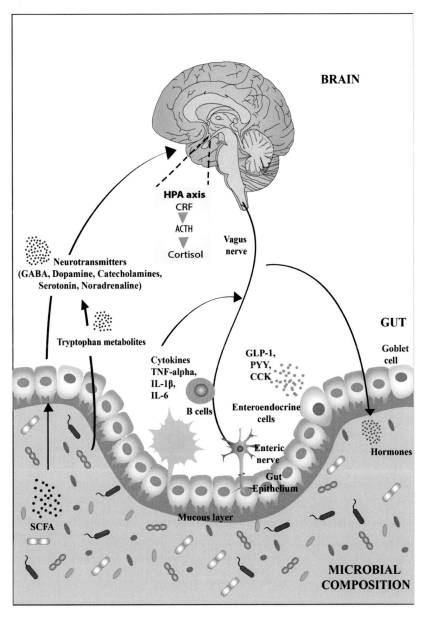

Figure 13.1 Key communicating pathways of the microbiome-gut-brain axis. There are different mechanisms via which the bacteria commensals in our gut signal to the brain. These include activation of the vagus nerve, production of microbial metabolites (short chain fatty acids: SCFA), immune mediators and endocrine cell signalling. Alteration in the gut microbiota subsequently results in the disruption in central processes. Numerous studies have shown alteration in the gut microbiota in neuropsychiatric conditions, which may account for the behaviour abnormalities. Normalization of the gut composition with microbial therapy (prebiotics or probiotics) may offer a viable treatment for neuropsychiatric conditions. ACTH Adrenocorticotropic hormone; CCK cholecystokinin; CRF Corticotropin-releasing factor; GABA γ-aminobutyric acid; GLP glucagon-like peptide; IL interleukin; PYY peptide YY; TNF tumour necrosis factor.

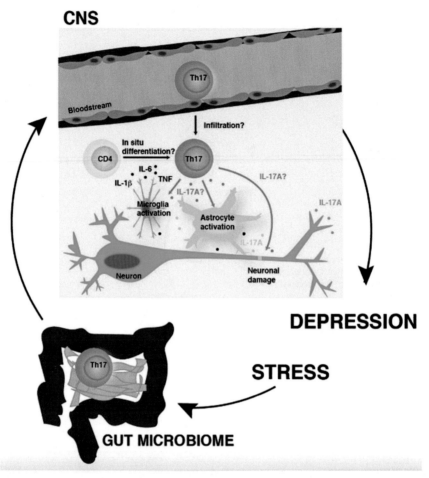

Figure 14.2 Potential mechanisms of action of Th17 cells in the brain during depression. In response to stress, peripheral Th17 cells (possibly released from the lamina propria of the small intestine) may infiltrate the brain parenchyma, or surveying CD4+T cells may differentiate into Th17 cells *in situ* after receiving signals from proinflammatory cytokines (e.g., IL-6, IL-1α, TNF) generated during the neuroinflammatory response to stress. Once in the brain parenchyma, Th17 cells may exert direct or indirect effects on the brain via production of IL-17A or other cytokines or factors produced by Th17 cells by either inducing activation of astrocytes and microglia, and/or by inducing neuronal damage, enhancing the neuroinflammatory response (including the production of IL-17A by CNS resident cells) and leading to increased susceptibility to depressive-like behaviours. Reproduced from Beurel E, Lowell JA. *Brain Behav Immun.* 2018; 69:28–34.

69. Cunningham C. Central and systemic endotoxin challenges exacerbate the local inflammatory response and increase neuronal death during chronic neurodegeneration. *J Neurosci*. 2005;25 (40):9275–84.

70. Perry VH, Cunningham C, Holmes C. Systemic infections and inflammation affect chronic neurodegeneration. *Nat Rev Immunol*. 2007;7(2):161–7.

71. Murray C, Sanderson DJ, Barkus C, et al. Systemic inflammation induces acute working memory deficits in the primed brain: Relevance for delirium. *Neurobiol Aging*. 2012;33(3):603–16.

72. Godbout JP. Exaggerated neuroinflammation and sickness behavior in aged mice after activation of the peripheral innate immune system. *FASEB J*. 2005;19(10):1329–31.

73. Frank MG, Barrientos RM, Watkins LR, Maier SF. Aging sensitizes rapidly isolated hippocampal microglia to LPS ex vivo. *J Neuroimmunol*. 2010 Sep 14;226 (1):181–4.

74. Pace JL, Russell SW, Torres BA, Johnson HM, Gray PW. Recombinant mouse gamma interferon induces the priming step in macrophage activation for tumor cell killing. *J Immunol*. 1983;130 (5):2011–3.

75. Walsh DT, Betmouni S, Perry VH. Absence of detectable IL-1β production in Murine Prion disease: a model of chronic neurodegeneration. *J Neuropathol Exp Neurol*. 2001 Feb 1;60(2): 173–82.

76. Holtman IR, Raj DD, Miller JA, et al. Induction of a common microglia gene expression signature by aging and neurodegenerative conditions: a co-expression meta-analysis. *Acta Neuropathol Commun*. 2015;3(1):31.

77. Mathys H, Adaikkan C, Gao F, et al. Temporal tracking of microglia activation in neurodegeneration at single-cell resolution article temporal tracking of microglia activation in neurodegeneration at single-cell resolution. *Cell Rep*. 2017;21 (2):366–80.

78. Keren-Shaul H, Spinrad A, Weiner A, et al. A unique microglia type associated with restricting development of Alzheimer's disease. *Cell*. 2017 Jun 15;169 (7):1276–90.e17.

79. Mrdjen D, Pavlovic A, Hartmann FJ, et al. High-dimensional single-cell mapping of central nervous system immune cells reveals distinct myeloid subsets in health, aging, and disease. *Immunity*. 2018 Feb 20;48(2):380–95.e6.

80. Deczkowska A, Keren-Shaul H, Weiner A, et al. Disease-associated microglia: a universal immune sensor of neurodegeneration. *Cell*. 2018;173 (5):1073–81.

81. Hughes MM, Field RH, Perry VH Microglia in the degenerating brain are capable of phagocytosis of beads and of apoptotic cells, but do not efficiently remove PrPSc, even upon LPS stimulation. *Glia*. 2010 Sep 27;58(16):2017–30.

82. Cunningham C. Microglia and neurodegeneration: the role of systemic inflammation. *Glia*. 2013;61(1):71–90.

83. Field R, Campion S, Warren C, Murray C, Cunningham C. Systemic challenge with the TLR3 agonist poly I:C induces amplified IFNα/β and IL-1β responses in the diseased brain and exacerbates chronic neurodegeneration. *Brain Behav Immun*. 2010;24(6):996–1007.

84. Yin Z, Raj D, Saiepour N, et al. Immune hyperreactivity of Aβ plaque-associated microglia in Alzheimer's disease. *Neurobiol Aging*. 2017;55:115–22.

85. Lopez-Rodriguez AB, Hennessy E, Murray C, et al. Microglial and Astrocyte priming in the APP/PS1 model of Alzheimer's Disease: increased vulnerability to acute inflammation and cognitive deficits. *bioRxiv*. 2018 Jan 1;344218.

86. Kyrkanides S, Tallents RH, Miller JNH, et al. Osteoarthritis accelerates and exacerbates Alzheimer's disease pathology in mice. *J Neuroinflammation*. 2011;8 (1):112.

87. Godoy MCP, Tarelli R, Ferrari CC, Sarchi MI, Pitossi FJ. Central and systemic

IL-1 exacerbates neurodegeneration and motor symptoms in a model of Parkinson's disease. *Brain.* 2008;131(7):1880–94.

88. Palin K, Cunningham C, Forse P, Perry VH, Platt N. Systemic inflammation switches the inflammatory cytokine profile in CNS Wallerian degeneration. *Neurobiol Dis.* 2008;30(1):19–29.

89. Cunningham C. Microglia and neurodegeneration. The role of systemic inflammation. *Glia.* 2013;61(1):71–90.

90. Saijo K, Glass CK. Microglial cell origin and phenotypes in health and disease. *Nat Rev Immunol.* 2011 Oct 25;11(11):775–87.

91. Couch Y, Alvarez-Erviti L, Sibson NR, Wood MJA, Anthony DC. The acute inflammatory response to intranigral α-synuclein differs significantly from intranigral lipopolysaccharide and is exacerbated by peripheral inflammation. *J Neuroinflammation.* 2011 Nov 28;8:166.

92. Andersson U, Tracey KJ. HMGB1 is a therapeutic target for sterile inflammation and infection. *Annu Rev Immunol.* 2011;29:139–62.

93. Paudel YN, Shaikh MF, Chakraborti A, et al. HMGB1: a common biomarker and potential target for TBI, neuroinflammation, epilepsy, and cognitive dysfunction. *Front Neurosci.* 2018 Sep 11;12:628.

94. Fonken LK, Frank MG, Kitt MM, et al. The alarmin HMGB1 mediates age-induced neuroinflammatory priming. *J Neurosci.* 2016 Jul 27;36(30):LP7946–56.

95. Weber MD, Frank MG, Tracey KJ, Watkins LR, Maier SF. Stress induces the danger-associated molecular pattern HMGB-1 in the hippocampus of male sprague dawley rats: a priming stimulus of microglia and the NLRP3 inflammasome. *J Neurosci.* 2015 Jan 7;35(1):316–24.

96. Barrientos RM, Frank MG, Hein AM, et al. Time course of hippocampal IL-1 β and memory consolidation impairments in aging rats following peripheral infection. *Brain Behav Immun.* 2009;23(1):46–54.

97. Hong S, Beja-Glasser VF, Nfonoyim BM, et al. Complement and microglia mediate early synapse loss in Alzheimer mouse models. *Science.* 2016 May 6;352 (6286):712–6.

98. Ramaglia V, Hughes TR, Donev RM, et al. C3-dependent mechanism of microglial priming relevant to multiple sclerosis. *Proc Natl Acad Sci USA.* 2012 Jan 17;109 (3):965–70.

99. Raj DDA, Jaarsma D, Holtman IR, et al. Priming of microglia in a DNA-repair deficient model of accelerated aging. *Neurobiol Aging.* 2014;35(9): 2147–60.

100. Lunnon K, Teeling JL, Tutt AL, et al. Systemic inflammation modulates Fc receptor expression on microglia during chronic neurodegeneration. *J Immunol.* 2011 Jun 15;186(12):7215–24.

101. Poliani PL, Wang Y, Fontana E, et al. TREM2 sustains microglial expansion during aging and response to demyelination. *J Clin Invest.* 2015 May 1;125(5):2161–70.

102. Lill CM, Rengmark A, Pihlstrøm L, et al. The role of TREM2 R47H as a risk factor for Alzheimer's disease, frontotemporal lobar degeneration, amyotrophic lateral sclerosis, and Parkinson's disease. *Alzheimer's Dement.* 2015 Dec 1;11 (12):1407–16.

103. Zhao Y, Wu X, Li X, et al. TREM2 is a receptor for β-amyloid that mediates microglial function. *Neuron.* 2018 Mar 7;97(5):1023–31.e7.

104. Fahrenhold M, Rakic S, Classey J, et al. TREM2 expression in the human brain: a marker of monocyte recruitment? *Brain Pathol.* 2018 Sep;28(5):595–602.

105. Vitek MP, Brown CM, Colton CA. APOE genotype-specific differences in the innate immune response. *Neurobiol Aging.* 2009 Sep;30(9):1350–60.

106. Gale SC, Gao L, Mikacenic C, et al. APOε4 is associated with enhanced in vivo innate immune responses in human subjects. *J Allergy Clin Immunol.* 2014 Jul;134 (1):127–34.

107. Bennett FC, Bennett ML, Yaqoob F, et al. A combination of ontogeny and CNS

environment establishes microglial identity. *Neuron*. 2018 Jun 27;98(6):1170–83e8.

108. Costello DA, Lyons A, Denieffe S, et al. Long term potentiation is impaired in membrane glycoprotein CD200-deficient mice: a role for Toll-like receptor activation. *J Biol Chem*. 2011 Oct 7;286 (40):34722–32.

109. Wynne AM, Henry CJ, Huang Y, Cleland A, Godbout JP. Protracted downregulation of CX3CR1 on microglia of aged mice after lipopolysaccharide challenge. *Brain Behav Immun*. 2010;24 (7):1190–201.

110. Lehrman EK, Wilton DK, Litvina EY, et al. CD47 protects synapses from excess microglia-mediated pruning during development. *Neuron*. 2018;100 (1):120–134.e6.

111. O'Sullivan JB, Ryan KM, Curtin NM, Harkin A, Connor TJ. Noradrenaline reuptake inhibitors limit neuroinflammation in rat cortex following a systemic inflammatory challenge: implications for depression and neurodegeneration. *Int J Neuropsychopharmacol*. 2009 Jun 1;12(5):687–99.

112. Heneka MT, Nadrigny F, Regen T, et al. Locus ceruleus controls Alzheimer's disease pathology by modulating microglial functions through norepinephrine. *Proc Natl Acad Sci USA*. 2010 Mar 30;107(13):6058–63.

113. Tracey KJ. Reflex control of immunity. *Nat Rev Immunol*. 2009;9(6):418–28.

114. Frank MG, Thompson BM, Watkins LR, Maier SF. Glucocorticoids mediate stress-induced priming of microglial pro-inflammatory responses. *Brain Behav Immun*. 2012 Feb 24;26(2):337–45.

115. Ros-Bernal F, Hunot S, Herrero MT, et al. Microglial glucocorticoid receptors play a pivotal role in regulating dopaminergic neurodegeneration in parkinsonism. *Proc Natl Acad Sci*. 2011 Apr 19;108(16):6632–37.

116. Munhoz CD, Sorrells SF, Caso JR, Scavone C, Sapolsky RM. Glucocorticoids exacerbate lipopolysaccharide-induced signaling in the frontal cortex and hippocampus in a dose-dependent manner. *J Neurosci*. 2010;30(41):13690–8.

117. Drake C, Boutin H, Jones MS, et al. Brain inflammation is induced by co-morbidities and risk factors for stroke. *Brain Behav Immun*. 2011 Aug 16;25 (6–4):1113–22.

118. Sheng JG, Bora SH, Xu G, et al. Lipopolysaccharide-induced-neuroinflammation increases intracellular accumulation of amyloid precursor protein and amyloid β peptide in APPswe transgenic mice. *Neurobiol Dis*. 2003;14(1):133–45.

119. Cunningham C, Hennessy E. Co-morbidity and systemic inflammation as drivers of cognitive decline: new experimental models adopting a broader paradigm in dementia research. *Alzheimer's Res Ther*. 2015;7(1):33.

120. Muccigrosso MM, Ford J, Benner B, et al. Cognitive deficits develop 1 month after diffuse brain injury and are exaggerated by microglia-associated reactivity to peripheral immune challenge. *Brain Behav Immun*. 2016 May 14;54:95–109.

121. Johnson VE, Stewart JE, Begbie FD, et al. Inflammation and white matter degeneration persist for years after a single traumatic brain injury. *Brain*, 2013 Jan 1;136(1):28–42.

122. Netea MG, Latz E, Mills KHG, O'Neill LAJ. Innate immune memory: a paradigm shift in understanding host defense. *Nat Immunol*. 2015 Jun 18;16 (7):675–9.

123. Püntener U, Booth SG, Perry VH, Teeling JL. Long-term impact of systemic bacterial infection on the cerebral vasculature and microglia. *J Neuroinflammation*. 2012 Jun 27;9:146.

124. Wendeln A-C, Degenhardt K, Kaurani L, et al. Innate immune memory in the brain shapes neurological disease hallmarks. *Nature*. 2018;556(7701):332–8.

125. Bodea L-G, Wang Y, Linnartz-Gerlach B, et al. Neurodegeneration by activation of the microglial complement–phagosome

pathway. *J Neurosci.* 2014 Jun 18;34(25): LP8546–56.

126. Askew K, Li K, Olmos-alonso A, et al. Coupled proliferation and apoptosis maintain the rapid turnover of microglia in the adult brain. *Cell Rep.* 2017;18 (2):391–405.

127. Füger P, Hefendehl JK, Veeraraghavalu K, et al. Microglia turnover with aging and in an Alzheimer's model via long-term in vivo single-cell imaging. *Nat Neurosci.* 2017 Aug 28;20(10):1371–6.

128. Hopperton KE, Mohammad D, Trépanier MO, Giuliano V, Bazinet RP. Markers of microglia in post-mortem brain samples from patients with Alzheimer's disease: a systematic review. *Mol Psychiatry.* 2017 Dec 12;23:177.

129. Minett T, Classey J, Matthews FE, et al. Microglial immunophenotype in dementia with Alzheimer's pathology. *J Neuroinflammation.* 2016; 13(1):135.

130. Griffin WST, Sheng JG, Roberts GW, Mrak RE. Interleukin-1 expression in different plaque types in Alzheimer's disease: significance in plaque evolution. *J Neuropathol Exp Neurol.* 1995 Mar 1;54 (2):276–81.

131. McGeer PL, Akiyama H, Itagaki S, McGeer EG. Activation of the classical complement pathway in brain tissue of Alzheimer patients. *Neurosci Lett.* 1989;107(1):341–6.

132. Lemstra AW, Groen in't Woud JCM, Hoozemans JJM, et al. Microglia activation in sepsis: a case-control study. *J Neuroinflammation.* 2007;4(1):4.

133. Gosselin D, Skola D, Coufal NG, et al. An environment-dependent transcriptional network specifics human microglia identity. *Science.* 2017 Jun 23;356(6344): eaal3222.

134. Galatro TF, Holtman IR, Lerario AM, et al. Transcriptomic analysis of purified human cortical microglia reveals age-associated changes. *Nat Neurosci.* 2017;20(8):1162–71.

135. Pugh CR, Kumagawa K, Fleshner M, et al. Selective effects of peripheral lipopolysaccharide administration on contextual and auditory-cue fear conditioning. *Brain Behav Immun.* 1998;12(3):212–29.

136. Katsuki H, Nakai S, Hirai Y, et al. Interleukin-1β inhibits long-term potentiation in the CA3 region of mouse hippocampal slices. *Eur J Pharmacol.* 1990;181(3):323–6.

137. Lynch MA. Long-term potentiation and memory. *Physiol Rev.* 2004 Jan 1;84 (1):87–136.

138. Frank MG, Barrientos RM, Hein AM, et al. IL-1RA blocks E. coli-induced suppression of Arc and long-term memory in aged F344 × BN F1 rats. *Brain Behav Immun.* 2010;24(2):254–62.

139. Cibelli M, Fidalgo AR, Terrando N, et al. Role of interleukin-1β in postoperative cognitive dysfunction. *Ann Neurol.* 2010;68(3):360–8.

140. Griffin EW, Skelly DT, Murray CL, Cunningham C. Cyclooxygenase-1-dependent prostaglandins mediate susceptibility to systemic inflammation-induced acute cognitive dysfunction. *J Neurosci.* 2013;33 (38):15248–58.

141. Skelly D, Griffin EW, Murray C, et al. Acute transient cognitive dysfunction and acute brain injury induced by systemic inflammation occur by dissociable IL-1-dependent mechanisms. *Mol Psychiatry.* 2019;24:1533–48.

142. Thygesen C, Ilkjær L, Kempf SJ, et al. Diverse protein profiles in CNS myeloid cells and CNS tissue from lipopolysaccharide- and vehicle-injected APPSWE/PS1ΔE9 transgenic mice implicate cathepsin Z in Alzheimer's disease. *Frontiers in Cellular Neuroscience.* 2018; 12:397.

143. Bhaskar K, Konerth M, Kokiko-Cochran ON, et al. Regulation of tau pathology by the microglial fractalkine receptor. *Neuron.* 2010 Oct 6;68(1):19–31.

144. Gao H-M, Zhang F, Zhou H, et al. Neuroinflammation and α-synuclein

dysfunction potentiate each other, driving chronic progression of neurodegeneration in a mouse model of Parkinson's disease. *Environ Health Perspect.* 2011 Jun 18;119(6):807–14.

145. Moreno B, Jukes JP, Vergara-Irigaray N, et al. Systemic inflammation induces axon injury during brain inflammation. *Ann Neurol.* 2011;70(6):932–42.

146. Sofroniew MV. Astrocyte barriers to neurotoxic inflammation. *Nat Rev Neurosci.* 2015 Apr 20;16(5):249–63.

147. Murray KN, Parry-Jones AR, Allan SM. Interleukin-1 and acute brain injury. *Frontiers in Cellular Neuroscience.* 2015;9:18.

148. Wang Y, Jin S, Sonobe Y, et al. Interleukin-1β induces blood–brain barrier disruption by downregulating sonic hedgehog in astrocytes. *PLoS One.* 2014 Oct 14;9(10):e110024.

149. Watanabe M, Masaki K, Yamasaki R, et al. Th1 cells downregulate connexin 43 gap junctions in astrocytes via microglial activation. *Sci Rep.* 2016 Dec 8;6: 38387.

150. D'Mello C, Le T, Swain MG. Cerebral microglia recruit monocytes into the brain in response to tumor necrosis factor signaling during peripheral organ inflammation. *J Neurosci.* 2009 Feb 18;29 (7):2089–102.

151. Vacas S, Degos V, Tracey KJ, Maze M. High-mobility group box 1 protein initiates postoperative cognitive decline by engaging bone marrow–derived macrophages. *Anesthesiology.* 2014 May 1;120(5):1160–7.

152. Andonegui G, Zelinski EL, Schubert CL, et al. Targeting inflammatory monocytes in sepsis-associated encephalopathy and long-term cognitive impairment. *JCI Insight.* 2018 May 3;3(9): e99364.

153. Waltl I, Käufer C, Bröer S, et al. Macrophage depletion by liposome-encapsulated clodronate suppresses seizures but not hippocampal damage after acute viral encephalitis. *Neurobiol Dis.* 2018;110:192–205.

154. Garré JM, Silva HM, Lafaille JJ, Yang G. CX3CR1+ monocytes modulate learning and learning-dependent dendritic spine remodeling via TNF-α. *Nat Med.* 2017 May 15;23:714.

155. McColl BW, Rothwell NJ, Allan SM. Systemic inflammatory stimulus potentiates the acute phase and CXC chemokine responses to experimental stroke and exacerbates brain damage via interleukin-1- and neutrophil-dependent mechanisms. *J Neurosci.* 2007;27 (16):4403–12.

156. Blank T, Detje CN, Spieß A, et al. Brain Endothelial- and Epithelial-Specific Interferon Receptor Chain 1 Drives Virus-Induced Sickness Behavior and Cognitive Impairment. *Immunity.* 2016;44(4):901–912.

157. Le Thuc O, Cansell C, Bourourou M, et al. Central CCL2 signaling onto MCH neurons mediates metabolic and behavioral adaptation to inflammation. *EMBO Rep.* 2016 Dec 1;17(12):LP1738–52.

158. Marciniak E, Faivre E, Dutar P, et al. The chemokine MIP-1α/CCL3 impairs mouse hippocampal synaptic transmission, plasticity and memory. *Sci Rep.* 2015 Oct 29;5:15862.

159. Hasegawa-Ishii S, Inaba M, Umegaki H, et al. Endotoxemia-induced cytokine-mediated responses of hippocampal astrocytes transmitted by cells of the brain–immune interface. *Sci Rep.* 2016 May 5;6:25457.

160. Villeda SA, Luo J, Mosher KI, et al. The ageing systemic milieu negatively regulates neurogenesis and cognitive function. *Nature.* 2011 Aug 31;477 (7362):90–6.

161. Kreisl WC, Lyoo CH, McGwier M, et al. In vivo radioligand binding to translocator protein correlates with severity of Alzheimer's disease. *Brain.* 2013 Jul 1;136(7):2228–38.

162. Sandiego CM, Gallezot J-D, Pittman B, et al. Imaging robust microglial activation after lipopolysaccharide administration in humans with PET. *Proc Natl Acad Sci.* 2015 Oct 6;112(40):LP12468LP–73.

163. Owen DR, Narayan N, Wells L, et al. Pro-inflammatory activation of primary microglia and macrophages increases 18 kDa translocator protein expression in rodents but not humans. *J Cereb Blood Flow Metab*. 2017 May 22;37(8):2679–90.

164. Notter T, Coughlin JM, Sawa A, Meyer U. Reconceptualization of translocator protein as a biomarker of neuroinflammation in psychiatry. *Mol Psychiatry*. 2017 Dec 5;23:36.

165. Tronel C, Largeau B, Santiago Ribeiro MJ, Guilloteau D, Dupont A-C, Arlicot N. Molecular targets for PET imaging of activated microglia: the current situation and future expectations. *Int J Mol Sci*. 2017 Apr 11;18(4):802.

166. Horti AG, Naik R, Foss CA, et al. PET imaging of microglia by targeting macrophage colony-stimulating factor 1 receptor (CSF1R). *Proc Natl Acad Sci*. 2019 Jan 11;201812155.

167. Harrison NA, Brydon L, Walker C, et al. Neural origins of human sickness in interoceptive responses to inflammation. *Biol Psychiatry*. 2009 Sep 1;66(5):415–22.

168. Harrison NA, Cooper E, Dowell NG, et al. Quantitative magnetization transfer imaging as a biomarker for effects of systemic inflammation on the brain. *Biol Psychiatry*. 2015 Jul 1;78(1):49–57.

169. Guldbrandsen A, Vethe H, Farag Y, et al. In-depth characterization of the cerebrospinal fluid (CSF) proteome displayed through the CSF proteome resource (CSF-PR). *Mol Cell Proteomics*. 2014 Nov;13(11):3152–63.

170. Guldbrandsen A, Farag Y, Kroksveen AC, et al. CSF-PR 2.0: an interactive literature guide to quantitative cerebrospinal fluid mass spectrometry data from neurodegenerative disorders. *Mol & Cell Proteomics*. 2017 Feb 1;16(2):LP300–9.

171. Cape E, Hall RJ, van Munster BC, et al. Cerebrospinal fluid markers of neuroinflammation in delirium: a role for interleukin-1β in delirium after hip fracture. *J Psychosom Res*. 2014;77 (3):219–25.

172. MacLullich AMJ, Edelshain BT, Hall RJ, et al. Cerebrospinal fluid interleukin-8 levels are higher in people with hip fracture with perioperative delirium than in controls. *J Am Geriatr Soc*. 2011;59 (6):1151–3.

173. Lind A-L, Wu D, Freyhult E, et al. A multiplex protein panel applied to cerebrospinal fluid reveals three new biomarker candidates in ALS but none in neuropathic pain patients. *PLoS One*. 2016 Feb 25;11(2):e0149821.

174. Coutinho LG, Grandgirard D, Leib SL, Agnez-Lima LF. Cerebrospinal-fluid cytokine and chemokine profile in patients with pneumococcal and meningococcal meningitis. *BMC Infect Dis*. 2013;13(1):326.

175. Pinheiro MAL, Kooij G, Mizee MR, et al. Immune cell trafficking across the barriers of the central nervous system in multiple sclerosis and stroke. *Biochim Biophys Acta (BBA)-Molecular Basis Dis*. 2016;1862 (3):461–71.

176. Rostami A, Ciric B. Role of Th17 cells in the pathogenesis of CNS inflammatory demyelination. *J Neurol Sci*. 2013;333 (1):76–87.

177. Bielekova B, Pranzatelli MR. Promise, progress, and pitfalls in the search for central nervous system biomarkers in neuroimmunological diseases: a role for cerebrospinal fluid immunophenotyping. *Semin Pediatr Neurol*. 2017;24(3):229–39.

178. Ajami B, Samusik N, Wieghofer P, et al. Single-cell mass cytometry reveals distinct populations of brain myeloid cells in mouse neuroinflammation and neurodegeneration models. *Nat Neurosci*. 2018;21(4):541–51.

179. Todorovic V. Single-cell RNA-seq – now with protein. *Nat Methods*. 2017 Oct 31;14:1028.

180. Blennow K, Hampel H, Weiner M, Zetterberg H. Cerebrospinal fluid and plasma biomarkers in Alzheimer disease. *Nat Rev Neurol*. 2010 Feb 16;6:131.

181. Blennow K, Zetterberg H. Biomarkers for Alzheimer's disease: current status and

prospects for the future. *J Intern Med.* 2018 Dec;284(6):643–63.

182. Felger JC, Haroon E, Patel TA, et al. What does plasma CRP tell us about peripheral and central inflammation in depression? *Mol Psychiatry.* 2020; Jun;25 (6):1301–1311.

183. Han S, Lin YC, Wu T, et al. Comprehensive immunophenotyping of cerebrospinal fluid cells in patients with neuroimmunological diseases. *J Immunol.* 2014 Mar 15;192(6):2551–63.

184. Franceschi C, Capri M, Monti D, et al. Inflammaging and anti-inflammaging: a systemic perspective on aging and longevity emerged from studies in humans. *Mech Ageing Dev.* 2007;128 (1):92–105.

185. Björkqvist M, Wild EJ, Thiele J, et al. A novel pathogenic pathway of immune activation detectable before clinical onset in Huntington's disease. *J Exp Med.* 2008 Aug 4;205(8):LP1869–77.

186. McGeer PL, Schulzer M, McGeer EG. Arthritis and anti-inflammatory agents as possible protective factors for Alzheimer's disease: a review of 17 epidemiologic studies. *Neurology.* 1996;47 (2):425–32.

187. Koychev I, Galna B, Zetterberg H, et al. Aβ42/Aβ40 and Aβ42/Aβ38 ratios are associated with measures of gait variability and activities of daily living in mild Alzheimer's disease: a pilot study. *J Alzheimer's Dis.* 2018 Sep 25;65(4):1377–83.

188. Davis D, Richardson S, Hornby J, et al. The delirium and population health informatics cohort study protocol: ascertaining the determinants and outcomes from delirium in a whole population. *BMC Geriatr.* 2018 Feb 9;18(1):45.

189. Schmitt EM, Saczynski JS, Kosar CM, et al. The successful aging after elective surgery (SAGES) study: cohort description and data quality procedures. *J Am Geriatr Soc.* 2015 Dec;63 (12):2463–71.

190. Butchart J, Brook L, Hopkins V, et al. Etanercept in Alzheimer disease: a randomized, placebo-controlled, double-blind, phase 2 trial. *Neurology.* 2015 May 26;84(21): 2161–8.

191. Clark IA, Vissel B. A neurologist's guide to TNF biology and to the principles behind the therapeutic removal of excess TNF in disease. *Neural Plast.* 2015;2015:358263.

192. Nazmi A, Griffin EW, Field RH, et al. Cholinergic signalling in the forebrain controls microglial phenotype and responses to systemic inflammation. *bioRxiv.* 2021. doi: https://doi.org/10.1101/2021.01.18.427123

Role of Inflammation in Lewy Body Dementia

Ajenthan Surendranathan and John T. O'Brien

10.1 Introduction

Lewy body dementia (LBD) is an umbrella term used to group together the two closely related conditions of dementia with Lewy bodies (DLB) and Parkinson's disease dementia (PDD). Cortical neuronal Lewy bodies and Lewy neurites are found in both conditions at autopsy. As well as dementia, DLB and PDD also share common clinical features including fluctuations in attention, visual hallucinations and parkinsonism (1,2). If parkinsonism is present one year before the onset of dementia, patients are diagnosed with PDD, if it is less than one year, or it is not present, the diagnosis is DLB.

DLB makes up about 5% of dementia cases as a whole clinically(3,4), while dementia also develops in over 80% of those with Parkinson's disease (PD)(5), with PDD forming 3.6% of all dementia cases (6). Pathological studies of dementia cases estimate the combined prevalence rate of PDD and DLB to be even higher, at over 15% (7).

The aetiology of DLB and PDD remains unclear, but a role for inflammation has been proposed, based on emerging evidence for inflammation in the aetiology of Alzheimer's disease (AD) and other neurodegenerative conditions. In AD neuropathological studies report evidence of brain inflammation (8), positron emission tomography (PET) imaging reveals microglial activation in vivo (9), genetic studies implicate polymorphisms in genes involved in the inflammatory response as risk factors (10), epidemiological studies indicate a protective effect of non-steroidal anti-inflammatory drugs (NSAIDs) and mouse models of AD suggest NSAIDs reduce neuroinflammation and protein deposition (11).

In light of the gathering evidence for neuroinflammation in AD, we reviewed the literature for evidence that inflammation also plays a role in the aetiology of LBD.

10.2 Literature Search Strategy

References were identified using searches of PubMed with key words. The following combinations were used in a search of titles and abstracts in June 2015 and updated in March 2018 (the number of articles yielded is noted in brackets):

1. 'Lewy' and ('inflammation' OR 'neuroinflammation') (186 articles)
2. ('Parkinson's disease dementia' OR 'PDD' OR 'DLB' OR ('Dementia AND Parkinson*')) AND ('neuroinflammation' OR 'inflammation') (361 articles)
3. 'synuclein' AND 'microglia' (295 articles)
4. 'synuclein' AND ('inflammation' OR 'neuroinflammation') (410 articles)

The abstracts of these articles were screened and full texts obtained of those articles which were potentially relevant to this review. In order to ensure that all relevant references were sourced, references were in turn reviewed for other relevant articles, supplemented by articles known to the authors.

10.3 Neuroinflammation

Neuroinflammation describes the response to injury within the central nervous system (CNS) leading to the activation of microglia and astrocytes, release of cytokines and chemokines, invasion of circulating immune cells and complement activation. Microglia are the resident macrophages of the CNS, originating from progenitors in the embryonic yolk sac (12). They provide the innate immune response to invading pathogens and also initiate the adaptive response through antigen presentation (13).

Microglia are resting or "inactivated" under physiological conditions with characteristic ramified morphology and distributed within brain regions, such that rami are close but not touching, implying each cell has its own distinctive territory. But even in this inactive state, they have been shown using two-photon microscopy to be vigilant: continuously monitoring the extracellular spaces with their processes and protrusions in adult mice (14). Activation can lead to morphological change with microglia assuming a more rounded amoeboid shape, with targeted movement of processes towards sites of injury or stimuli to initiate phagocytosis (14) and can also lead to production of chemokines, that amplify the response by recruiting other microglia, plus cytokines, free radicals and proteases which destroy infectious organisms and infected neurons.

The potential role of microglia as primary contributors to neurodegeneration was highlighted by the discovery that null mutations of triggering receptor expressed on myeloid cells 2 (TREM2), which is only expressed in microglia within the CNS, cause Nasu-Hakola disease, a rare condition leading to a degenerative midlife dementia, amongst other impairments (15). TREM2 suppresses inflammatory processes and promotes phagocytosis of cell debris and bacteria, lending support for a generally protective function (16). TREM2 variants have been associated with increased risk of developing a number of degenerative conditions including AD, frontotemporal dementia and PD (17). Intriguingly, ApoE has been found to be a high affinity ligand to TREM2 and can coat apoptotic neurons to promote phagocytosis through this interaction, though there was no variation in binding based on the different isoforms of ApoE, which can alter risk of developing AD. However certain mutations in TREM2 that are associated with AD can block the binding between TREM2 and ApoE (irrespective of isoform) (18).

Microglia appear to have an important part both in MPTP (1-methyl-4-phenyl-1,2,3,6-tetrahydropyridine, a neurotoxin that leads to parkinsonism) disease progression and idiopathic PD (19), suggesting a central role in nigrostriatal degeneration, irrespective of aetiology. Microglia may be especially susceptible to mechanisms of ageing as their maintenance is proposed to be dependent on self-renewal rather than replenishment by peripheral blood precursors (20), and their phagocytic function could diminish with age (21), which could be highly significant in age dependent neurodegenerative conditions such as LBD. Systemic infections or disease, which rise in number with age, could also lead to priming of microglia, such that their response is exaggerated and damaging to nearby neurons leading to cognitive decline (22). It has also been proposed that an initial stimulus that triggers microglial activation could persist in neurodegenerative disorders leading to repeated cyclical chronic neuroinflammation causing neuronal dysfunction and cell death (23). The specificity of these changes to LBDs is unclear.

Astrocytes are the primary glial cells of the CNS, involved in brain homeostasis: supporting neurons and regulating the extracellular balance of fluid, ions and neurotransmitters. They also have an inflammatory response, with an ability to secrete cytokines and chemokines and activate the adaptive immune system. In comparison to microglia, astrocytes have been less well studied in neurodegeneration, however evidence is emerging of their potential as regulators of inflammation, in both protective and detrimental roles (24).

10.4 α-Synuclein and Neuroinflammation

α-synuclein is the main component of Lewy bodies which characterize LBDs pathologically, and the likely driving force behind the disease process, hence its interaction with microglia appears to be critical (25). α-synuclein inclusions in neurons and glia are associated with DLB and PDD, as well as PD and multiple system atrophy. In DLB and PDD, the inclusions are in the form of neuronal cytoplasmic Lewy bodies (25) or Lewy neurites consisting of coarse dystrophic neurites. With 140 amino acids, α-synuclein's possible intracellular forms include monomeric (26) or a relatively stable folded tetramer (27).

Many studies have found evidence of α-synuclein's ability to activate microglia and induce dopamine cell loss (28–31), including monomeric wild-type and mutant forms as well as extracellular oligomeric conformations and fibrils. Indeed, neuron-glia cultures depleted of microglia have been shown to be resistant to α-synuclein induced dopaminergic neurotoxicity (28). The initiation of the innate response occurs through pattern-recognition receptors (PRRs) expressed on CNS cells (for example the Toll-like receptor (TLR)) through activation by pathogen associated molecular patterns or danger associated molecular patterns.

Recently the focus has shifted to possible mechanisms of interaction, with models of PD being used to study this relationship rather than models of DLB – most commonly with overexpression of α-synuclein in the substantia nigra using viral vectors. A survey of the literature shows several potential mechanisms (see Table 10.1).

10.4.1 Toll-Like Receptors

A number of immunomodulatory proteins and compounds are implicated in α-synuclein microglial recognition, chemotaxis, activation and response. TLRs 1, 2 and 4 are PRRs key to the innate response machinery and have been reported as having a role in recognition of α-synuclein by microglia (32–34). Microglia exposed to higher-ordered oligomers (but not monomers) of α-synuclein changed to an amoeboid, phagocytic morphology with increased secretion of tumour necrosis factor α (TNF-α) that was reduced by inhibition of the TLR 1/2 complex (32). A separate study found only β-sheet rich oligomeric conformations of α-synuclein could activate microglia via TLR 2, but both aggregated and non-aggregated forms could activate microglia through TLR 4. Furthermore pro-inflammatory cytokine/chemokine release was completely eliminated in TLR 2 knockout mouse microglia exposed to α-synuclein, but remained unaffected in TLR 4 knockout mouse microglia (35). Selective activation of TLR 4 rather than TLR 2 receptors in transgenic α-synuclein mouse models also led to increased clearance of α-synuclein, improved motor performance and rescue of nigrostriatal neurons (36). In addition, human oligomeric α-synuclein injected into mouse hippocampi inhibited memory function, which was prevented by TLR 2 inhibition but not TLR 4 knockout (37). This suggests recognition of oligomeric α-synuclein by TLR 2 leads to inflammation and dysfunction, whereas TLR 4 receptors respond with phagocytosis and cellular protection.

Table 10.1 Potential mechanisms of interaction between α-synuclein and microglia

INTERACTION/ RECEPTOR	PROPOSED MECHANISM OF MICROGLIAL INTERACTION WITH α-SYNUCLEIN	PD MODEL	REFERENCES
TLR 1&2 complex	**Oligomeric α-synuclein induces a pro-inflammatory microglial phenotype through TLR 1/2 complex:** microglia exposed to oligomers of α-synuclein changed to an amoeboid, phagocytic shape, with increased secretion of TNF-α and interleukin-1b. TNF-α secretion was reduced by the addition of a TLR-1/2 complex inhibitor or by a MyD88 inhibitor	Primary microglia cultures derived from mouse cortices were exposed to high-order oligomeric forms of purified human wild-type α-synuclein	(32)
Fractalkine (FKN) receptor	**Fractalkine receptor required for α-synuclein phagocytosis and inflammatory response:** MHCII expression and IgG deposition in response to α-synuclein overexpression is attenuated by deletion of FKN	Mouse model using overexpression of human α-synuclein via viral vector in wild-type and FKN knockout mice	(39)
Secreted fractalkine receptor (sFKN)	**Secreted form of fractalkine is neuro-protective:** soluble sFKN prevents reduction in tyrosine hydroxylase cell staining compared to controls and membrane bound fractalkine models when exposed to overexpression of α-synuclein, despite increased MHCII expression on microglia	Overexpression of human α-synuclein via viral vector combined with a variety of viral constructs of fractalkine	(38)
CD11b receptor	**[β]α-synuclein[/β] binds to CD11b on microglia to direct microglial migration:** neuronal α-synuclein overexpression led to microglial migration toward neurons, which was reduced by antibodies to the CD11b receptor and diminished in CD11b knockout mice	Overexpression of human α-synuclein via viral vector in rat primary neuron-enriched cultures	(54)

Table 10.1 (cont.)

INTERACTION/ RECEPTOR	PROPOSED MECHANISM OF MICROGLIAL INTERACTION WITH α-SYNUCLEIN	PD MODEL	REFERENCES
Galectin-3 (carbohydrate-binding protein and inflammatory mediator)	**Galectin 3 mediates microglial cytokine release:** release of Interleukin-2 and Interleukin-12 after exposure to monomeric and aggregated forms of recombinant α-synuclein reduced by genetic down regulation or pharmacological inhibition of galectin-3	Microglia from wild-type and galectin-3 knockout mice	(56)
Leucine-rich repeat kinase 2 (LRRK2)	**LRRK2 required for microglial activation and dopaminergic degeneration:** rats lacking LRRK2 demonstrated a significant reduction in microglial activation compared to wild-type mice rats, when exposed to lipopolysaccharide (LPS) and were protected from dopaminergic neurodegeneration from α-synuclein overexpression	Rats exposed to intracranial LPS injection or overexpression of human α-synuclein via viral vector	(45)
β1-integrin	**Migration of microglia to disease affected regions is via β1-integrin:** β1-integrin inhibition reduced microglial morphological changes and motility (as shown by reduced wound healing)	Rat primary microglia exposed to α-synuclein conditioned medium (αSCM)	(55)
Interleukin-1 (IL-1)	**IL-1 is required for microglial activation:** behavioural deficiencies that occurred in wild-type mice, following LPS administration did not occur in IL-1 knockout mice. Tyrosine Hydroxylase gene expression was similarly preserved in IL-1 knockout but not wild-type mice	Mouse model using intracranial LPS injection into wild-type and IL-1 (α and β) knockout mice	(43)
MHCII Complex	**MHCII complex mediates microglial activation and dopaminergic cell loss:** overexpression of synuclein leads to induction of	Mouse model using overexpression of human α-synuclein via viral vector in wild-type and MHCII knockout mice	(50)

	MHCII expression on microglia and genetic knockout of MHCII prevents microglial activation, IgG deposition and dopaminergic cell loss in vivo	
TLR 4	**TLR 4 mediates microglial phagocytic activity and cytokine release in the presence of α-synuclein:** microglia phagocytic activity was significantly reduced in TLR4 knockout microglia mice after treatment with different forms of α-synuclein; knockout mice also showed significantly reduced TNF-α production following treatment with α-synuclein	Mouse primary microglia from wild-type and TLR4 knockout mice challenged with cloned human α-synuclein from spinal cord cDNA (34)
TLR 2	**TLR 2 mediates microglial activation by oligomeric α-synuclein:** TLR2 knockout mice exhibited significantly lowered microglial activation compared with wild-type mice when exposed to α-synuclein overexpression; cytokine/chemokine gene induction following exposure to αSCM, was prevented by antagonizing TLR2 and by depletion of the TLR2 gene; and TLR2 was only activated by oligomeric α-synuclein not the dimer or monomer forms	Mouse model using overexpression of human α-synuclein via viral vector in wild-type and TLR 2 knockout mice; oligomeric human α-synuclein proteins released from dSY5Y cells (33)
Fc gamma receptors (FcγR)	**FcγR mediates α-synuclein intracellular localization to autophagosomes and NF-κB pro-inflammatory signalling:** microglia internalized α-synuclein in a dense aggregated form in wild-type mice but a diffuse manner in FcγR knockout mice; FcγR knockout mice treated with α-synuclein also failed to trigger the	Primary microglial cultures from wild-type and FcγR knockout mice, treated with human α-synuclein (48)

Table 10.1 (cont.)

INTERACTION/ RECEPTOR	PROPOSED MECHANISM OF MICROGLIAL INTERACTION WITH α-SYNUCLEIN	PD MODEL	REFERENCES
	enhancement of nuclear NFκB p65 seen when wild-type mice are exposed to α-synuclein		
NRF2 (NF-E2-related factor 2), a transcription factor	**NRF2 protects against α-synuclein mediated microglial activation and dopaminergic cell loss:** NRF2 knockout mice showed increased microglial activation and greater nigral dopaminergic neuronal loss than wild-type mice when exposed to α-synuclein overexpression; NRF2 knockout neurons were characterized by thick dendrites loaded with α-synuclein, similar in appearance to Lewy neurites and this was associated with reduced levels of the beta subunit (PSMB7) of the catalytic core 20S proteasome compared to wild-type mice	Mouse model using overexpression of human α-synuclein via viral vector in wild-type and NRF2 knockout mice	(40)
Prostaglandin E2 receptor subtype 2 (PGE2)	**PGE2 is key to regulation of aggregated α-synuclein levels:** microglia isolated from PGE2 knockout mice exhibited enhanced clearance of aggregated α-synuc ein and showed increased resistance to MPTP with less aggregated α-synuclein in the substantia nigra and striatum	Aggregated α-synuclein from human DLB cases incubated with wild-type and PGE2 knockout mice microglia	(52)

10.4.2   Fractalkine and NRF2

Another molecule which could feature in the initiation of microglia activation is fractalkine, a membrane bound chemokine which acts on its receptor (CX3CR1) on microglia to suppress production of inflammatory molecules. The soluble secreted form of fractalkine had a protective function in an animal model of α-synuclein overexpression, suggesting loss of this membrane bound chemokine could lead to neuronal loss through microglia mediated cell damage (38). Deletion of CX3CR1 reduces microglial phagocytosis and MHC class II (MHC-II) expression in response to α-synuclein, and prevented increased neuronal loss again in mouse models of α-synuclein overexpression (39). Another protein involved is NRF2, a transcription factor for a number of cell protection proteins that appears to have a protective role in the interaction (40) – activation leads to protection from α-synuclein toxicity (41).

10.4.3   Interleukin-1 and TNF-α

Once microglia are activated, interleukin-1 (IL-1) appears to promote an inflammatory response. IL-1α and β knockout mice did not show loss of dopamine neurons or behavioural deficits seen in wild-type mice in a PD model, utilizing lipopolysaccharide (LPS) injections into the substantia nigra. LPS injections are reported to produce microglial activation, cytokine release and subsequent dopaminergic cell loss in the substantia nigra (42). TNF-α knockout mice however showed similar results to wild-type mice (43), indeed TNF-α may have a role in promoting α-synuclein accumulation (44).

10.4.4   LRRK2

Leucine-rich repeat kinase 2 (LRRK2) is a protein expressed on microglia when they are in their inflammatory state and has been shown to have a significant role in α-synuclein mediated microglial activation and subsequent cell loss, with LRRK2 knockout mice being protected from α-synuclein overexpression (45) as were mice treated with LRRK2 inhibitors (46). LRRK2 knockout mice also exhibited increased clearance of α-synuclein compared to wild-type mice (47). Yet mutations in LRRK2 are associated with PD (see Section 10.7), suggesting the contribution of this kinase to PD pathology is unclear.

10.4.5   Adaptive Immune System Mechanisms

Several studies suggest the adaptive immune response is engaged by microglia following their activation. Knockout mice without Fc gamma receptors (FcγR), which are found on microglia and involved in facilitating phagocytosis through binding of IgG, showed reduced pro-inflammatory signalling in the presence of aggregated α-synuclein. Suggesting the latter could be triggering inflammation and antibody mediated cell damage through FcγR (48). However, one specific subtype FcγRIIB, in the presence of aggregated α-synuclein, inhibits microglial phagocytosis, suggesting an alternative means of microglial dysfunction through these receptors in synucleinopathies (49).

A knockout of all four murine MHCII complex genes prevented α-synuclein induced dopaminergic cell loss in a mouse model, strongly suggesting that CD4 T lymphocytes are critical to α-synuclein cell damage. Microglia, as the only resident cells expressing MHCII in the CNS, would be candidates for their recruitment, although infiltrating antigen presenting cells such as macrophages (or their precursors, monocytes) may also be involved (50,51).

Furthermore, mice with microglia deficient in prostaglandin E2, which is thought to have a role in lymphocyte proliferation, have increased resistance to MPTP mediated pathology (52). In addition, inhibiting the JAK/STAT pathway that is known to underlie many aspects of the immune response, suppresses microglial activation, T-cell infiltration in the substantia nigra and neurodegeneration in mouse models of α-synuclein overexpression (53).

10.4.6 Other Mechanisms

Alpha-synuclein, in extracellular aggregated form, has been shown to be a chemoattractant through CD11b receptors on microglia (54). Also, the β1-integrin subunit, which forms transmembrane adhesion molecules has been reported as being required for the morphological changes and migration of microglia seen in the presence of extracellular α-synuclein (55).

Galectin-3 has been shown to be important for the inflammatory effect of α-synuclein. Its inhibition significantly reduced cytokine release by microglia in response to aggregated α-synuclein (56).

Inflammatory stimuli can also lead to truncation of α-synuclein, through activation of an inflammatory enzyme – caspase 1, and subsequent aggregation and neurotoxicity in neuronal cell cultures (57). Such a pathway could lead to cell death independently or synergistically with microglial activation.

In summary, misfolded α-synuclein recognition by TLRs could lead to deleterious or protective downstream effects on neurons, the former possibly mediated through IL-1, LRRK2 and an antibody or cell mediated acquired immune system response and the latter possibly through fractalkine and NRF2 (see Figure 10.1).

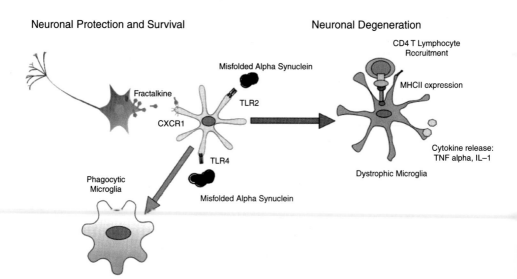

Figure 10.1 Possible mechanisms of microglial activation. Studies of mouse models suggest misfolded α-synuclein can activate microglia through a number of pathways. TLR2 and TLR4 may trigger different microglial phenotypes resulting in detrimental or beneficial effects respectively, on the surrounding cells.

Table 10.2 All studies used 11C-PK11195 except Terada et a. (64) which used 11C-DPA713. * Note no assessment was made of participants and controls as to whether they were low, mixed or high affinity binders, despite the use of 11C-DPA713 which has variable affinity to TSPO dependent on a person's genotype. 11C-PK11195 binding is insensitive to genotype (65)

STUDY	PARTICIPANT NUMBERS (controls)	PARTICIPANT AGE (years)	PARTICIPANT MMSE	DISEASE DURATION (years)	REGIONS WITH INCREASED MICROGLIAL ACTIVATION COMPARED TO CONTROLS
(61)	10 PD (10 controls)	Range: 43–72; Mean: 59.6	Range: 26–30; Mean: 28.3	Range: 0.4–2.5; Mean: 1.4	Midbrain contralateral to the clinically affected side
(68)	6 PD (11 controls)	Range: 60–74 ; Mean: 70.2	Range: 27–30; Mean: 29	Range: 0.6–1; Mean: 0.8	Putamen, substantia nigra
(62)	18 PD (11 controls)	Range: 50–69; Mean: 59.2	Not specifically stated, screening tests normal in PD group	Range: 0.5–21; Mean: 8.6	Striatum, pallidum, thalamus, cortex (precentral gyrus, frontal lobe, anterior cingulate gyrus, posterior cingulate gyrus) and pons
(67)	8 PD (10 controls)	Range: 58–75; Mean: 68.2	Range: 27–30; Mean: 28.8	Mean: 9.2	Cortex (temporal, parietal, and occipital regions)
(64)	11 PD (12 controls)	Range: 62–80; Mean: 68.1	Range: 24–30; Mean: 26.3	Range: 1–8; Mean 3.1	*Cortex (initial scan: left fusiform and precentral gyrus; one year follow-up scan: left middle frontal, left precuneus, left inferior temporal, left parahippocampus, right inferior occipital, right postcentral gyrus, right superior parietal gyrus)

Table 10.2 (cont.)

STUDY	PARTICIPANT NUMBERS (controls)	PARTICIPANT AGE (years)	PARTICIPANT MMSE	DISEASE DURATION (years)	REGIONS WITH INCREASED MICROGLIAL ACTIVATION COMPARED TO CONTROLS
(69)	9 PDD (8 controls)	Range: 64–79; Mean: 69.3	Range: 18–25; Mean: 21.3	Not stated	Striatum, cortex (anterior cingulate gyrus, posterior cingulate gyrus, frontal lobe, temporal lobe, parietal lobe, occipital lobe)
(58)	11 PDC (8 controls)	Range: 55–75; Mean: 68.4	Range: not stated; Mean: 22.1	Not stated	Anterior cingulate gyrus, posterior cingulate gyrus, frontal lobe, temporal lobe, parietal lobe, occipital lobe, medial temporal lobe, amygdala and hippocampus
(67)	11 PDD (10 controls)	Range: 56–80; Mean: 69.3	Range: 16–26; Mean: 21.8	PD duration mean: 10.6; Dementia duration mean: 3.5	Striatum, cortex (frontal, temporal, parietal, anterior and posterior cingulate gyrus, and occipital cortical regions)
(68)	6 DLB (11 controls)	Range: 62–82 ; Mean: 72	Range: 19–30; Mean: 24	Range: 0.7–1; Mean: 0.8	Caudate, putamen, thalamus, substantia nigra, cortex (frontal lateral, parietal lateral, temporal lateral, temporal pole, precuneus, occipital medial, occipital lateral, anterior cingulate, posterior cingulate) and cerebellum

10.5 Imaging of Neuroinflammation and Neuronal Dysfunction

Imaging studies have shown an association between neuroinflammation in vivo and cognitive dysfunction. Microglial activation has been identified in PD and PDD (58) (see Table 10.2), in the majority of cases using 11C-*R*PK11195 (PK11195), a PET ligand that binds to a translocator protein (TSPO) found on microglia in their activated state. Extensive microglial activation has similarly been identified in another α-synucleinopathy: multiple systems atrophy (59), as well as other degenerative conditions, including AD, a condition which shares some of the pathological features of LBD (60).

An association between microglial activation in the midbrain and dopaminergic loss in the dorsal putamen has been found in the early stages of PD (disease duration less than 2.5 years), both contralateral to the clinically affected side, with levels of activation correlating with severity of motor impairment measured by the Unified Parkinson's Disease Rating Scale (UPDRS) (61). In the later stages of disease (disease duration range 0.5–21 years), there is extensive microglial activation, with the basal ganglia, cortex and pons (but not the substantia nigra) all showing significantly increased levels. Follow-up scans in eight of these subjects (after 18–28 months) showed no significant change in microglial activation from baseline despite a clear deterioration in disability as measured using the UPDRS. Cognition was however not assessed longitudinally (62). The authors also noted a clear overlap in the areas of microglial activation and the regions proposed by Braak et al. (63) in their study of PD pathology. Another longitudinal study, this time with a second generation TSPO ligand [11C]-DPA713, found increased microglial activation, compared to controls, spreading in cortical regions (temporal and occipital) in the same subjects over one year, despite no change in mini mental state examination (MMSE) scores (64). Second generation ligands are reported to have a higher sensitivity to TSPO (65), however their affinity to TSPO depends on the expression of a polymorphism in the gene for this receptor unlike PK11195 (66). Yet participants in this latter study were not assessed for genotype, calling into question the validity of the results.

In PDD subjects, there is increased cortical microglial activation compared to control subjects, however levels of activation were also increased in comparison to PD cases, but just in the left parietal lobe (67).

In DLB, increased microglial activation in the substantia nigra and putamen, plus several cortical regions was found in a pilot imaging study of six cases of less than one year's disease duration (68). That microglial activation occurs in more widespread regions in early DLB, where there is greater cognitive dysfunction compared to early PD, strengthens the link between microglial activation and cognitive function.

A relationship between microglial activation and cognitive function has been found in PDD, where cortical activation levels inversely correlated with MMSE in temporo-parietal, occipital, and frontal cortical regions (58,67). Fan et al. also demonstrated a significant negative correlation between whole brain levels of microglial activation and glucose metabolism (58). Femminella et al. went further and demonstrated microglial activation within cortical and subcortical areas in PDD subjects correlated inversely with hippocampal volume and negatively with hippocampal glucose metabolism (69).

Small clusters of positive correlations were also found between PK11195 binding and amyloid load (as determined by [11C]Pittsburgh compound B, a marker of fibrillary amyloid load) in PDD subjects, but this was not as strong as found in AD subjects. There was also little amyloid deposition found in PDD cases overall (58). Proteins other than amyloid, such as α-synuclein or tau, could be triggering microglial activation in PDD, however currently there are no α-synuclein PET ligands available and studies are yet to investigate the relationship between tau and inflammation.

Overall small-scale studies with in vivo imaging have suggested that in PD, PDD and DLB, there is early microglial activation. But, this does not appear to increase over time in regions once it is established. Early microglial activation in synucleinopathies is further supported by PK11195 studies in patients with rapid eye movement sleep behaviour disorder – a condition now considered to be a prodromal stage of synucleinopathies (70), which show increased binding in the substantia nigra (71) and occipital cortex (72), prior to any motor or cognitive impairment .

The evidence for extensive microglial activation in LBDs, in an immunologically privileged site such as the brain, is highly significant. Immune responses are tightly controlled and yet there is widespread inflammatory cell activation, starting early and present chronically during the disease.

10.6 Pathological Studies

Pathological studies further support a role for inflammation. Large numbers of microglia were reported to be HLA-DR-positive, which can indicate activation, in the substantia nigra of PD and PDD cases together with Lewy bodies in association with a reduction in dopaminergic cells. In the PDD cases HLA-DR positive microglia were also found in the hippocampus, though this was associated with neuritic plaques and tangles suggestive of AD pathology (73). Increased microglial expression of MHCII has also been reported in transentorhinal, cingulate and temporal cortices in PD (74).

In a post-mortem study of controls, idiopathic Lewy body disease patients and PD subjects, different patterns of inflammatory cytokine changes were found in the substantia nigra and striatum. Microglial HLA-DR expression in the substantia nigra was found to be both intense and reduced in PD cases. In the striatum, tyrosine hydroxylase fibres were lower in PD compared to controls, but those which survived had particularly intense microglial HLA-DR staining (75).

The presence of CD4 (as well as CD8) T lymphocytes within the substantia nigra of PD cases at post-mortem has also been found (76). In addition, concentrations of interleukin-1β, interleukin-6 and transforming growth factor-α were higher in the striatal regions of post-mortem PD brains compared to controls (77). Complement proteins were also found with Lewy bodies within this region in PD (78). Furthermore TLR 2 expression is increased in PD brains and correlate with α-synuclein deposits. TLR 2 was found on neurons and microglia, the former correlating with disease duration (79). α-synuclein deposits have also been reported in the astrocytes of PD patients within the brainstem and cortex, adjacent to Lewy bodies and Lewy neurites (80,81).

In DLB cases, both complement proteins and MHCII positive microglia are associated with Lewy body containing degenerated neurons on autopsy, suggesting microglial involvement (82). An increase in MHCII positive microglia has also been reported, positively correlating with the number of Lewy bodies regionally (83). However this was not as high as in those cases with concomitant senile plaques and a second study has shown a lack of MHCII positive microglia in the absence of neuritic plaques in DLB (84). Streit and Xue report that Iba1 staining which identifies all microglia, did not find microglia to be hypertrophic, which they consider a clearer indication of activation than MHCII positivity, in DLB compared to controls in the frontal or temporal cortices. CD68 staining was however raised in DLB cases, though this is a label for lipofuscin deposits in microglial cells, that could indicate either activated phagocytic microglia or senescent microglia that have accumulated lipofuscin with age (85). Bachstetter and colleagues found that dystrophic microglia, rather than hypertrophic microglia were the predominant subtype in the hippocampus of DLB cases, suggesting hypofunction rather than a pro-inflammatory role (86).

In addition a correlation between changes in the anti-inflammatory marker CD200 or pro-inflammatory marker intercellular adhesion molecule-1 with amyloid plaques and tau tangles but not Lewy bodies in patients with DLB has also been reported (87). A comparison of middle-aged healthy controls, rapidly progressive (less than two years between first symptom and death) DLB and other DLB cases, found no change in expression of a limited set of inflammatory genes between groups, but did find TNF-α protein levels were higher in the rapidly progressive group compared to controls (88).

Hence, there is some evidence of inflammation but so far there is an absence of a link between microglia and pathological protein deposition in both PDD and DLB. Pathological studies in DLB vary in their findings dependent on the marker used to identify microglia. While there is no evidence of hypertrophic change, MHCII expression and possibly phagocytosis and dystrophic changes appear to be increased in patients with DLB. It should however be noted that autopsy studies are by definition at the end-stage of the disease process and may not be reflective of active disease mechanisms, especially those relevant at early stage of disease.

10.7 Genetic Studies

Genetic studies have identified polymorphisms in genes coding IL-1β, TNF-α and TREM2 as risk factors for PD. Up to a doubling of risk has been reported amongst carriers of a genotype of IL-1β that is associated with increased gene expression (89,90). Those carrying the homozygous variant genotype TNF-α-308, which is thought to be a stronger transcriptional activator, experience doubled risk (89). Overall the results are consistent with a gene dosing effect for these two powerful cytokines. A rare variant of the microglial receptor TREM2, that leads to loss of function, was found to be another risk factor for PD (91). Missense mutations in the LRRK2 gene are found in 1–2% of patients with PD. As mentioned, LRRK2 is highly expressed in immune cells, and could also play a role in the formation of the inflammasome – signalling complexes that play an important part of the inflammatory response (92).

Genome-wide association studies (GWAS) provide further evidence for inflammatory pathology in PD. Polymorphisms in HLA regions that code segments of the MHCII molecule present increased risk. A strong association was found within non-coding intron 1 of HLA-DRA by Hamza and colleagues (93), with subsequent large-scale meta-analyses of single nucleotide polymorphisms (SNP) confirming associations amid the HLA-DR locus, with both HLA-DRB5 and HLA-DQB1 identified (94,95). Wissemann and colleagues found loci that predisposed to, as well as protected from, PD within the same dataset initially analyzed by Hamza et al. (93), and replicated these in a subsequent study (96). The strongest association was again intron 1 of the HLA-DRA region, which regulates gene expression and linked to increased risk. This suggests HLA expression levels may play a role in determining risk for PD. Indeed subjects homozygous for the G allele in this SNP, were found to have significantly increased MHCII expression, compared to subjects who did not have a single G allele. In addition, exposure to a common insecticide, pyrethroid, when combined with possession of the GG allele, significantly increased PD risk (97).

Polymorphisms in genes associated with inflammation are yet to be identified as risk factors for PDD specifically, though ApoE, which may be involved in immune signalling (see above), has been identified as increasing risk (98,99).

10.8 Blood Biomarkers

Elevated peripheral inflammatory markers both before and after the onset of PD, suggest inflammation is concurrent with the disease. Increased plasma interleukin-6 (IL-6), measured on average 4.3 years before diagnosis, is associated with increased risk of developing PD, with higher levels associated with higher risk. After disease onset, levels of IL-6, IL-1β and TNF-α are elevated in PD, as are RANTES (regulated on activation, normal T cell expressed and secreted), a chemokine which attracts T cells, and high sensitivity CRP (100–102). RANTES levels also correlated with motor symptom severity (103) and CRP with subsequent progression of motor impairment (104).

A decrease in the overall level of T-helper CD4 cells but a rise in the subset of activated T-helper cells is reported in PD cases compared to controls, suggesting adaptive immune system involvement (105).

In PDD, high sensitivity CRP is increased compared to controls, but a significant elevation was not found in PDD compared to PD (106). In DLB, one study has assessed inflammatory blood biomarkers in DLB and prodromal DLB, the latter defined as the presence of two core or suggestive features of DLB, in the absence of dementia. While no changes were found in established disease, interleukin-10, interleukin-1β, interleukin-4 and interleukin-2 were higher in prodromal DLB than in controls (107).

10.9 Cerebrospinal Fluid (CSF) Biomarkers

The inflammatory cytokines TNF-α (108,109), IL-6 (110,111) and IL-1β (102,110) have been investigated in PD with raised levels seen in the CSF of PD cases compared to controls. IL-1β levels in the CSF were associated with raised α-synuclein oligomers also in the CSF, suggesting a direct link with protein deposition (102).

In a study of 22 cases of PD, IL-6 was found to associate inversely with disease severity as assessed by the UPDRS (111). In a larger study of 62 cases, IL-6 was elevated in cases of PD with cognitive impairment compared to those without, the levels being negatively correlated to cognitive function. TNF-α and Interferon γ levels were however reduced in those with cognitive impairment in PD compared to control subjects (112). A rise in the fractalkine: Aβ42 ratio in CSF is also associated with motor severity of PD (again measured by UPDRS) but not with disease duration (113). An increase in this ratio could suggest increased inflammatory signalling and microglial activation.

An increase in leucine-rich α2-glycoprotein (LRG), thought to be a marker of inflammation, is reported in the CSF and post-mortem tissue of PDD and DLB cases, compared to controls (114). In addition, the inflammatory marker procalcitonin has been found to be significantly raised in dementia subjects within the CSF, compared to controls, with the highest median level found in DLB cases (115). In addition, in a longitudinal study of PD cases, the inflammatory protein YKL-40 was found to rise over two years in the CSF (116).

Though, when compared to AD cases, DLB and PDD subjects have lower levels of YKL-40 in their CSF (117,118).

10.10   Epidemiological Studies

There is limited support for neuroinflammation in PD from epidemiology studies. A meta-analysis of the association of NSAIDs and the risk of developing PD, showed a 15% reduction in incidence among users of non-aspirin NSAIDS, which was more pronounced among regular users, and those taking ibuprofen (119). A further meta-analysis showed no overall protective effect, however there were methodological differences including the inclusion of aspirin and studies where NSAID exposure was entirely within a year of the diagnosis of PD. Nevertheless a slight protective effect for ibuprofen in lowering the risk of PD was still confirmed (120). The evidence from these studies is however difficult to interpret because of variations in the drugs investigated, the duration of the drug treatment and the timing of administration in relation to disease onset.

Whether NSAIDs could reduce the risk of developing DLB or PDD has not yet been established.

10.11   A Role for the Adaptive Immune System

Despite the evidence of microglial activation and an interaction between α-synuclein and microglia, the precise mechanism and whether it is always detrimental to neurons remains unclear. A paucity of the relationship between Lewy bodies and antigen presenting activated microglia in post-mortem studies was reported by Imamura et al. (74), indeed there was only a 20% association. This would suggest that Lewy bodies alone are not sufficient in themselves to trigger antigen presentation by microglia. In addition, increasing neuronal loss in the substantia nigra with lengthening disease duration was not associated with an increase in microglial activation, which is also reflected by in vivo PET studies (see above), implying a steady rather than escalating inflammatory response (121).

Orr and colleagues (121) also demonstrated that substantia nigra neurons were immuno-positive for IgG in PD, whereas control cases' substantia nigra neurons as well as the visual cortex of PD cases showed negative immunoreactivity. Neuronal IgG labelling related to the degree of neuronal loss and microglial activation.

The MHCII complex is also reported to be key in dopamine neuronal cell loss in mouse models (50), suggesting an adaptive immune response may be the final path to neuronal loss. Consistent with this theory is the genetic risk associated with HLA class II gene variation previously described, as well as the alteration in peripheral lymphocyte subsets found in PD cases (105), and the evidence that T lymphocyte infiltration of the substantia nigra is found at post-mortem in PD subjects (76) and in a mouse model of α-synuclein overexpression (30). In addition α-synuclein fibrils lead to striatal degeneration and invasion of MHCII positive monocytes in mouse models (122) and increased microglial MHCII expression has been repeatedly found at post-mortem in Lewy body disorders (83,84).

It is possible initial protein clearance by microglia could be switched to a more harmful toxic function through initiation of the adaptive response leading to neuronal degeneration. Triggers for this switch may be peripheral inflammation or increased vulnerability of microglia through ageing, the latter supported by the identification of increased dystrophic microglia in DLB (86). The timing of treatment initiation would be key in such circumstances.

10.12 Conclusion

Evidence for the role of neuroinflammation in LBDs continues to accumulate, building on the evidence of neuroinflammation in AD and PD. Imaging studies lead the way in supporting neuroinflammation as a key part of the pathogen process in LBDs, supported by pathological and biomarker evidence. Future studies are required to further establish the presence of inflammation in DLB including imaging and peripheral biomarker studies.

Involvement of microglia in LBDs is signified by the presence of activation years before neuronal death as revealed by in vivo imaging. Microglial involvement is also supported by evidence of the activation of microglia by α-synuclein. Levels of activation however appear to remain relatively stable, which could indicate initiation and propagation of the disease process by microglia or alternatively a protective function that is eventually overcome. In order to understand how inflammation affects disease progression in LBD, studies need to try and link the nature and extent of microglial activation with peripheral markers and important indicators of disease severity such as protein deposition and the onset and progression of key cognitive and non-cognitive symptoms through longitudinal studies in established disease and in those at risk. A better understanding of these mechanisms and the stage within the disease at which they operate, could potentially lead the way to trials of novel immunomodulatory therapies.

10.13 Acknowledgements

This research was supported by the National Institute for Health Research (NIHR) Cambridge Dementia Biomedical Research Unit based at the Cambridge Biomedical Campus.

This review was adapted from the paper published in Parkinsonism and Related Disorders in October 2015 (123) where AS was lead author and wrote the manuscript.

References

1. McKeith IG, Boeve BF, Dickson DW, et al. Diagnosis and management of dementia with Lewy bodics: fourth consensus report of the DLB Consortium. *Neurology.* 2017;89 (1):88–100.

2. Emre M, Aarsland D, Brown R, et al. Clinical diagnostic criteria for dementia associated with Parkinson's disease. *Mov Disord.* 2007;22(12):1689–707.

3. Hogan D, Fiest KM, Roberts JI, et al. The prevalence and incidence of dementia with Lewy bodies: a systematic review. *Can J Neurol Sci.* 2016;43(S1):S83–95.

4. Vann Jones SA, O'Brien JT. The prevalence and incidence of dementia with Lewy bodies: a systematic review of population and clinical studies. *Psychol Med.* 2014;44 (4):673–83.

5. Hely MA, Reid WGJ, Adena MA, Halliday GM, Morris JGL. The Sydney multicenter study of Parkinson's disease: the inevitability of dementia at 20 years. *Mov Disord.* 2008;23(6): 837–44.

6. Aarsland D, Zaccai J, Brayne C. A systematic review of prevalence studies of dementia in Parkinson's disease. *Mov Disord.* 2005;20 (10):1255–63.

7. Fujimi K, Sasaki K, Noda K, et al. Clinicopathological outline of dementia with Lewy bodies applying the revised criteria: the Hisayama study. *Brain Pathol.* 2008;18(3):317–25.

8. McGeer PL, McGeer EG. The amyloid cascade-inflammatory hypothesis of Alzheimer disease: Implications for therapy. *Acta Neuropathol.* 2013;126(4):479–97.

9. Hamelin L, Lagarde J, Dorothé G, et al. Early and protective microglial activation in Alzheimer's disease: a prospective study using 18 F-DPA-714 PET imaging. *Brain.* 2016;139(4):1252–64.

10. Lambert JC, Ibrahim-Verbaas CA, Harold D, et al. Meta-analysis of 74,046 individuals identifies 11 new susceptibility loci for Alzheimer's disease. *Nat Genet.* 2013;45(12):1452–8.

11. Lee Y-J, Han SB, Nam S-Y, Oh K-W, Hong JT. Inflammation and Alzheimer's disease. *Arch Pharm Res.* 2010;33 (10):1539–56.

12. Ginhoux F, Lim S, Hoeffel G, Low D, Huber T. Origin and differentiation of microglia. *Front Cell Neurosci.* 2013;7 (April):1–14.

13. Nayak D, Roth TL, McGavern DB. Microglia development and function. *Annu Rev Immunol.* 2014;32:367–402.

14. Nimmerjahn A, Kirchhoff F, Helmchen F. Resting microglial cells are highly dynamic surveillants of brain parenchyma in vivo. *Science.* 2005;308(5726):1314–8.

15. Dardiotis E, Siokas V, Pantazi E, et al. A novel mutation in TREM2 gene causing Nasu-Hakola disease and review of the literature. *Neurobiol Aging.* 2017;53:194. e13–194.e22.

16. Ransohoff RM. How neuroinflammation contributes to neurodegeneration. *Science.* 2016;353(6301):777–83.

17. Yeh FL, Hansen D V., Sheng M. TREM2, microglia, and neurodegenerative diseases. *Trends Mol Med.* 2017;23 (6):512–33.

18. Atagi Y, Liu C-C, Painter MM, et al. Apolipoprotein E is a ligand for triggering receptor expressed on myeloid cells 2 (TREM2). *J Biol Chem.* 2015;290 (43):26043–50.

19. Gao H, Liu B, Zhang W, Hong J. Critical role of microglial NADPH oxidase-derived free radicals in the in vitro MPTP model of Parkinson's disease. *FASEB J.* 2003;17 (13):1954–6.

20. Prinz M, Priller J. Microglia and brain macrophages in the molecular age: from origin to neuropsychiatric disease. *Nat Rev Neurosci.* 2014;15(5):300–12.

21. Bliederhaeuser C, Grozdanov V, Speidel A, et al. Age-dependent defects of alpha-synuclein oligomer uptake in microglia and monocytes. *Acta Neuropathol.* 2016;131(3):379–91.

22. Perry VH, Holmes C. Microglial priming in neurodegenerative disease. *Nat Rev Neurol.* 2014;10(4):217–24.

23. Gao H-M, Hong J-S. Why neurodegenerative diseases are progressive: uncontrolled inflammation drives disease progression. *Trends Immunol.* 2008;29(8):357–65.

24. Colombo E, Farina C. Astrocytes: key regulators of neuroinflammation. *Trends Immunol.* 2016;37(9):608–20.

25. Spillantini MG, Schmidt ML, Lee VM, et al. Alpha-synuclein in Lewy bodies. *Nature.* 1997;388(6645):839–40.

26. Lashuel H a, Overk CR, Oueslati A, Masliah E. The many faces of α-synuclein: from structure and toxicity to therapeutic target. *Nat Rev Neurosci.* 2013;14(1):38–48.

27. Bartels T, Choi JG, Selkoe DJ. α-Synuclein occurs physiologically as a helically folded tetramer that resists aggregation. *Nature.* 2011;477(7362):107–10.

28. Zhang WW, Wang T, Pei Z, et al. Aggregated alpha-synuclein activates microglia: a process leading to disease progression in Parkinson's disease. *FASEB J.* 2005;19(6):533–42.

29. Zhang W, Dallas S, Zhang D, et al. Microglial PHOX and Mac 1 are essential to the enhanced dopaminergic neurodegeneration elicited by A30P and A53T mutant alpha-synuclein. *Glia.* 2007;55(11):1178–88.

30. Theodore S, Cao S, McLean PJ, Standaert DG. Targeted overexpression of human alpha-synuclein triggers microglial activation and an adaptive immune response in a mouse model of Parkinson disease. *J Neuropathol Exp Neurol.* 2008;67 (12):1149–58.

31. Hoffmann A, Ettle B, Bruno A, et al. Alpha-synuclein activates BV2 microglia dependent on its aggregation state. *Biochem Biophys Res Commun.* 2016;479 (4):881–6.

32. Daniele SG, Béraud D, Davenport C, et al. Activation of MyD88-dependent TLR1/2

signaling by misfolded α-synuclein, a protein linked to neurodegenerative disorders. *Sci Signal.* 2015;8(376):ra45.

33. Kim WS, Kågedal K, Halliday GM. Alpha-synuclein biology in Lewy body diseases. *Alzheimers Res Ther.* 2014;6(5):73.

34. Fellner L, Irschick R, Schanda K, et al. Toll-like receptor 4 is required for α-synuclein dependent activation of microglia and astroglia. *Glia.* 2013;61 (3):349–60.

35. Kim C, Ho D-H, Suk J-E, et al. Neuron-released oligomeric α-synuclein is an endogenous agonist of TLR2 for paracrine activation of microglia. *Nat Commun.* 2013;4:1562.

36. Venezia S, Refolo V, Polissidis A, et al. Toll-like receptor 4 stimulation with monophosphoryl lipid A ameliorates motor deficits and nigral neurodegeneration triggered by extraneuronal α-synucleinopathy. *Mol Neurodegener.* 2017;12(1):1–13.

37. La Vitola P, Balducci C, Cerovic M, et al. Alpha-synuclein oligomers impair memory through glial cell activation and via Toll-like receptor 2. *Brain Behav Immun.* 2018;69:591–602.

38. Nash KR, Moran P, Finneran DJ, et al. Fractalkine over expression suppresses α-synuclein-mediated neurodegeneration. *Mol Ther.* 2015;23(1):17–23.

39. Thome AD, Standaert DG, Harms AS. Fractalkine signaling regulates the inflammatory response in an α-synuclein model of Parkinson disease. *PLoS One.* 2015;10(10):1–13.

40. Lastres-Becker I, Ulusoy A, Innamorato NG, et al. α-Synuclein expression and Nrf2 deficiency cooperate to aggravate protein aggregation, neuronal death and inflammation in early-stage Parkinson's disease. *Hum Mol Genet.* 2012;21(14):3173–92.

41. Lastres-Becker I, García-Yagüe AJ, Scannevin RH, et al. Repurposing the NRF2 activator dimethyl fumarate as therapy against synucleinopathy in Parkinson's disease. *Antioxid Redox Signal.* 2016;25(2):61–77.

42. Sharma N, Nehru B. Characterization of the lipopolysaccharide induced model of Parkinson's disease: role of oxidative stress and neuroinflammation. *Neurochem Int.* 2015;87:92–105.

43. Tanaka S, Ishii A, Ohtaki H, et al. Activation of microglia induces symptoms of Parkinson's disease in wild-type, but not in IL-1 knockout mice. *J Neuroinflammation.* 2013;10:143.

44. Wang M-X, Cheng X-Y, Jin M, et al. TNF compromises lysosome acidification and reduces α-synuclein degradation via autophagy in dopaminergic cells. *Exp Neurol.* 2015;271:112–21.

45. Daher JPL, Volpicelli-Daley LA, Blackburn JP, Moehle MS, West AB. Abrogation of α-synuclein-mediated dopaminergic neurodegeneration in LRRK2-deficient rats. *Proc Natl Acad Sci USA.* 2014;111(25):9289–94.

46. Daher JPL, Abdelmotilib HA, Hu X, et al. Leucine-rich repeat kinase 2 (LRRK2) pharmacological inhibition abates α-synuclein gene-induced neurodegeneration. *J Biol Chem.* 2015;290 (32):19433–44.

47. Maekawa T, Sasaoka T, Azuma S, et al. Leucine-rich repeat kinase 2 (LRRK2) regulates α-synuclein clearance in microglia. *BMC Neurosci.* 2016;17(1):1–12.

48. Cao S, Standaert DG, Harms AS. The gamma chain subunit of Fc receptors is required for alpha-synuclein-induced pro-inflammatory signaling in microglia. *J Neuroinflammation.* 2012;9(1):259.

49. Choi YR, Kang SJ, Kim JM, et al. FcγRIIB mediates the inhibitory effect of aggregated α-synuclein on microglial phagocytosis. *Neurobiol Dis.* 2015;83:90–9.

50. Harms AS, Cao S, Rowse AL, et al. MHCII is required for α-synuclein-induced activation of microglia, CD4 T cell proliferation, and dopaminergic neurodegeneration. *J Neurosci.* 2013;33 (23):9592–600.

51. Harms AS, Thome AD, Yan Z, et al. Peripheral monocyte entry is required for alpha-synuclein induced inflammation and neurodegeneration in a model of

Parkinson disease. *Exp Neurol.* 2018;300 (August2017):179–87.

52. Jin J, Shie F-S, Liu J, et al. Prostaglandin E2 receptor subtype 2 (EP2) regulates microglial activation and associated neurotoxicity induced by aggregated alpha-synuclein. *J Neuroinflammation.* 2007;4:2.

53. Qin H, Buckley JA, Li X, et al. Inhibition of the JAK/STAT pathway protects against α-synuclein-induced neuroinflammation and dopaminergic neurodegeneration. *J Neurosci.* 2016;36(18):5144–59.

54. Wang S, Chu C-H, Stewart T, et al. α-Synuclein, a chemoattractant, directs microglial migration via H2O2-dependent Lyn phosphorylation. *Proc Natl Acad Sci USA.* 2015;112(15):E1926–35.

55. Kim C, Cho E-D, Kim H-K, et al. B1-integrin-dependent migration of microglia in response to neuron-released a-synuclein. *Exp Mol Med.* 2014;46(4):e91.

56. Boza-Serrano A, Reyes JF, Rey NL, et al. The role of Galectin-3 in α-synuclein-induced microglial activation. *Acta Neuropathol Commun.* 2014;2(1):156.

57. Wang W, Nguyen LTT, Burlak C, et al. Caspase-1 causes truncation and aggregation of the Parkinson's disease-associated protein α-synuclein. *Proc Natl Acad Sci.* 2016;113(34):9587–92.

58. Fan Z, Aman Y, Ahmed I, et al. Influence of microglial activation on neuronal function in Alzheimer's and Parkinson's disease dementia. *Alzheimers Dement.* 2015;11 (6):608–21.e7.

59. Gerhard A, Banati RB, Goerres GB, et al. [11C](R)-PK11195 PET imaging of microglial activation in multiple system atrophy. *Neurology.* 2003;61(5):686–9.

60. Edison P, Archer HA, Gerhard A, et al. Microglia, amyloid, and cognition in Alzheimer's disease: an [11C](R)PK11195-PET and [11C]PIB-PET study. *Neurobiol Dis.* 2008;32(3):412–9.

61. Ouchi Y, Yoshikawa E, Sekine Y, et al. Microglial activation and dopamine terminal loss in early Parkinson's disease. *Ann Neurol.* 2005;57(2):168–75.

62. Gerhard A, Pavese N, Hotton G, et al. In vivo imaging of microglial activation with [11C](R)-PK11195 PET in idiopathic Parkinson's disease. *Neurobiol Dis.* 2006;21 (2):404–12.

63. Braak H, Tredici K Del, Rüb U, et al. Staging of brain pathology related to sporadic Parkinson's disease. *Neurobiol Aging.* 2003;24(2):197–211.

64. Terada T, Yokokura M, Yoshikawa E, et al. Extrastriatal spreading of microglial activation in Parkinson's disease: a positron emission tomography study. *Ann Nucl Med.* 2016;30(8):579–87.

65. Kobayashi M, Jiang T, Telu S, et al. 11C-DPA-713 has much greater specific binding to translocator protein 18 kDa (TSPO) in human brain than11C-(R)-PK11195. *J Cereb Blood Flow Metab.* 2018;38(3):393–403.

66. Owen DR, Yeo AJ, Gunn RN, et al. An 18-kDa Translocator Protein (TSPO) polymorphism explains differences in binding affinity of the PET radioligand PBR28. *J Cereb Blood Flow Metab.* 2012;32(1):1–5.

67. Edison P, Ahmed I, Fan Z, et al. Microglia, amyloid, and glucose metabolism in Parkinson's disease with and without dementia. *Neuropsychopharmacology.* 2013;38(6):938–49.

68. Iannaccone S, Cerami C, Alessio M, et al. In vivo microglia activation in very early dementia with Lewy bodies, comparison with Parkinson's disease. *Parkinsonism Relat Disord.* 2013;19(1):47–52.

69. Femminella GD, Ninan S, Atkinson R, et al. Does microglial activation influence hippocampal volume and neuronal function in Alzheimer's disease and Parkinson's disease dementia? *J Alzheimer's Dis.* 2016;51(4):1275–89.

70. Högl B, Stefani A, Videnovic A. Idiopathic REM sleep behaviour disorder and neurodegeneration – an update. *Nat Rev Neurol.* 2018;14(1):40–56.

71. Stokholm MG, Iranzo A, Østergaard K, et al. Assessment of neuroinflammation in patients with idiopathic rapid-eye-movement sleep behaviour disorder: a

case-control study. *Lancet Neurol.* 2017;16 (10):789–96.

72. Stokholm MG, Iranzo A, Østergaard K, et al. Extrastriatal monoaminergic dysfunction and enhanced microglial activation in idiopathic rapid eye movement sleep behaviour disorder. *Neurobiol Dis.* 2018;115(January):9–16.

73. McGeer PL, Itagaki S, Boyes BE, McGeer EG. Reactive microglia are positive for HLA-DR in the substantia nigra of Parkinson's and Alzheimer's disease brains. *Neurology.* 1988;38(8):1285–91.

74. Imamura K, Hishikawa N, Sawada M, et al. Distribution of major histocompatibility complex class II-positive microglia and cytokine profile of Parkinson's disease brains. *Acta Neuropathol.* 2003;106 (6):518–26.

75. Walker DG, Lue LF, Serrano G, et al. Altered expression patterns of inflammation-associated and trophic molecules in substantia nigra and striatum brain samples from Parkinson's disease, incidental Lewy body disease and normal control cases. *Front Neurosci.* 2016;9 (Jan):1–18.

76. Brochard V, Combadière B, Prigent A, et al. Infiltration of CD4+ lymphocytes into the brain contributes to neurodegeneration in a mouse model of Parkinson disease. *J Clin Invest.* 2009;119(1):182–92.

77. Mogi M, Harada M, Kondo T, et al. Interleukin-1 beta, interleukin-6, epidermal growth factor and transforming growth factor-alpha are elevated in the brain from parkinsonian patients. *Neurosci Lett.* 1994;180(2):147–50.

78. Loeffler DA, Camp DM, Conant SB. Complement activation in the Parkinson's disease substantia nigra: an immunocytochemical study. *J Neuroinflammation.* 2006;3:29.

79. Dzamko N, Gysbers A, Perera G, et al. Toll-like receptor 2 is increased in neurons in Parkinson's disease brain and may contribute to alpha-synuclein pathology. *Acta Neuropathol.* 2017;133(2):303–19.

80. Wakabayashi K, Hayashi S, Yoshimoto M, Kudo H, Takahashi H. NACP/alpha-synuclein-positive filamentous inclusions in astrocytes and oligodendrocytes of Parkinson's disease brains. *Acta Neuropathol.* 2000;99(1):14–20.

81. Braak H, Sastre M, Del Tredici K. Development of α-synuclein immunoreactive astrocytes in the forebrain parallels stages of intraneuronal pathology in sporadic Parkinson's disease. *Acta Neuropathol.* 2007;114(3): 231–41.

82. Togo T, Iseki E, Marui W, et al. Glial involvement in the degeneration process of Lewy body-bearing neurons and the degradation process of Lewy bodies in brains of dementia with Lewy bodies. *J Neurol Sci.* 2001;184(1):71–5.

83. Mackenzie IR. Activated microglia in dementia with Lewy bodies. *Neurology.* 2000;55:132–4.

84. Shepherd CE, Thiel E, Mccann H, Harding AJ, Halliday GM. Cortical inflammation in Alzheimer disease but not dementia with Lewy bodies. *Arch Neurol.* 2015;57(6):817–22.

85. Streit WJ, Xue QS. Microglia in dementia with Lewy bodies. *Brain Behav Immun.* 2016;55:191–201.

86. Bachstetter AD, Van Eldik LJ, Schmitt FA, et al. Disease-related microglia heterogeneity in the hippocampus of Alzheimer's disease, dementia with Lewy bodies, and hippocampal sclerosis of aging. *Acta Neuropathol Commun.* 2015;3 (1):1–16.

87. Walker DG, Lue LF, Tang TM, et al. Changes in CD200 and intercellular adhesion molecule-1 (ICAM-1) levels in brains of Lewy body disorder cases are associated with amounts of Alzheimer's pathology not α-synuclein pathology. *Neurobiol Aging.* 2017;54:175–86.

88. Garcia-Esparcia P, López-González I, Grau-Rivera O, et al. Dementia with Lewy bodies: molecular pathology in the frontal cortex in typical and rapidly progressive forms. *Front Neurol.* 2017;8:89.

89. Wahner AD, Sinsheimer JS, Bronstein JM, Ritz B. Inflammatory cytokine gene polymorphisms and increased risk of

Parkinson disease. *Arch Neurol.* 2007;64 (6):836–40.

90. McGeer PL, Yasojima K, McGeer EG. Association of interleukin-1β polymorphisms with idiopathic Parkinson's disease. *Neurosci Lett.* 2002;326(1):67–9.

91. Rayaprolu S, Mullen B, Baker M, et al. TREM2 in neurodegeneration: evidence for association of the p.R47H variant with frontotemporal dementia and Parkinson's disease. *Mol Neurodegener.* 2013;8(1):19.

92. Alessi DR, Sammler E. LRRK2 kinase in Parkinson's disease. *Science.* 2018;360 (6384):36–7.

93. Hamza TH, Zabetian CP, Tenesa A, et al. Common genetic variation in the HLA region is associated with late-onset sporadic Parkinson's disease. *Nat Genet.* 2010;42(9):781–5.

94. Nalls MA, Plagnol V, Hernandez DG, et al. Imputation of sequence variants for identification of genetic risks for Parkinson's disease: a meta-analysis of genome-wide association studies. *Lancet.* 2011;377(9766):641–9.

95. Nalls MA, Pankratz N, Lill CM, et al. Large-scale meta-analysis of genome-wide association data identifies six new risk loci for Parkinson's disease. *Nat Genet.* 2014;46 (9):989–93.

96. Wissemann WT, Hill-Burns EM, Zabetian CP, et al. Association of Parkinson disease with structural and regulatory variants in the HLA region. *Am J Hum Genet.* 2013;93(5):984–93.

97. Kannarkat GT, Cook DA, Lee J-K, et al. Common genetic variant association with altered HLA expression, synergy with pyrethroid exposure, and risk for Parkinson's disease: an observational and case–control study. *NPJ Park Dis.* 2015;1 (January):15002.

98. Guerreiro R, Ross OA, Kun-Rodrigues C, et al. Investigating the genetic architecture of dementia with Lewy bodies: a two-stage genome-wide association study. *Lancet Neurol.* 2018;17(1):64–74.

99. Guerreiro R, Ross OA, Kun-Rodrigues C, et al. Investigating the genetic architecture of dementia with Lewy bodies: a two-stage genome-wide association study. *Lancet Neurol.* 2018;17(1):64–74.

100. Chen H, O'Reilly EJ, Schwarzschild MA, Ascherio A. Peripheral inflammatory biomarkers and risk of Parkinson's disease. *Am J Epidemiol.* 2008;167 (1):90–5.

101. Dobbs RJ, Charlett A, Purkiss AG, et al. Association of circulating TNF-alpha and IL-6 with ageing and parkinsonism. *Acta Neurol Scand.* 1999;100(1):34–41.

102. Hu Y, Yu S, Zuo L, et al. Parkinson disease with REM sleep behavior disorder: Features, α-synuclein, and inflammation. *Neurology.* 2015;84(9):888–94.

103. Rentzos M, Nikolaou C, Andreadou E, et al. Circulating interleukin-15 and RANTES chemokine in Parkinson's disease. *Acta Neurol Scand.* 2007;116 (6):374–9.

104. Umemura A, Oeda T, Yamamoto K, et al. Baseline plasma C-reactive protein concentrations and motor prognosis in Parkinson disease. *PLoS One.* 2015;10 (8):1–12.

105. Bas J, Calopa M, Mestre M, et al. Lymphocyte populations in Parkinson's disease and in rat models of parkinsonism. *J Neuroimmunol.* 2001;113:146–52.

106. Song I-U, Kim Y-D, Cho H-J, Chung S-W. Is Neuroinflammation Involved in the Development of Dementia in Patients with Parkinson's Disease? *Intern Med.* 2013;52(16):1787–92.

107. King E, O'Brien JT, Donaghy P, et al. Peripheral inflammation in prodromal Alzheimer's and Lewy body dementias. *J Neurol Neurosurg Psychiatry.* 2018;89:339–45.

108. Mogi M, Harada M, Riederer P, et al. Tumor necrosis factor-alpha (TNF-alpha) increases both in the brain and in the cerebrospinal fluid from parkinsonian patients. *Neurosci Lett.* 1994;165 (1–2):208–10.

109. Delgado-Alvarado M, Gago B, Gorostidi A, et al. Tau/α-synuclein ratio and inflammatory proteins in Parkinson's disease: An exploratory study. *Mov Disord.* 2017;32(7):1066–73.

110. Blum-Degen D, Müller T, Kuhn W, et al. Interleukin-1β and interleukin-6 are elevated in the cerebrospinal fluid of Alzheimer's and de novo Parkinson's disease patients. *Neurosci Lett.* 1995;202 (1–2):17–20.

111. Müller T, Blum-Degen D, Przuntek H, Kuhn W. Interleukin-6 levels in cerebrospinal fluid inversely correlate to severity of Parkinson's disease. *Acta Neurol Scand.* 1998;98(2):142–4.

112. Yu S-Y, Zuo L-J, Wang F, et al. Potential biomarkers relating pathological proteins, neuroinflammatory factors and free radicals in PD patients with cognitive impairment: a cross-sectional study. *BMC Neurol.* 2014;14(1):113.

113. Shi M, Bradner J, Hancock AM, et al. Cerebrospinal fluid biomarkers for Parkinson disease diagnosis and progression. *Ann Neurol.* 2011;69 (3):570–80.

114. Miyajima M, Nakajima M, Motoi Y, et al. Leucine-rich α2-glycoprotein is a novel biomarker of neurodegenerative disease in human cerebrospinal fluid and causes neurodegeneration in mouse cerebral cortex. *PLoS One.* 2013;8(9): e74453.

115. Ernst A, Morgenthaler NG, Buerger K, et al. Procalcitonin is elevated in the cerebrospinal fluid of patients with dementia and acute neuroinflammation. *J Neuroimmunol.* 2007;189(1–2):169–74.

116. Hall S, Surova Y, Öhrfelt A, et al. Longitudinal Measurements of Cerebrospinal Fluid Biomarkers in Parkinson's Disease. *Mov Disord.* 2016;31 (6):898–905.

117. Wennström M, Surova Y, Hall S, et al. The inflammatory marker YKL-40 is elevated in cerebrospinal fluid from patients with Alzheimer's but not Parkinson's disease or dementia with Lewy bodies. *PLoS One.* 2015;10(8):1–13.

118. Janelidze S, Hertze J, Zetterberg H, et al. Cerebrospinal fluid neurogranin and YKL-40 as biomarkers of Alzheimer's disease. *Ann Clin Transl Neurol.* 2016;3 (1):12–20.

119. Gagne JJ, Power MC. Anti-inflammatory drugs and risk of Parkinson disease: a meta-analysis. *Neurology.* 2010;74 (12):995–1002.

120. Samii A, Etminan M, Wiens MO, Jafari S. NSAID use and the risk of Parkinson's disease: systematic review and meta-analysis of observational studies. *Drugs Aging.* 2009;26(9):769–79.

121. Orr CF, Rowe DB, Mizuno Y, Mori H, Halliday GM. A possible role for humoral immunity in the pathogenesis of Parkinson's disease. *Brain.* 2005;128(Pt 11):2665–74.

122. Harms AS, Delic V, Thome AD, et al. α-Synuclein fibrils recruit peripheral immune cells in the rat brain prior to neurodegeneration. *Acta Neuropathol Commun.* 2017;5(1):85.

123. Surendranathan A, Rowe JB, O'Brien JT. Neuroinflammation in Lewy body dementia. *Park Relat Disord.* 2015;21 (12):1398–406.

The Role of Adaptive and Innate Immunity in Alzheimer's Disease

Clive Holmes

11.1 Introduction

In the past the role of neuroinflammation in Alzheimer's disease (AD) was considered to be a simple response to the established neuropathological features (e.g., the extracellular deposits of amyloid beta: neuritic plaques) of the disease. However, emerging evidence now shows it is a major contributor to the progression and development of the disease. Indeed, both preclinical and clinical research supports an early and substantial involvement of neuroinflammation in AD pathogenesis that changes in character as the disease progresses. Here, the term 'neuroinflammation', is used in its broadest sense to encompass any inflammatory process, whether acute or chronic, involving the nervous system. Depending on the nature of the inflammatory process diverse cell types may be involved. The central nervous system (CNS) resident cells (microglia and astrocytes) are a major component of this inflammatory response. However, in some circumstances e.g., where the blood-brain-barrier (BBB) is damaged or in areas surrounding the vasculature of the brain, other peripherally derived cells (e.g., lymphocytes, macrophages and monocytes) may also be involved. In AD the key cellular players are thought to be the CNS resident cells with its key mediators being cytokines but also chemokines, nitric oxide, hydrogen peroxide, complement and anti-microbial peptides (AMPS). However, there is also a developing interest in the potential role of adaptive immunity in the development of AD. In addition, there is increasing recognition that the neuroinflammatory processes within the AD brain are markedly influenced by genetic factors and by inflammatory processes that occur outside the CNS. A better understanding of the central and peripheral inflammatory processes involved in AD will undoubtedly enable the development of clinical tools allowing the early detection of the disease but will, most importantly, lead to new preventative strategies and treatment approaches.

11.2 CNS Resident Cells

11.2.1 Microglia

Microglia are unique among the major cell types of the CNS in that they are not derived from the neuroectoderm (1). These resident CNS cells were originally derived from myeloid precursors, and are representatives of the early migration of monocytes from the periphery into the brain (2).

In AD microglia are ubiquitously distributed throughout the brain and constantly survey their environment for the presence of pathogens, protein aggregates and evidence of neuronal cell death or synaptic damage. Detection of these triggers is mediated by receptors that recognize pathogen-associated molecular patterns (PAMPs); danger-associated molecular patterns (DAMPs) and other cell surface receptors including cluster of differentiation (CD) 33, CD36, CD40 and Toll-like (TL) receptors (e.g., TLR3, TLR4 and TLR6) that drive the activation of these microglial cells (3–6).

Activation of microglia to these triggers is a complex process and our understanding is largely based on models of activated macrophages outside the CNS. Although simplified, activated macrophages can be considered to be in two broad phenotypes. The first phenotype M1 or classical activation is defined by the response of macrophages to challenge by the cytokine interferon γ, a cytokine usually associated with host defence to intracellular pathogens. M1 is pro-inflammatory and is characterized by increases in pro-inflammatory cytokines including interleukin (IL)-1, IL-6, IL-12 and tumour necrosis factor (TNF)-α and is associated with tissue damage caused by increases in nitric oxide and reactive oxygen species. The second major phenotype M2 or alternative activation phenotype is defined by the response to the cytokine IL-4, a cytokine associated with the host defence to extracellular pathogens and is associated with the upregulation of the mannose receptor which binds to the surface of bacteria, fungi enabling their phagocytosis. M2 is characterized by secretion of anti-inflammatory cytokines IL-4, IL-10, IL-13 and transforming growth factor (TGF)β and is also associated with tissue repair and remodelling. A third type of activation, acquired deactivation (considered a subtype of M2) is defined by the response to the cytokine IL-10, a cytokine associated with the presence of apoptotic cells. Acquired deactivation is associated with removal of apoptotic cells, a strong immunosuppressive profile and by an increase in the cytokine TGFβ (7,8).

Whether this simplified polarized view of MI and M2 activation states described in the macrophage population is relevant or helpful in our understanding of microglial cell function is contentious (9). Thus, microglial cells and macrophages have very different environments; microglial cells and infiltrating macrophages show widely different expression profiles and functions and studies of infiltrating macrophages show that these divergent polarisation states are co-expressed within the same cells (10). Against this complex background is the finding that microglial cells show enhanced sensitivity to inflammatory stimuli with ageing with an upregulation of a range of cell surface receptors and an exaggerated microglial response to a second inflammatory stimulus. This phenomena is called priming and its exact causes are unknown. It might be caused by microglial senescence or by prolonged exposure to the aged neuronal environment including the presence of protein such as amyloid (Aβ) protein. The result is that in aged animal or AD mouse models, priming results in microglial cells that show a markedly increased production of pro-inflammatory cytokines, enhanced phagocytic activity and an increased production of reactive oxygen species by microglia following a second stimuli. Thus priming results in a microglial state that once activated cuts across the simple classification of M1 or M2 states by having elements of both (11,12). Thus, within the brain it might be best to think of these polarized states as examples of 'outlying states' with the true physiological position lying somewhere in between.

It is clear from the above description that the activation of microglial cells can have both beneficial and detrimental effects. Classical activation of microglia (e.g., following traumatic brain injury and stroke) is associated with persistent microglial activation, neuronal damage and reduced phagocytic removal of Aβ and detrimental outcomes on disease progression. However, activation of the alternative pathway might be considered to have potentially positive effects by increasing phagocytosis of Aβ (13–15). Cellular studies have shown that microglia bind to soluble Aβ oligomers and Aβ fibrils through the cell surface CD33 receptors (16). This results in activation of microglia with extracellular enzymatic degradation of soluble Aβ and the phagocytosis of Aβ fibrils and degradation in the endolysosomal pathway. Here deficits in the alternative pathway, caused in part by down regulation of CD33 receptors, may lead to inefficient clearance of Aβ by microglia and to the accumulation of Aβ. In support of this hypothesis peripheral macrophages isolated from subjects carrying the single nucleotide polymorphism (SNP) in CD33, an established risk factor for the development of AD, have been shown to have reduced Aβ phagocytosis (17).

The time course of classical versus alternate microglial activation states as the disease progresses remains unclear. Human imaging studies have focused on the direct examination of microglial activation using translocator protein (TSPO) ligands. These studies suggest an early M1 state leading to dementia. Thus, in amnestic mild cognitive impairment (aMCI), considered to be an early form of AD, a study using ^{11}C-PK11195 detected an increase in TSPO uptake (indicative of inflammation) in 40% of aMCI subjects (18). An aMCI study using ^{11}C-DAA1106 showed a 30% increase in uptake in the lateral temporal cortex, compared with controls (19). In this study around 70% patients with MCI with high ^{11}C-DAA1106 uptake, progressed to dementia during a two-year follow-up period. In AD cross-sectional PET studies support evidence of an up to 50% increased binding of ^{11}C-PK11195 in the frontal and temporal cortex of AD (18,20–24) and an increase uptake of up to 33% of ^{11}C-DAA1106 in patients with AD (19). Interestingly, AD studies that have examined both microglial and Aβ markers have found significant correlations between cognitive scores and both TSPO ligands ^{11}C-PK11195 and ^{11}C-PBR28 (25) but not with the amyloid ligand Pittsburgh compound B (^{11}C-PIB) binding(23,26) supporting the view that microglial activation rather than Aβ alone may be a key change leading to neurodegeneration. The lack of correlation of ^{11}C-PIB binding and cognitive scores together with the failure to find a strong relationship between the ^{11}C-PK11195 microglial activation marker and ^{11}C-PIB binding (18,23,24,26) is supportive of the hypothesis that microglial activation is independent of the continued presence of Aβ.

Post-mortem studies, which are largely focussed on the later stages of the disease, emphasic the appearance of an M2 activation state as the disease progresses. Thus, early stage AD brain samples appear to show microglial markers characteristic of an early M1-like population and a separate, more pathologically advanced, M2-like population (27). Other AD post-mortem brain studies have also emphasized elements of M2 activation states in late stage AD with dementia being associated with increased markers of phagocytosis (CD68); macrophage scavenger receptor-A but, interestingly, also markers of reduced motility (Iba1) (28).

11.2.2 Astrocytes

Astrocytes, unlike microglial cells, are ectodermally derived (29). Their role in mediating CNS inflammation has been relatively neglected but they also have an important role in innate immunity, including cytokine production, complement and nitric oxide production (30). In AD astrocytes, like microglia, are found around Aβ plaques in a hypertrophic reactive state and, like microglia, they have also a role in internalization and degradation of fibrillar Aβ (31). In addition, astrocytes have a role in clearance of soluble Aβ from the parenchyma to cerebral blood vessels a process that requires the presence of apolipoprotein E (ApoE) (32). In addition, astrocytes are central to the maintenance of synaptic transmission and because of their location in close contact with neurons and cerebral blood vessels (the neurovascular unit) they can also act to modify BBB permeability (33).

11.3 Non-Resident Cells

11.3.1 Lymphocytes

Some human post-mortem studies have described increased intracerebral T cell infiltration in AD (34). T cell infiltration has been hypothesized to occur due to the activation of microglial cells by Aβ1–42 leading to the release of TNF-α, which then promotes transendothelial migration of T cells (35). AD treatment studies (36) using active immunisation against Aβ are known to give rise to vaccine-induced T cell responses against amyloid-β (37). Whether the consequences of T cell infiltration are beneficial or detrimental is complex. Thus, in animal studies Aβ reactive T cells are able to target Aβ plaque in the brain and to enhance phagocytic activity of Aβ by local microglial cells (38). IFN-γ additionally facilitates T cell migration into and within the brain parenchyma (39) promoting neuronal repair. However, Aβ reactive T cells can also lead to increased levels of pro-inflammatory cytokines which in turn enhances neurotoxicity and impairs neuronal function and repair (40). The differences in outcomes is likely to depend on the different functionality of the T cells (e.g., T helper cells (Th)1; Th2 or regulatory T cell (Tregs)). Thus, infiltrating Th1 cells are usually considered to be detrimental with increased pro-inflammatory responses, increased amyloid production and impaired cognitive function, while Th2 cells are usually considered to be beneficial with reduced pro-inflammatory responses, lower amyloid production and improved cognitive function (41,42). Treg cells, like Th2 cells may also play a beneficial role in the pathophysiology of AD, by slowing disease progression and modulating microglial response to amyloid-β deposition. Thus, in APPPS1 mice depletion of Tregs appears to accelerate the onset of cognitive deficits triggered by Aβ deposition with reduced recruitment of microglia towards Aβ deposits, while selective amplification of Tregs, using low-dose IL-2 treatment, increases numbers of plaque-associated microglia, and is results in improved cognitive function (43).

11.3.2 Mononuclear Cells

In humans it is known that sepsis (44) and persistent peripheral inflammatory stimuli may compromise the BBB because of a breakdown of the intercellular tight junctions caused by lipopolysaccharide (LPS) and peptidoglycans (45). In these situations, a compromised BBB may lead to direct entry of mononuclear cells (monocytes, macrophages) from the periphery into the brain. However, while there is little evidence of this process in human AD, mouse models have shown infiltration of peripheral mononuclear cells associated with amyloid plaques (46). Furthermore prevention of the entry of blood-derived mononuclear cells into the brain, by deletion of the chemokine (C-C motif) receptor (CCR)2 which mediates the accumulation of microglia at sites of neuroinflammation leads to an increased plaque load (47). However, most of these studies used bone marrow irradiation and irradiation of whole animals is likely to cause damage to the BBB. A further study in which the brain was shielded, thereby limiting irradiation to the rest of the body, did not report any cerebral infiltration by peripheral macrophages, but concluded that perivascular macrophages, protected by shielding of the brain, were able to modulate Aβ deposition depending on the presence of CCR2 (48). Involvement of perivascular macrophages has also been shown for removal of Aβ in a mouse model of cerebral amyloid angiopathy (49). Thus these studies support the idea that perivascular macrophages have some effect on removal of CNS Aβ depositions but do not support a substantial contribution of blood-derived monocytes.

11.3.3 Blood and Cerebrospinal Fluid Markers

A number of cross-sectional studies have tried to establish differences in serum or plasma markers of inflammation between AD populations and aged matched control groups. A meta-analysis of these studies (50) suggests that overall there are increases in pro-inflammatory cytokines in AD compared with control groups, although clearly cross-sectional studies cannot establish whether this is cause or effect. More informative data comes from longitudinal studies. Thus, C-reactive protein (CRP) and IL-6, have been found to be elevated five years before the clinical onset of dementia (51–53). Indeed, a raised CRP in midlife has been associated with a threefold increased risk of developing AD up to 25 years later (54) and has been shown to be raised in prodromal AD (55). Another study has found that higher levels of serum soluble TNF receptors (TNFR1 and TNFR2) in MCI subjects are also associated with an increase in the development of dementia over a four- to six-year follow-up period (56). Furthermore, a proteomics study that had not a priori identified inflammatory protein candidates as potential markers of disease development reported the presence of a number of plasma inflammatory proteins including complement factors and clusterin to be associated with hippocampal atrophy and clinical progression in MCI and AD (57). In another AD cohort evidence of acute and chronic systemic inflammatory diseases were associated with raised serum TNF-α levels and an exacerbation of sickness behaviour like symptoms and increased cognitive decline (58,59).

Several studies have also examined concentrations of cytokines in the cerebrospinal fluid (CSF) of patients with MCI and AD. Here increased concentrations of the pro-inflammatory cytokine TNF-α and decreased levels of the anti-inflammatory cytokine TGFβ have been shown to be risk factors for increased rates of cognitive decline as well as conversion of MCI to AD (60,61).

11.4 Molecular Mediators of CNS Inflammation

Both astrocytes and microglial cells are sources of a variety of molecules that orchestrate the inflammatory response. These include cytokines, chemokines, nitric oxide, hydrogen peroxide, complement and AMPS.

Cytokines in the brain are produced largely by microglia and astrocytes. There is increasing evidence from animal studies to suggest that the development of AD is preceded by a relative increase in the pro-inflammatory cytokine response (M1) e.g., TNF-α, IL-6 and IL-1β and a reduced anti-inflammatory cytokine response (M2) e.g., IL-4, IL-10, IL-13. Thus, both cellular and animal studies of amyloid precursor protein (APP) transgenic mice show that pro-inflammatory cytokine expression increases with increasing Aβ levels (62). Several other interactions, also suggest an M1-like activation state to exist in early AD. For example, in neuron–microglia co-cultures, the synergistic action of Aβ with either IFN-γ or cluster of differentiation (CD)40 ligand triggers TNF-α secretion and production of neurotoxic reactive oxygen species (63–65). Additionally, the innate immune receptor Toll-like receptor (TLR)4 is responsible for increased concentrations of TNF-α in mouse models of AD (66). However, although a pro-inflammatory drive may drive the development of the disease, once there is appreciable cell death, mouse models show that the inflammatory response more closely resembles an acquired deactivation state becoming more muted and with active apoptosis (40,67).

Interestingly, and consistent with the priming hypothesis, in a mouse APP/ Presenilin (PS)1 model of AD where microglial are primed by the presence of Aβ, the additional transgenic expression of a second pro-inflammatory stimulus (IL-1β) leads to a robust inflammatory state and a reduction of amyloid plaque pathology (68). In another study, expression of IFN-γ in the brains of another amyloid mouse model showed the ability of this pro-inflammatory cytokine to enhance clearance of amyloid plaques, with a widespread increase in astrogliosis and microgliosis (69). Additionally, these mice had decreased concentrations of soluble Aβ and Aβ plaque burden, without altered APP processing. Similar results were obtained following the expression of the pro-inflammatory cytokines IL-6 and TNF-α (70,71) and conversely, the expression of the anti-inflammatory cytokine IL-4 resulted in an exacerbation of Aβ deposition (72).

In addition to their direct actions via surface receptors, cytokines also stimulate nitric oxide synthase (iNOS) in microglia and astroglia cells, producing high concentrations of nitric oxide that is toxic to neurons, whereas genetic knockouts of iNOS are protective in mouse models of AD (73). Likewise, nicotinamide adenine dinucleotide phosphate (NADPH) oxidase is highly expressed by microglia, and rapidly activated by inflammatory stimuli such as Aβ, resulting in production of hydrogen peroxide, which further promotes microglia activation (74,75).

Chemokines have a role to play in microglial migration to areas of neuroinflammation, thereby potentially enhancing local inflammation in AD (76). In AD, upregulation of the chemokines CCL2, CCR3, CCL4 and CCR5 has been reported in reactive microglia and astrocytes (77,78). In in vitro studies of human post-mortem tissue, Aβ has been shown to lead to the generation of CXCL8 (also known as IL-8), CCL2, CCL3 in human macrophages and astrocytes(79,80).

The complement system is another major constituent of the innate immune system, mainly involved in the defence against pathogens. Activation of the proteolytic complement cascade results in opsonization and in lysis of microorganisms. In the brain, the major cells that contribute to production of proteins of the complement system are microglia and, to a lesser extent, astrocytes (81). Activated factors of the complement system are associated with Aβ deposits (82) and a number of genetic variants of complement are associated with the development of AD providing strong evidence for the importance of the complement system in disease pathogenesis (83,84).

AMPS are produced by a large number of cells including microglia and other phagocytes and endothelial cells in the defence against pathogens (85). AMPS are small proteins, usually less than 50 amino acids long, which interact with the outer membrane of pathogens leading to pore formation and the destabilisation of the membrane (86,87). Oligomerization of AMPS is key to the targeting and increased permeability of membranes (88) with non-oligomerized fibrils having little anti-microbial properties. AMPS also trigger the upregulation of TNF-α. A number of cerebral AMPS are known to exist including neuro-AMP but it has recently been suggested that $A\beta_{1-42}$ is an AMP (89). Thus it has been hypothesized that the development of Aβ deposits in AD may be initiated by pathogens originating in the periphery and entering the brain following altered BBB permeability (90). Whether the signalling mechanisms communicating the presence of systemic inflammation to the brain are also associated with increased brain AMPS is not known, but animal studies have shown that peripheral infections in animal with an intact BBB are associated with the deposition of amyloid (91).

11.5 Modulators of CNS Inflammation

11.5.1 Genetic Factors

In a small number of individuals, less than 0.1% of the total AD population, mutations in one of three genes, Presenilin 1; Presenilin 2 and APP or a duplication of the APP gene (92,93) are directly responsible for the development of early onset AD by altering amyloid processing so that Aβ deposition is greatly enhanced (94). However, the majority of the cases of AD are of late onset. Genome-wide association studies (GWAS) have now established that, in addition to the established common genetic risk factor ApoE ε4 with its large size effect, a large number of less common genetic polymorphisms are also associated with increased risk of developing late onset AD (see Table 11.1). Of the genetic variants identified by GWAS the immune and complement system/inflammatory response pathway is the most substantial accounting for around half of the genes identified. Thus the first two large-scale GWAS (83,84) both identified polymorphisms in the genes encoding complement receptor 1 (CR1) and clusterin. CR1 has binding sites for complement factors C3b and C4b. Like ApoE, clusterin is involved in lipid transport, but it has also been hypothesized to influence receptor-mediated clearance of Aβ from the brain by microglial endocytosis (95). Two subsequent studies (96,97) identified six additional genes (CD33, the MS4A6–MS4A4 cluster, ABCA7, CD2AP, BIN1 and EPHA1), the products of which are all postulated to be involved in immune system activation. A further large, two stage meta-analysis of AD (98) has identified three further genes involved in inflammatory processes including HLA-DRB5-CDRB1, INPP5D, and MEF2C and more recently other protein altering genetic variants highly expressed in microglial cells including PLCG2, AB13 have been identified (99). More recently, in the largest GWAS study to date, of around 90 thousand individuals, four new genome-wide loci have been identified (IQCK, ACE, ADAM10 and ADAMTS1) all of which contain genes that are implicated in the immune system (100). Other genetic approaches have included an attempt at identifying pleiotropic variants (i.e., analysing genetic variants that link to two separate disorders, e.g., autoimmune disorders and Alzheimer's disease). Here research has shown that patients with SNPs for autoimmune disorders are more likely to have SNPs associated with AD that might be expected by chance and that patients with known SNPs for AD are also more likely to have SNPs associated with autoimmune disorders that might be expected by chance (101). More recent research (102) has suggested that innate immunity may play an even more central role than previously thought. This study identified a polymorphism that lowers expression of microglial transcription factor PU.1 and delays the onset of AD. PU.1 controls microglial differentiation and function with a number of downstream targets which have been previously identified as AD RISK genes including triggering receptor expressed on myeloid cells (TREM)2, CD33, MS4A cluster that are mostly expressed in microglial cells rather than neurons. This finding puts the microglial response as key in AD pathogenesis. Interestingly, mice knock outs of PU.1 had microglia with reduced pro-inflammatory cytokines and decreased phagocytic properties. While these new risk alleles have a much smaller individual effect on AD susceptibility than ApoE ε4, in combination they have a substantial impact on AD predisposition. Thus, estimates of the population-attributable fractions for these individual

Table 11.1 Summary of major genetic risk factors for late onset AD

Variant	Chromosome	Closest gene	Odds ratio
rs429358	19	ApoE	3.32
rs75932628	6	TREM-2	2.01
rs616338	17	AB13	1.43
rs138190086	17	ACE	1.29
rs6733839	2	BIN1	1.18
rs4844610	1	CR1	1.16
rs62039712	16	WWOX	1.16
rs17125924	14	FERMT2	1.13
rs3752246	19	ABCA7	1.13
rs9271058	6	HLA-DRB1	1.10
rs73223431	8	PTK28	1.10
rs9473117	6	CD2AP	1.09
rs7920721	10	ECHDC3	1.08
rs190982	5	MEF2C	0.95
rs4723711	7	NME8	0.95
rs12539172	7	NYAP1	0.93
rs593742	15	ADAM10	0.93
rs2830500	21	ADAMTS1	0.93
rs12881735	14	SLC24A4	0.92
rs7185636	16	IQCK	0.92
rs3740688	11	SPI1	0.91
rs10933431	2	INPP5D	0.90
rs10808026	7	EPHA1	0.90
rs7933202	11	MS4A2	0.89
rs3851179	11	PICALM	0.89
rs3865444	19	CD33	0.89
rs9331896	8	CLU	0.88
rs6024870	20	CASS4	0.88
rs11218343	11	SORL1	0.81
rs72824905	16	PLG2	0.68

new loci are smaller than for ApoE ε4 (in the range 1–8.1% c.f. 27.3%) but the cumulative population-attributable fraction effect is 31.7% and is therefore comparable (98).

In addition to relatively common genetic variants with small effect sizes, a rare genetic variant involved in innate immunity with an effect size comparable to ApoE ε4 has also been identified. Thus, two independent data sets have identified a rare missense mutation in TREM2, which gives rise to a threefold increase in the risk of AD (103,104). TREM2 is highly expressed on microglial cells and its expression is thought to suppress pro-inflammatory cytokine production (105) suggesting that these variants confer a heightened risk of AD by increasing the pro-inflammatory response. TREM2 protein can be measured as a soluble variant in CSF where it is found to be increased in early AD probably reflecting a microglial activation response to neuronal death (106,107).

Thus, in summary while early genetic studies found variation in genes affecting amyloid metabolism as being the key genetic component of early onset AD, more recent studies have now identified inflammatory pathways as a major component of late onset AD.

11.5.2 Systemic Inflammation

In the past the parenchyma of the CNS was considered an 'immunologically privileged site' because the BBB was thought to prevent the entry, or exit, of many molecules including antibodies from the periphery and was largely devoid of peripheral immune cells such as macrophages, neutrophils and lymphocytes. This historical concept has led to research on CNS inflammation being viewed in isolation and independent of systemic inflammation occurring outside the CNS. However, communication of the presence of systemic inflammation to the brain is clearly supported by the constellation of centrally derived symptoms that occur in animals following an acute systemic bacterial or viral infection. This syndrome is known as 'sickness behaviour' and includes anorexia; depression; somnolence; decreased social interaction; decreased concentration and fever, and is an evolutionary conserved, homeostatic mechanism that allows the body to adapt to an insult (108). The state of the BBB in AD is still uncertain and, although controversial, it is possible that there may, in limited circumstances, be some direct entry of lymphocytes and mononuclear cells (monocytes, macrophages) from the periphery into the brain. However, as previously stated, in AD evidence of infiltration of blood-derived mononuclear cells is restricted to animal studies and the evidence for this as being an important route of communication of systemic inflammation to the brain is limited. However, there are a number of other communication routes from the periphery to the brain that occur despite the presence of an intact BBB. These include:

1. Stimulation of peripheral nerves (e.g., the vagus) by cytokines and prostaglandin which signal to the medulla oblongata and are relayed to the hypothalamus (109,110).
2. Direct actions of LPS or pro-inflammatory cytokines at brain areas lacking a BBB e.g., the circumventricular organs (111).
3. Direct action of LPS or pro-inflammatory cytokines of perivascular macrophages in the neurovascular unit of the BBB (112).

In animals, unless the peripheral inflammatory event is extreme, sickness behaviour is a relatively benign and transient phenomenon (113). Damage limitation in the brain is in part due to the wide number of the regulatory molecules, as previously discussed, that reduce the pro-inflammatory response to an acute challenge within the brain. Thus, following a peripheral signal the pro-inflammatory response in the brain appears to be suppressed by the increased production of a large variety of proteins from microglial cells including anti-inflammatory cytokines IL-10; TGFβ and other cytokine signalling protein suppressors (114). However, in circumstances, as previously stated, where microglial cells are primed the response of these cells to even a very modest peripheral inflammatory event is very different. Here the largely down regulation state is rapidly changed to a damaging phenotype with increased pro-inflammatory cytokine productive and oxidative stress and neuronal damage (11). Figure 11.1 This hypothesis is supported by animal studies showing an exaggerated inflammatory and oxidative stress response to peripheral stimuli in aged mice (115), increased concentrations of interleukin 1β in the CNS and neuronal apoptosis in the ME7 prion mouse after peripheral challenge with the bacterial mimic LPS or the viral mimic polyinosinic-polycytidylic acid (116–118).

In humans a range of inflammatory conditions outside the CNS are also known to act as risk factors for the development of AD. Delirium, a condition largely attributed to the presence of a variety of acute systemic infections, is associated with an increased risk of developing dementia. Thus, the increased risk of developing dementia in cognitively intact individuals following a delirium is substantial with a cumulative incidence of 55% after one-year follow-up (119). In addition, the risk of developing AD appears increased following the development of an acute infection in the absence of an obvious delirium. Thus, in a retrospective general practitioner database the presence of one or more infections over a five-year follow-up period increased the odds of developing AD by around twofold with increased risk increasing with age (120). In addition to acute infections there is also increasing evidence for a role for low grade chronic peripheral infections being associated with increased risk. Thus there has been an increased focus on the role of the microbiome in AD (121) with a number of studies suggesting an association of gut dysbiosis (122,123) and periodontitis (124,125) with AD. In addition to infective agents, aseptic chronic inflammatory conditions including atherosclerosis (126) and diabetes (127) have a robust epidemiological basis for being proposed as risk factors in the development of AD. For all of these risk factors their individual attributable risk is likely to be small (128). However, their combined cumulative effects over time might be considerable.

Importantly there are a number of modifying factors that can influence the onset of this systemic pro-inflammatory environment as we age, also known as 'inflammaging'. One important modifying factor is age-related endocrine dyscrasia. Thus, the loss of sex steroids and associated elevation of gonadotrophins as we age is associated with an increase in the pro-inflammatory state and is also associated with the development of AD pathology (129,130). Likewise lifestyle factors may also modify inflammaging and delay the onset of AD including exercise and calorific restriction (131).

11.6 Therapeutic Strategies

Given the increasing evidence for a role for inflammation in the development and progression of AD it is disappointing to see mixed findings from a wide range of treatment studies aimed at modulating inflammatory pathways.

Table 11.2 shows a summary of randomized placebo-controlled trials in AD, preventative trials in MCI and in asymptomatic at-risk individuals. In AD small early trials with indomethacin suggested some evidence of reduced cognitive decline (132). However, this study was not replicated in a later follow-up study (133). Large-scale studies of other NSAIDs including napoxen (134) and rofecoxib (135) in AD have also been unsuccessful. Randomized trials with a range of other anti-inflammatory drugs, including prednisone (136), hydroxychloroquine (137), simvastatin (138) atorvastatin (139,140), aspirin (141) and rosiglitazone (142) have also shown no clinically significant changes in primary cognitive outcomes in patients with AD. More recently, a small study of AD subjects using the

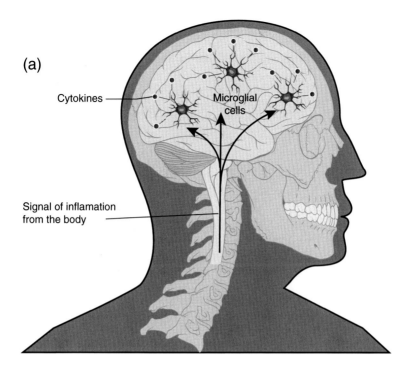

(a)

Cytokines

Microglial cells

Signal of inflamation from the body

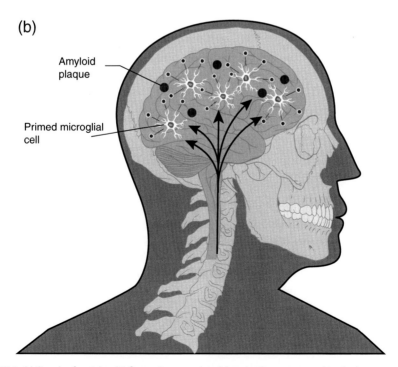

(b)

Amyloid plaque

Primed microglial cell

Figure 11.1 (a) Signals of peripheral inflammation are relayed (e.g., by the vagus nerve) to the immune cells of the brain. In turn, these cells produce cytokines that signal to different areas of the brain to bring about specific sickness behaviours (e.g., lethargy, loss of appetite, depression etc.) (b) In AD the presence of amyloid deposits 'prime' immune cells such as microglial cells causes them to respond more aggressively to the peripheral inflammatory signal with a greater cytokine response resulting in detrimental downstream changes including neuronal degeneration. (A black and white version of this figure will appear in some formats. For the colour version, please refer to the plate section.)

Table 11.2 Randomized placebo-controlled trials using ant-inflammatory agents in AD; MCI and asymptomatic at-risk individuals

Drug vs placebo	Participants	Treatment duration	Cognitive findings
Indometacin 100–150 mg o.d.(132)	28 AD	6 months	Positive effects
Indometacin 100 mg o.d. (133)	51 AD	1 year	Neutral effects
Prednisone 10 mg o.d.(136)	138 AD	1 year	Neutral effect
Naproxen 220 mg b.d. or rofecoxib 25 mg o.d. (134)	351 AD	1 year	Neutral (naproxen) to negative (rofecoxib) effect
Naproxen 220 mg b.d. (152)	195 healthy FH positive subjects	2 years	Neutral effects
Rofecoxib 25 mg o.d. (135)	692 AD	1 year	Negative effects
Rofecoxib 25 mg o.d. (148)	1457 MCI	3–5 years	Negative effects
Hydroxychloroquine 200–400 mg o.d. (137)	168 AD	1.5 years	Neutral effects
Celocoxib 100 mg b.d. or Naproxen 220 mg b.d. (150)	2528 healthy FH positive subjects	5 to 7 years	Neutral effects
Simvastatin 80 mg o.d. (138)	44 AD	26 weeks	Neutral effects
Atorvastatin 80 mg o.d. (139)	67 AD	1 year	Positive effects
Atorvastatin 80 mg o.d. (140)	640 AD	72 weeks	Neutral effects
Rosiglitazone 2 mg or 8 mg o.d. (142)	2981 AD	48 weeks	Neutral effects
Etanercept 50 mg weekly (130)	21 AD	26 weeks	Positive effects

TNF-α inhibiting agent etanercept in AD does show some evidence of a reduction of decline on a number of clinical outcomes but it has yet to be replicated (143).

Epidemiological studies of the protective effects of NSAIDs are more positive. Thus, the incidence of AD in cohorts of older people taking NSAIDs has been examined in several large prospective studies (143,144). The largest of these prospective studies, the Baltimore Longitudinal study of Ageing, found a relative risk of AD of 0.35 for ten years of NSAID use (145). A meta-analysis of case-control studies found that regular NSAID use was associated with a two-fold reduction in the odds of developing AD (OR = 0.5; p = 0.0002) (146) and, not included in this analysis, the largest case-control study to date (49,349 cases and 196,850 matched controls) (147) also showed a significant reduction in odds of developing AD after five years of regular use, with a combined OR of 0.76. However, randomized placebo control trials examining the possible protective effects seen in these epidemiological studies are more mixed. Thus a large trial of rofecoxib examining conversion of MCI subjects to AD found an increased risk of conversion in the MCI treated group (148). Likewise a large randomized study of the NSAIDs naproxen and celecoxib in asymptomatic individuals with a family history of AD initially reported an increased risk of increased cognitive decline or development of AD for both drugs (149). However, a longer-term follow-up of these patients suggests that careful selection of asymptomatic patients and the choice of the specific NSAID is important (150). Thus, the early detrimental effects were mostly in a small group of patients with early cognitive impairment and naproxen seemed thereafter to be protective in patients for up to four years in those who had been asymptomatic at baseline (150,151).

Although speculative, the reasons for these mixed findings are likely to be found in the variability in the inflammatory state as the disease progresses and in the ability of agents to target the key pathways. Thus, early interventions prior to development of Aβ may benefit from approaches aimed at dampening down the largely peripherally driven M1 activation state seen in inflammaging and thus reducing the drive towards Aβ deposition. However, once Aβ is deposited and microglial cells are primed the high sensitivity of these cells to central and systemic pro-inflammatory signals and the damaging nature of the activated primed microglial cell response is likely to require a peripheral and/or centrally targeted robust suppression of the pro-inflammatory pathway to reduce neuronal damage at the potential expense of reducing Aβ phagocytosis.

References

1. Chan WY, Kohsaka S, Rezaie P. The origin and cell lineage of microglia: new concepts. *Brain Res Rev.* 2007;53(2):344–54.

2. Ginhoux F, Greter M, Leboeuf M, et al. Fate mapping analysis reveals that adult microglia derive from primitive macrophages. *Science.* 2010;330 (6005):841–5.

3. Bianchi ME. DAMPs, PAMPs and alarmins: all we need to know about danger. *J Leukoc Biol.* 2007;81(1):1–5.

4. Kono H, Rock KL. How dying cells alert the immune system to danger. *Nat Rev Immunol.* 2008;8(4):279–89.

5. Medzhitov R. Recognition of microorganisms and activation of the immune response. *Nature.* 2007;449 (7164):819–26.

6. Stewart CR, Stuart LM, Wilkinson K, et al. CD36 ligands promote sterile inflammation through assembly of a Toll-like receptor 4 and 6 heterodimer. *Nat Immunol.* 2010;11 (2):155–61.

7. Colton CA. Heterogeneity of microglial activation in the innate immune response in the brain. *J Neuroimmune Pharmacol.* 2009;4(4):399–418.

8. Boche D, Perry VH, Nicoll JA. Review: activation patterns of microglia and their identification in the human brain. *Neuropathol Appl Neurobiol.* 2013;39 (1):3–18.

9. Ransohoff RM. A polarizing question: do M1 and M2 microglia exist? *Nat Neurosci.* 2016;19(8):987–91.

10. Yamasaki R, Lu H, Butovsky O, et al. Differential roles of microglia and monocytes in the inflamed central nervous system. *J Exp Med.* 2014;211(8):1533–49.

11. Perry VH, Holmes C. Microglial priming in neurodegenerative disease. *Nat Rev Neurol.* 2014;10(4):217–24.

12. Perry VH, Nicoll JA, Holmes C. Microglia in neurodegenerative disease. *Nat Rev Neurol.* 2010;6(4):193–201.

13. Tajiri N, Kellogg SL, Shimizu T, Arendash GW, Borlongan CV. Traumatic brain injury precipitates cognitive impairment and extracellular Aβ aggregation in Alzheimer's disease transgenic mice. *PLoS One.* 2013;8(11): e78851.

14. Koshinaga M, Katayama Y, Fukushima M, et al. Rapid and widespread microglial activation induced by traumatic brain

injury in rat brain slices. *J Neurotrauma.* 2000;17(3):185–92.

15. Gentleman SM, Leclercq PD, Moyes L, et al. Long-term intracerebral inflammatory response after traumatic brain injury. *Forensic Sci Int.* 2004;146 (2–3):97–104.

16. Griciuc A, Serrano-Pozo A, Parrado AR, et al. Alzheimer's disease risk gene CD33 inhibits microglial uptake of amyloid beta. *Neuron.* 2013;78(4):631–43.

17. Bradshaw EM, Chibnik LB, Keenan BT, et al. CD33 Alzheimer's disease locus: altered monocyte function and amyloid biology. *Nat Neurosci.* 2013;16(7):848–50.

18. Okello A, Edison P, Archer HA, et al. Microglial activation and amyloid deposition in mild cognitive impairment: a PET study. *Neurology.* 2009;72(1):56–62.

19. Yasuno F, Kosaka J, Ota M, et al. Increased binding of peripheral benzodiazepine receptor in mild cognitive impairment-dementia converters measured by positron emission tomography with [(1)(1)C]DAA1106. *Psychiatry Res.* 2012;203(1):67–74.

20. Diorio D, Welner SA, Butterworth RF, Meaney MJ, Suranyi-Cadotte BE. Peripheral benzodiazepine binding sites in Alzheimer's disease frontal and temporal cortex. *Neurobiol Aging.* 1991;12(3):255–8.

21. Cagnin A, Brooks DJ, Kennedy AM, et al. In-vivo measurement of activated microglia in dementia. *Lancet.* 2001;358 (9280):461–7.

22. Venneti S, Lopresti BJ, Wang G, et al. PK11195 labels activated microglia in Alzheimer's disease and in vivo in a mouse model using PET. *Neurobiol Aging.* 2009;30 (8):1217–26.

23. Edison P, Archer HA, Gerhard A, et al. Microglia, amyloid, and cognition in Alzheimer's disease: An [11C](R) PK11195-PET and [11C]PIB-PET study. *Neurobiol Dis.* 2008;32(3):412–9.

24. Wiley CA, Lopresti BJ, Venneti S, et al. Carbon 11-labeled Pittsburgh Compound B and carbon 11-labeled (R)-PK11195 positron emission tomographic imaging in

Alzheimer disease. *Arch Neurol.* 2009;66 (1):60–7.

25. Kreisl WC, Lyoo CH, McGwier M, et al. In vivo radioligand binding to translocator protein correlates with severity of Alzheimer's disease. *Brain.* 2013;136(Pt 7):2228–38.

26. Yokokura M, Mori N, Yagi S, et al. In vivo changes in microglial activation and amyloid deposits in brain regions with hypometabolism in Alzheimer's disease. *Eur J Nucl Med Mol Imaging.* 2011;38 (2):343–51.

27. Sudduth TL, Schmitt FA, Nelson PT, Wilcock DM. Neuroinflammatory phenotype in early Alzheimer's disease. *Neurobiol Aging.* 2013;34(4):1051–9.

28. Minett T, Classey J, Matthews FE, et al. Microglial immunophenotype in dementia with Alzheimer's pathology. *J Neuroinflammation.* 2016;13(1):135.

29. Campbell GL, Williams MP. In vitro growth of glial cell-enriched and depleted populations from mouse cerebellum. *Brain Res.* 1978;156(2):227–39.

30. Sofroniew MV, Vinters HV. Astrocytes: biology and pathology. *Acta Neuropathol.* 2010;119(1):7–35.

31. Medeiros R, LaFerla FM. Astrocytes: conductors of the Alzheimer disease neuroinflammatory symphony. *Exp Neurol.* 2013;239:133–8.

32. Koistinaho M, Lin S, Wu X, et al. Apolipoprotein E promotes astrocyte colocalization and degradation of deposited amyloid-beta peptides. *Nat Med.* 2004;10(7):719–26.

33. Farina C, Aloisi F, Meinl E. Astrocytes are active players in cerebral innate immunity. *Trends Immunol.* 2007;28(3):138–45.

34. Togo T, Akiyama H, Iseki E, et al. Occurrence of T cells in the brain of Alzheimer's disease and other neurological diseases. *J Neuroimmunol.* 2002;124 (1–2):83–92.

35. Yang YM, Shang DS, Zhao WD, Fang WG, Chen YH. Microglial TNF-alpha-dependent elevation of MHC class I expression on brain endothelium induced

by amyloid-beta promotes T cell transendothelial migration. *Neurochem Res.* 2013;38(11):2295-304.

36. Schenk D, Barbour R, Dunn W, et al. Immunization with amyloid-beta attenuates Alzheimer-disease-like pathology in the PDAPP mouse. *Nature.* 1999;400(6740):173-7.

37. Nicoll JA, Wilkinson D, Holmes C, et al. Neuropathology of human Alzheimer disease after immunization with amyloid-beta peptide: a case report. *Nat Med.* 2003;9(4):448-52.

38. Monsonego A, Imitola J, Petrovic S, et al. Abeta-induced meningoencephalitis is IFN-gamma-dependent and is associated with T cell-dependent clearance of Abeta in a mouse model of Alzheimer's disease. *Proc Natl Acad Sci USA.* 2006;103(13):5048-53.

39. Pierson E, Simmons SB, Castelli L, Goverman JM. Mechanisms regulating regional localization of inflammation during CNS autoimmunity. *Immunol Rev.* 2012;248(1):205-15.

40. Streit WJ, Sammons NW, Kuhns AJ, Sparks DL. Dystrophic microglia in the aging human brain. *Glia.* 2004;45(2):208-12.

41. Ethell DW, Shippy D, Cao C, et al. Abeta-specific T-cells reverse cognitive decline and synaptic loss in Alzheimer's mice. *Neurobiol Dis.* 2006;23(2):351-61.

42. Cao C, Arendash GW, Dickson A, et al. Abeta-specific Th2 cells provide cognitive and pathological benefits to Alzheimer's mice without infiltrating the CNS. *Neurobiol Dis.* 2009;34(1):63-70.

43. Dansokho C, Ait Ahmed D, Aid S, et al. Regulatory T cells delay disease progression in Alzheimer-like pathology. *Brain.* 2016;139(Pt 4):1237-51.

44. Lee WL, Slutsky AS. Sepsis and endothelial permeability. *N Engl J Med.* 2010;363(7):689-91.

45. Nau R, Sorgel F, Eiffert H. Penetration of drugs through the blood-cerebrospinal fluid/blood-brain barrier for treatment of central nervous system infections. *Clin Microbiol Rev.* 2010;23(4):858-83.

46. Simard AR, Soulet D, Gowing G, Julien JP, Rivest S. Bone marrow-derived microglia play a critical role in restricting senile plaque formation in Alzheimer's disease. *Neuron.* 2006;49(4):489-502.

47. El Khoury J, Toft M, Hickman SE, et al. Ccr2 deficiency impairs microglial accumulation and accelerates progression of Alzheimer-like disease. *Nat Med.* 2007;13(4):432-8.

48. Mildner A, Schlevogt B, Kierdorf K, et al. Distinct and non-redundant roles of microglia and myeloid subsets in mouse models of Alzheimer's disease. *J Neurosci.* 2011;31(31):11159-71.

49. Hawkes CA, McLaurin J. Selective targeting of perivascular macrophages for clearance of beta-amyloid in cerebral amyloid angiopathy. *Proc Natl Acad Sci USA.* 2009;106(4):1261-6.

50. Swardfager W, Lanctot K, Rothenburg L, et al. A meta-analysis of cytokines in Alzheimer's disease. *Biol Psychiatry.* 2010;68(10):930-41.

51. Engelhart MJ, Geerlings MI, Meijer J, et al. Inflammatory proteins in plasma and the risk of dementia: the rotterdam study. *Arch Neurol.* 2004;61(5):668-72.

52. Tilvis RS, Kahonen-Vare MH, Jolkkonen J, et al. Predictors of cognitive decline and mortality of aged people over a 10-year period. *J Gerontol A Biol Sci Med Sci.* 2004;59(3):268-74.

53. Kuo HK, Yen CJ, Chang CH, et al. Relation of C-reactive protein to stroke, cognitive disorders, and depression in the general population: systematic review and meta-analysis. *Lancet Neurol.* 2005;4(6):371-80.

54. Laurin D, David Curb J, Masaki KH, White LR, Launer LJ. Midlife C-reactive protein and risk of cognitive decline: a 31-year follow-up. *Neurobiol Aging.* 2009;30(11):1724-7.

55. Hu WT, Holtzman DM, Fagan AM, et al. Plasma multianalyte profiling in mild cognitive impairment and Alzheimer disease. *Neurology.* 2012;79(9):897-905.

56. Buchhave P, Zetterberg H, Blennow K, et al. Soluble TNF receptors are associated with Abeta metabolism and conversion to dementia in subjects with mild cognitive impairment. *Neurobiol Aging*. 2010;31 (11):1877–84.

57. Thambisetty M, Lovestone S. Blood-based biomarkers of Alzheimer's disease: challenging but feasible. *Biomark Med*. 2010;4(1):65–79.

58. Holmes C, Cunningham C, Zotova E, et al. Systemic inflammation and disease progression in Alzheimer disease. *Neurology*. 2009;73(10):768–74.

59. Holmes C, Cunningham C, Zotova E, Culliford D, Perry VH. Proinflammatory cytokines, sickness behavior, and Alzheimer disease. *Neurology*. 2011;77 (3):212–8.

60. Tarkowski E, Andreasen N, Tarkowski A, Blennow K. Intrathecal inflammation precedes development of Alzheimer's disease. *J Neurol Neurosurg Psychiatry*. 2003;74(9):1200–5.

61. Galimberti D, Fenoglio C, Scarpini E. Inflammation in neurodegenerative disorders: friend or foe? *Curr Aging Sci*. 2008;1(1):30–41.

62. Patel NS, Paris D, Mathura V, et al. Inflammatory cytokine levels correlate with amyloid load in transgenic mouse models of Alzheimer's disease. *J Neuroinflammation*. 2005;2(1):9.

63. Meda L, Cassatella MA, Szendrei GI, et al. Activation of microglial cells by beta-amyloid protein and interferon-gamma. *Nature*. 1995;374 (6523):647–50.

64. Tan J, Town T, Paris D, et al. Microglial activation resulting from CD40-CD40L interaction after beta-amyloid stimulation. *Science*. 1999;286(5448):2352–5.

65. Tan J, Town T, Crawford F, et al. Role of CD40 ligand in amyloidosis in transgenic Alzheimer's mice. *Nat Neurosci*. 2002;5 (12):1288–93.

66. Jin JJ, Kim HD, Maxwell JA, Li L, Fukuchi K. Toll-like receptor 4-dependent upregulation of cytokines in a transgenic mouse model of Alzheimer's disease. *J Neuroinflammation*. 2008;5:23.

67. Streit WJ. Microglial senescence: does the brain's immune system have an expiration date? *Trends Neurosci*. 2006;29(9):506–10.

68. Ghosh S, Wu MD, Shaftel SS, et al. Sustained interleukin-1beta overexpression exacerbates tau pathology despite reduced amyloid burden in an Alzheimer's mouse model. *J Neurosci*. 2013;33(11):5053–64.

69. Chakrabarty P, Ceballos-Diaz C, Beccard A, et al. IFN-gamma promotes complement expression and attenuates amyloid plaque deposition in amyloid beta precursor protein transgenic mice. *J Immunol*. 2010;184(9):5333–43.

70. Chakrabarty P, Jansen-West K, Beccard A, et al. Massive gliosis induced by interleukin-6 suppresses Abeta deposition in vivo: evidence against inflammation as a driving force for amyloid deposition. *FASEB J*. 2010;24(2):548–59.

71. Chakrabarty P, Herring A, Ceballos-Diaz C, Das P, Golde TE. Hippocampal expression of murine TNFalpha results in attenuation of amyloid deposition in vivo. *Mol Neurodegener*. 2011;6:16.

72. Chakrabarty P, Tianbai L, Herring A, et al. Hippocampal expression of murine IL-4 results in exacerbation of amyloid deposition. *Mol Neurodegener*. 2012;7:36.

73. Nathan C, Calingasan N, Nezezon J, et al. Protection from Alzheimer's-like disease in the mouse by genetic ablation of inducible nitric oxide synthase. *J Exp Med*. 2005;202 (9):1163–9.

74. Jekabsone A, Mander PK, Tickler A, Sharpe M, Brown GC. Fibrillar beta-amyloid peptide Abeta1-40 activates microglial proliferation via stimulating TNF-alpha release and H2O2 derived from NADPH oxidase: a cell culture study. *J Neuroinflammation*. 2006;3:24.

75. Choi SH, Aid S, Kim HW, Jackson SH, Bosetti F. Inhibition of NADPH oxidase promotes alternative and anti-inflammatory microglial activation during neuroinflammation. *J Neurochem*. 2012;120(2):292–301.

76. Savarin-Vuaillat C, Ransohoff RM. Chemokines and chemokine receptors in neurological disease: raise, retain, or reduce? *Neurotherapeutics*. 2007;4 (4):590–601.

77. Xia MQ, Qin SX, Wu LJ, Mackay CR, Hyman BT. Immunohistochemical study of the beta-chemokine receptors CCR3 and CCR5 and their ligands in normal and Alzheimer's disease brains. *Am J Pathol*. 1998;153(1):31–7.

78. Ishizuka K, Kimura T, Igata-yi R, et al. Identification of monocyte chemoattractant protein-1 in senile plaques and reactive microglia of Alzheimer's disease. *Psychiatry Clin Neurosci*. 1997;51(3):135–8.

79. Smits HA, Rijsmus A, van Loon JH, et al. Amyloid-beta-induced chemokine production in primary human macrophages and astrocytes. *J Neuroimmunol*. 2002;127(1–2):160–8.

80. Lue LF, Walker DG, Rogers J. Modeling microglial activation in Alzheimer's disease with human postmortem microglial cultures. *Neurobiol Aging*. 2001;22 (6):945–56.

81. Veerhuis R, Nielsen HM, Tenner AJ. Complement in the brain. *Mol Immunol*. 2011;48(14):1592–603.

82. Strohmeyer R, Ramirez M, Cole GJ, Mueller K, Rogers J. Association of factor H of the alternative pathway of complement with agrin and complement receptor 3 in the Alzheimer's disease brain. *J Neuroimmunol*. 2002;131(1–2):135–46.

83. Lambert JC, Heath S, Even G, et al. Genome-wide association study identifies variants at CLU and CR1 associated with Alzheimer's disease. *Nat Genet*. 2009;41 (10):1094–9.

84. Harold D, Abraham R, Hollingworth P, et al. Genome-wide association study identifies variants at CLU and PICALM associated with Alzheimer's disease. *Nat Genet*. 2009;41(10):1088–93.

85. Lupetti A, Nibbering PH, Welling MM, Pauwels EK. Radiopharmaceuticals: new antimicrobial agents. *Trends Biotechnol*. 2003;21(2):70–3.

86. Cudic M, Otvos L, Jr. Intracellular targets of antibacterial peptides. *Curr Drug Targets*. 2002;3(2):101–6.

87. Radek K, Gallo R. Antimicrobial peptides: natural effectors of the innate immune system. *Semin Immunopathol*. 2007;29 (1):27–43.

88. Kourie JI, Shorthouse AA. Properties of cytotoxic peptide-formed ion channels. *Am J Physiol Cell Physiol*. 2000;278(6): C1063–87.

89. Soscia SJ, Kirby JE, Washicosky KJ, et al. The Alzheimer's disease-associated amyloid beta-protein is an antimicrobial peptide. *PLoS One*. 2010;5(3):e9505.

90. Welling MM, Nabuurs RJ, van der Weerd L. Potential role of antimicrobial peptides in the early onset of Alzheimer's disease. *Alzheimer's & Dementia : The Journal of the Alzheimer's Association*. 2015;11(1):51–7.

91. Krstic D, Madhusudan A, Doehner J, et al. Systemic immune challenges trigger and drive Alzheimer-like neuropathology in mice. *J Neuroinflammation*. 2012;9:151.

92. Campion D, Dumanchin C, Hannequin D, et al. Early-onset autosomal dominant Alzheimer disease: prevalence, genetic heterogeneity, and mutation spectrum. *Am J Hum Genet*. 1999;65(3):664–70.

93. Rovelet-Lecrux A, Hannequin D, Raux G, et al. APP locus duplication causes autosomal dominant early-onset Alzheimer disease with cerebral amyloid angiopathy. *Nat Genet*. 2006;38(1):24–6.

94. Hardy J. Alzheimer's disease: the amyloid cascade hypothesis: an update and reappraisal. *J Alzheimers Dis*. 2006;9(3 Suppl):151–3.

95. Nuutinen T, Suuronen T, Kauppinen A, Salminen A. Clusterin: a forgotten player in Alzheimer's disease. *Brain Res Rev*. 2009;61 (2):89–104.

96. Hollingworth P, Harold D, Sims R, et al. Common variants at ABCA7, MS4A6A/ MS4A4E, EPHA1, CD33 and CD2AP are associated with Alzheimer's disease. *Nat Genet*. 2011;43(5):429–35.

97. Naj AC, Jun G, Beecham GW, et al. Common variants at MS4A4/MS4A6E, CD2AP, CD33 and EPHA1 are associated with late-onset Alzheimer's disease. *Nat Genet.* 2011;43(5):436–41.

98. Lambert JC, Ibrahim-Verbaas CA, Harold D, et al. Meta-analysis of 74,046 individuals identifies 11 new susceptibility loci for Alzheimer's disease. *Nat Genet.* 2013;45(12):1452–8.

99. Sims R, van der Lee SJ, Naj AC, et al. Rare coding variants in PLCG2, ABI3, and TREM2 implicate microglial-mediated innate immunity in Alzheimer's disease. *Nat Genet.* 2017;49(9):1373–84.

100. Kunkle BW, Grenier-Boley B, Sims R, et al. Genetic meta-analysis of diagnosed Alzheimer's disease identifies new risk loci and implicates Abeta, tau, immunity and lipid processing. *Nat Genet.* 2019;51 (3):414–30.

101. Yokoyama JS, Desikan RS. Association of Alzheimer Disease Susceptibility Variants and Gene Expression in the Human Brain-Reply. *JAMA Neurol.* 2016;73 (10):1255.

102. Huang KL, Marcora E, Pimenova AA, et al. A common haplotype lowers PU.1 expression in myeloid cells and delays onset of Alzheimer's disease. *Nat Neurosci.* 2017;20(8):1052–61.

103. Guerreiro R, Wojtas A, Bras J, et al. TREM2 variants in Alzheimer's disease. *N Engl J Med.* 2013;368(2):117–27.

104. Jonsson T, Stefansson H, Steinberg S, et al. Variant of TREM2 associated with the risk of Alzheimer's disease. *N Engl J Med.* 2013;368(2):107–16.

105. Neumann H, Takahashi K. Essential role of the microglial triggering receptor expressed on myeloid cells-2 (TREM2) for central nervous tissue immune homeostasis. *J Neuroimmunol.* 2007;184 (1–2):92–9.

106. Heslegrave A, Heywood W, Paterson R, et al. Increased cerebrospinal fluid soluble TREM2 concentration in Alzheimer's disease. *Mol Neurodegener.* 2016;11:3.

107. Suarez-Calvet M, Kleinberger G, Araque Caballero MA, et al. sTREM2 cerebrospinal fluid levels are a potential biomarker for microglia activity in early-stage Alzheimer's disease and associate with neuronal injury markers. *EMBO Mol Med.* 2016;8(5):466–76.

108. Hart BL. Biological basis of the behavior of sick animals. *Neurosci Biobehav Rev.* 1988;12(2):123–37.

109. Dantzer R, Konsman JP, Bluthe RM, Kelley KW. Neural and humoral pathways of communication from the immune system to the brain: parallel or convergent? *Auton Neurosci.* 2000;85 (1–3):60–5.

110. Ek M, Kurosawa M, Lundeberg T, Ericsson A. Activation of vagal afferents after intravenous injection of interleukin-1beta: role of endogenous prostaglandins. *J Neurosci.* 1998;18 (22):9471–9.

111. Blatteis CM, Bealer SL, Hunter WS, et al. Suppression of fever after lesions of the anteroventral third ventricle in guinea pigs. *Brain Res Bull.* 1983;11(5):519–26.

112. Matsumura K, Kobayashi S. Signaling the brain in inflammation: the role of endothelial cells. *Front Biosci.* 2004;9:2819–26.

113. Perry VH. Contribution of systemic inflammation to chronic neurodegeneration. *Acta Neuropathol.* 2010;120(3):277–86.

114. Rivest S. Regulation of innate immune responses in the brain. *Nat Rev Immunol.* 2009;9(6):429–39.

115. Godbout JP, Johnson RW. Age and neuroinflammation: a lifetime of psychoneuroimmune consequences. *Immunol Allergy Clin North Am.* 2009;29 (2):321–37.

116. Cunningham C, Wilcockson DC, Campion S, Lunnon K, Perry VH. Central and systemic endotoxin challenges exacerbate the local inflammatory response and increase neuronal death during chronic neurodegeneration. *J Neurosci.* 2005;25(40):9275–84.

117. Cunningham C, Campion S, Lunnon K, et al. Systemic inflammation induces acute behavioral and cognitive changes and accelerates neurodegenerative disease. *Biol Psychiatry*. 2009;65 (4):304–12.

118. Field R, Campion S, Warren C, Murray C, Cunningham C. Systemic challenge with the TLR3 agonist poly I:C induces amplified IFNalpha/beta and IL-1beta responses in the diseased brain and exacerbates chronic neurodegeneration. *Brain Behav Immun*. 2010;24 (6):996–1007.

119. Rahkonen T, Luukkainen-Markkula R, Paanila S, Sivenius J, Sulkava R. Delirium episode as a sign of undetected dementia among community dwelling elderly subjects: a 2 year follow up study. *J Neurol Neurosurg Psychiatry*. 2000;69(4):519–21.

120. Dunn N, Mullee M, Perry VH, Holmes C. Association between dementia and infectious disease: evidence from a case-control study. *Alzheimer Dis Assoc Disord*. 2005;19(2):91–4.

121. Calvani R, Picca A, Lo Monaco MR, et al. Of Microbes and Minds: A Narrative Review on the Second Brain Aging. *Front Med (Lausanne)*. 2018;5:53.

122. Vogt NM, Kerby RL, Dill-McFarland KA, et al. Gut microbiome alterations in Alzheimer's disease. *Sci Rep*. 2017;7 (1):13537.

123. Cattaneo A, Cattane N, Galluzzi S, et al. Association of brain amyloidosis with pro-inflammatory gut bacterial taxa and peripheral inflammation markers in cognitively impaired elderly. *Neurobiol Aging*. 2017;49:60–8.

124. Riviere GR, Riviere KH, Smith KS. Molecular and immunological evidence of oral Treponema in the human brain and their association with Alzheimer's disease. *Oral Microbiol Immunol*. 2002;17 (2):113–8.

125. Ide M, Harris M, Stevens A, et al. Periodontitis and Cognitive Decline in Alzheimer's Disease. *PLoS One*. 2016;11 (3):e0151081.

126. Casserly I, Topol E. Convergence of atherosclerosis and Alzheimer's disease: inflammation, cholesterol, and misfolded proteins. *Lancet*. 2004;363 (9415):1139–46.

127. Donath MY, Shoelson SE. Type 2 diabetes as an inflammatory disease. *Nat Rev Immunol*. 2011;11(2):98–107.

128. Launer LJ, Andersen K, Dewey ME, et al. Rates and risk factors for dementia and Alzheimer's disease: results from EURODEM pooled analyses. EURODEM Incidence Research Group and Work Groups. *European Studies of Dementia*. *Neurology*. 1999;52(1):78–84.

129. Clark IA, Atwood CS. Is TNF a link between aging-related reproductive endocrine dyscrasia and Alzheimer's disease? *J Alzheimers Dis*. 2011;27 (4):691–9.

130. Butchart J, Birch B, Bassily R, Wolfe L, Holmes C. Male sex hormones and systemic inflammation in Alzheimer disease. *Alzheimer Dis Assoc Disord*. 2013;27(2):153–6.

131. Ngandu T, Lehtisalo J, Solomon A, et al. A 2-year multidomain intervention of diet, exercise, cognitive training, and vascular risk monitoring versus control to prevent cognitive decline in at-risk elderly people (FINGER): a randomised controlled trial. *Lancet*. 2015;385(9984):2255–63.

132. Rogers J, Kirby LC, Hempelman SR, et al. Clinical trial of indomethacin in Alzheimer's disease. *Neurology*. 1993;43 (8):1609–11.

133. de Jong D, Jansen R, Hoefnagels W, et al. No effect of one-year treatment with indomethacin on Alzheimer's disease progression: a randomized controlled trial. *PLoS One*. 2008;3(1):e1475.

134. Aisen PS, Schafer KA, Grundman M, et al. Effects of rofecoxib or naproxen vs placebo on Alzheimer disease progression: a randomized controlled trial. *JAMA*. 2003;289(21):2819–26.

135. Reines SA, Block GA, Morris JC, et al. Rofecoxib: no effect on Alzheimer's disease in a 1-year, randomized, blinded,

controlled study. *Neurology*. 2004;62
(1):66–71.

136. Aisen PS, Davis KL, Berg JD, et al.
A randomized controlled trial of
prednisone in Alzheimer's disease.
Alzheimer's Disease Cooperative
Study. *Neurology*. 2000;54(3):
588–93.

137. Van Gool WA, Weinstein HC,
Scheltens P, Walstra GJ. Effect of
hydroxychloroquine on progression of
dementia in early Alzheimer's disease: an
18-month randomised, double-blind,
placebo-controlled study. *Lancet*.
2001;358(9280):455–60.

138. Simons M, Schwarzler F, Lutjohann D,
et al. Treatment with simvastatin in
normocholesterolemic patients with
Alzheimer's disease: A 26-week
randomized, placebo-controlled, double-
blind trial. *Ann Neurol*. 2002;52
(3):346–50.

139. Sparks DL, Sabbagh MN, Connor DJ,
et al. Atorvastatin for the treatment of
mild to moderate Alzheimer disease:
preliminary results. *Arch Neurol*. 2005;62
(5):753–7.

140. Feldman HH, Doody RS, Kivipelto M,
et al. Randomized controlled trial of
atorvastatin in mild to moderate
Alzheimer disease: LEADe. *Neurology*.
2010;74(12):956–64.

141. Bentham P, Gray R, Sellwood E, et al.
Aspirin in Alzheimer's disease (AD2000):
a randomised open-label trial. *Lancet
Neurol*. 2008;7(1):41–9.

142. Harrington C, Sawchak S, Chiang C, et al.
Rosiglitazone does not improve cognition
or global function when used as
adjunctive therapy to AChE inhibitors in
mild-to-moderate Alzheimer's disease:
two phase 3 studies. *Curr Alzheimer Res*.
2011;8(5):592–606.

143. Butchart J, Brook L, Hopkins V, et al.
Etanercept in Alzheimer disease:
A randomized, placebo-controlled,
double-blind, phase 2 trial. *Neurology*.
2015;84(21):2161–8.

144. McGeer PL, McGeer EG. NSAIDs and
Alzheimer disease: epidemiological,
animal model and clinical studies.
Neurobiol Aging. 2007;28(5):639–47.

145. Stewart WF, Kawas C, Corrada M,
Metter EJ. Risk of Alzheimer's disease and
duration of NSAID use. *Neurology*.
1997;48(3):626–32.

146. McGeer PL, Schulzer M, McGeer EG.
Arthritis and anti-inflammatory agents as
possible protective factors for Alzheimer's
disease: a review of 17 epidemiologic
studies. *Neurology*. 1996;47(2):425–32.

147. Vlad SC, Miller DR, Kowall NW,
Felson DT. Protective effects of NSAIDs
on the development of Alzheimer disease.
Neurology. 2008;70(19):1672–7.

148. Thal LJ, Ferris SH, Kirby L, et al.
A randomized, double-blind, study of
rofecoxib in patients with mild cognitive
impairment. *Neuropsychopharmacology :
Official Publication of the American
College of Neuropsychopharmacology*.
2005;30(6):1204–15.

149. Group AR, Lyketsos CG, Breitner JC, et al.
Naproxen and celecoxib do not
prevent AD in early results from
a randomized controlled trial. *Neurology*.
2007;68(21):1800–8.

150. Breitner JC, Baker LD, Montine TJ, et al.
Extended results of the Alzheimer's
disease anti-inflammatory prevention
trial. *Alzheimer's & Dementia : The
Journal of the Alzheimer's Association*.
2011;7(4):402–11.

151. Alzheimer's Disease Anti-inflammatory
Prevention Trial Research G. Results of
a follow-up study to the randomized
Alzheimer's Disease Anti-inflammatory
Prevention Trial (ADAPT). *Alzheimer's &
Dementia : The Journal of the Alzheimer's
Association*. 2013;9(6):714–23.

152. Meyer PF, Tremblay-Mercier J,
Leoutsakos J, et al. INTREPAD:
a randomized trial of naproxen to slow
progress of presymptomatic Alzheimer
disease. *Neurology*. 2019;92(18):
e2070–e80.

The Immune System and Anxiety Disorders

Vasiliki Michopoulos and Tanja Jovanovic

12.1 Introduction

Anxiety disorders, including post-traumatic stress disorder (PTSD), generalized anxiety disorder (GAD), panic disorder (PD) and phobias (including social phobia and agoraphobia), are the most common (1) and most economically costly psychiatric conditions (2). All anxiety disorders are characterized by pathological fear reactions and/or anxiety (3) in response to stimuli specific to each disorder in the absence of danger (4). Impairments in the ability to extinguish learned fear in response to specific stimuli and to learn safety behaviours are also cardinal characteristics of anxiety disorders (4). Because anxiety disorders are highly comorbid with other psychiatric conditions and adverse physical health conditions that increase mortality, including cardiovascular disease, obesity and diabetes (1,5), biomedical research has focused on defining the mechanisms underlying anxiety disorders.

The role of the immune system in the aetiology and maintenance of anxiety disorders has recently garnered much interest in psychiatry, as exposure to fear- and anxiety-provoking stimuli (including stressors and trauma) activates the hypothalamic-pituitary-adrenal (HPA) axis and stimulates the release of pro-inflammatory cytokines from the immune system (6). Importantly, repeated exposure to fear- and anxiety-provoking stimuli results in the dysregulation of the HPA and immune axes (6). In this chapter, we will highlight recent cross-sectional data linking anxiety disorders to increased systemic inflammation, and discuss how the dysregulation of the HPA and immune axes can contribute to the maintenance of anxiety-related symptoms in PTSD and other Diagnostic and Statistical Manual of Mental Disorders (DSM-5) anxiety disorders (3), including GAD, PD and phobias. We will also discuss the limited prospective data supporting the notion that heightened systemic inflammation may increase individual risk for the development of PTSD and other anxiety disorders.

12.2 The Immune System and PTSD

PTSD is a psychological disorder that can result from exposure to a life-threatening event (7). While PTSD has traditionally been categorized as a military disorder resulting from combat exposure, 70% of the general population in the United States will experience a traumatic event in their lifetime, and 7.8% will develop PTSD (7). The cardinal symptoms of PTSD include re-experiencing, avoidance/numbing, negative cognitions and hyperarousal symptoms (3). Individuals with PTSD also have an exaggerated fear response (8) that occurs concomitantly with deficits in fear extinction (9) and impairments in conditioned fear responses (10). Importantly, the neuroendocrine dysregulation of the HPA axis implicated in the pathophysiology of PTSD (11) and the high comorbidity of PTSD with cardiometabolic disorders (5) highlights a need to better understand the immune system in the context of PTSD.

An array of cross-sectional, association studies indicates that PTSD is associated with heightened basal concentrations of CRP and pro-inflammatory cytokines (Table 12.1). The high CRP concentrations that have been described in PTSD have also been associated with impaired fear inhibition (12) and threat sensitivity (13). Increased peripheral concentrations of interleukin (IL)-6, and IL-2 (14), tumour necrosis factor (TNF)-α and its receptor, interferon (INF)-γ (15) and intercellular adhesion molecule-1 (ICAM-1) (16,17) are also associated PTSD (Table 12.1). Peripheral TNF-α concentrations predict avoidance, re-experiencing and hyperarousal symptom sub-clusters (18). Elevated levels of chemokines and their receptors, including CXCL-12, CCL-5, CXCR-4, and CCR-5 (19), and elevated MCP4 (CCL13)/MCP1(CCL2) ratio (20) have also been associated with PTSD. Finally, a greater pro-inflammatory score based on circulating IL-1β, IL-6, TNF-α, IFN-γ, and CRP, is also associated with PTSD (21,22). While the above-summarized data indicate that PTSD is associated with immune system dysfunction, the cross-sectional nature of the studies limits our ability to determine whether PTSD is the cause or consequence of increased systemic inflammation. Furthermore, published findings from other studies suggest that this relationship between inflammation and PTSD is equivocal (Table 12.1), suggesting that other factors may contribute to inflammation in the context of PTSD and confound the relationship between inflammation and PTSD, such as age (23), race (23), sex (24), socioeconomic status (25) and the presence of psychiatric comorbidity (26). Furthermore, it is important to note that trauma exposure itself (particularly during childhood) has been associated with heightened inflammation in adulthood (27), including elevated CRP, IL-6, IL-1β, and TNF-α (28–38).

Although systematic reviews of the current literature suggest significant elevations of TNF-α (39) and IL-1β (40) in individuals with PTSD, meta-analyses may prove to be more powerful for

Table 12.1 Summary of the associations between PTSD with inflammatory signals. ↑ denotes increased concentrations in the majority of studies; ↓ denotes increased concentrations in the majority of studies; ↑↓ denotes mixed results; – no studies that have assessed the relationship

Signal	PTSD			
	Increased	**Decreased**	**Negative**	**Majority**
C-reactive protein (CRP)	(12,13,16,17,21, 22,59,217-221)	(222)	(18,223,224)	↑
Interleukin-6 (IL-6)	(14,21,22,219, 225-227)	(23)	(43)	↑
Interleukin-1β (IL-1β)	(18,19,21,22,210, 227,228)	–	–	↑
Tumour necrosis factor (TNF-α)	(17,18,51,219, 227)	–	–	↑
Interferon-γ (IFN-γ)	(15,21,22)	↑		↑

characterizing the relationship between the immune system and PTSD, as they overcome problems arising from small sample sizes and distinct samples. A meta-analysis was conducted to systematically address whether PTSD is associated with alterations in inflammatory signals across 20 independent studies (41). Results showed that individuals with PTSD had significantly higher peripheral IL-1β, IL-6, TNF-α, and IFN-γ concentrations compared to healthy, non-traumatized controls (41). A similar approach needs to be undertaken to assess the relationship between PTSD and anti-inflammatory makers, as current findings are limited in number and are equivocal in nature. Concentrations of IL-4, IL-8 and IL-10 have been reported to be both lower (18,30,42–44) and higher in individuals with PTSD (14).

One mechanism by which PTSD may contribute to increased circulating concentrations of inflammatory signals is by altering immune cell distribution and function (45). Specifically, immune responses to challenge differ, as individuals with PTSD show enhanced cell-mediated immunity in response to an in vivo hypersensitivity skin test (46,47). Furthermore, immune challenge in individuals with PTSD using in vivo endotoxin administration results in augmented IL-6 response (48). Ex vivo phytohemagglutinin (PHA) stimulation in peripheral blood mononuclear cells (PBMCs) results in greater IL-6 and TNF-α secretion (49), as well as lower production of anti-inflammatory IL-4 compared to controls (50). Several studies show greater overall numbers of T cells, leukocytes and lymphocytes in individuals with PTSD (51,52). PTSD has also been associated with higher numbers of PBMCs, pro-inflammatory Th1 and Th17 cells, and decreased T-regulatory (Treg) cells (15) that regulate and activate pro-inflammatory responses (53).

Changes in immune system signalling and function in PTSD may also be a consequence of epigenetic changes that influence gene transcription and expression (54,55). A recent epigenome-wide analysis revealed significant associations between PTSD and differential methylation in gene pathways implicated in inflammation (56). Earlier methylation studies implicated immune system genes, including Toll-like receptor (TLR)8, TLR1, TLR3, mannosidase alpha class 2C member 1 (MAN2C1), acid phosphatase 5 (ACP5), and absent in melanoma 2 (AIM2) in PTSD (30,57–59). Furthermore, the activity of transcription factors critical for immune cell function, such as nuclear factor-kappa B (NFκB), signal transducer and activator of transcription 5B (STAT5B) and nuclear factor I/A (NFIA), is increased in PTSD (60–63). Alterations in methylation and NFκB function can lead to the alterations in gene expression that have also been described in PTSD (64–66). Specifically, expression of the pro-inflammatory cytokine IL-18 and its receptor IL-18R1 and IL-16 are decreased, and the IL-8 receptor is increased in individuals with PTSD (64,65,67). Gene expression of IL-15 has also been shown to be increased in PTSD (68).

The expression of microRNAs (miRNAs) is also different in PTSD (55) in a manner that may contribute to increased inflammation and altered gene expression of inflammatory signals (69,70). For instance, greater peripheral concentrations of INF-γ in PTSD are associated with lower levels of expression of microRNA-125a (miR-125a), whose function is to attenuate IFN-γ secretion from PBMCs (15). Furthermore, increased levels of IL-12 in individuals with PTSD have been linked to attenuated expression of miR-193a-5p in PBMCs (71). Recent work has shown that decreased expression of miRNAs in PTSD is linked to a downregulation of AGO2 (Argonaute 2) and DCR1 (Dicer1), factors that are critical for the generation of mature miRNAs (69). More specifically, decreased DCR1 expression in PTSD is associated with lower level of miR-3130-5p (70). Importantly, activation of monocytes or CD4+ T cells leads to reduced availability of mature miRNAs and this downregulation of miRNAs in PTSD is associated with a pro-inflammatory state (69).

Variability in the genome has also been linked to increased individual vulnerability to a pro-inflammatory state in PTSD. Enrichment of immune signalling genes has been implicated in PTSD by a genome-wide association study (GWAS) in women (72). Single nucleotide polymorphisms (SNPs) in the gene encoding CRP have also been associated with heightened inflammation and PTSD in both civilian (12) and veteran (59) samples. For example, an SNP in the *CRP* gene (rs1130864) is associated with greater CRP concentrations, greater PTSD symptoms, and an increased likelihood of a PTSD diagnosis in traumatized individuals (12). Two other SNPs within the *CRP* gene (rs1295 and rs2794529) influence CRP concentrations in individuals with PTSD (59). Similarly, a SNP within the *TNF-α* gene (rs1800629) has been associated with PTSD severity (73). Taken together, these data indicate that genomic factors may influence inflammatory tone and confer individual risk for increased PTSD severity in traumatized individuals.

12.3 Inflammation and GAD, PD and Agoraphobias

Other anxiety disorders, as defined by the DSM-5, including GAD, PD and agoraphobia, share commonalities with PTSD, namely increased anxiety and arousal in response to specific stimuli, as well as common underlying neurobiological phenotypes. These other anxiety disorders have also been associated with alterations in the immune system that result in increased inflammation (74). Furthermore, anxiety in non-patient populations has also been associated with greater peripheral CRP and cytokine concentrations (75–77). However, the number of studies assessing the relationship between GAD, PD, agoraphobia and the immune system is much smaller than those described above in the context of PTSD (78).

Increased CRP, TNF-α and interleukin concentrations in the periphery have been associated with anxiety disorders (Table 12.2), and have been associated with greater symptom severity (79,80). Current anxiety disorders, including agoraphobia, have also been associated with steeper increases in CRP concentrations over time (81). It is important to note that for every

Table 12.2 Summary of the associations between GAD, PD and phobias with inflammatory signals. ↑ denotes increased concentrations in the majority of studies; ↓ denotes increased concentrations in the majority of studies; ↑↓ denotes mixed results; – no studies that have described the relationship

Signal	GAD, PD, phobias			
	Increased	Decreased	Negative	Majority
C-reactive protein (CRP)	(74,80,229-232)	–	(233)	↑
Interleukin-6 (IL-6)	(79,80,83)	–	(86)	↑
Interleukin-1β (IL-1β)	(83,234)	–	(84,86)	↑↓
Tumour necrosis factor (TNF-α)	(82,83)	–	(74,79,233, 235)	↑↓
Interferon-γ (IFN-γ)	(80)	(82,86)	–	↑↓

study showing an association between the pro-inflammatory markers and anxiety disorders, there is another study to suggest there is no relationship or a relationship in the opposite direction (Table 12.2). The same equivocal findings surround anti-inflammatory markers, as concentrations of IL-2 and IL-4 have been described as lower in GAD patients (82), greater (83–85) or no different from controls in PD (86). While recent meta-analyses support that notion that GAD and other anxiety disorders are associated with heightened systemic inflammation (87,88), the contradictory nature of the results from these studies underscores the need for better clarification of the relationship between the immune system and GAD, PD and agoraphobia (89). Capturing potential factors that may confound the relationship, including the type of assessment used to capture anxiety disorder diagnoses (self-report vs clinician administered measures), the population studied, sex and other sociodemographic factors, and the presence of comorbid physical and mental health disorder that have also been associated with a pro-inflammatory states, is also critical in future studies. One particularly important factor, which has typically not been considered in studies of inflammation and anxiety disorders, is depression. Depression is highly comorbid with anxiety disorders and has also been associated with increased systemic inflammation and alterations in immune function (90).

12.4 Processes Implicated in Systemic Inflammation in Anxiety Disorders

The heightened inflammatory state that has been described in PTSD and the other anxiety disorders discussed above likely arises by activation and dysregulation of stress responses in the body. Exposure to stimuli that elicit fear and anxiety in PTSD, GAD, PD and phobias not only directly induces the release of pro-inflammatory cytokines (91,92) via NFκB (93) and danger associated molecular patterns (DAMPs) (94,95), but also elicits activation of the autonomic nervous system and HPA axis. Upon stress exposure, there is an immediate activation of the sympathetic nervous system that facilitates release of norepinephrine (NE) into the vasculature, which in turn activates the innate immune system to stimulate the synthesis and release of cytokines (93,96,97). Activation of the HPA axis upon stressor exposure and subsequent synthesis and release of glucocorticoids, such as cortisol, act on a slower timeline to attenuate the release of stress-induced cytokines by inhibiting the NFκB pathway (98). Thus, this neuroendocrine feedback mechanism of the HPA axis functions to maintain immune homeostasis following exposure to threatening stimuli (Figure 12.1A).

Importantly, chronic, unpredictable and repeated exposure to threatening stimuli (stressors) associated with PTSD, GAD, PD and phobias results in the dysregulation of the HPA axis, such that this glucocorticoid negative feedback inhibition of the immune system is impaired, facilitating a pro-inflammatory state (Figure 12.1B). Individuals with PTSD show enhanced glucocorticoid negative feedback inhibition of the HPA axis as evidenced by increased suppression of cortisol levels following a dexamethasone suppression test (99), greater concentrations of peripheral and central corticotropin-releasing hormone (CRH) (100,101), and decreased levels of cortisol (102,103). Similar perturbations in HPA axis function have been described across the anxiety disorders. More specifically, hair and salivary cortisol are elevated in individuals with GAD and PD (104,105), and a heightened cortisol awaking response has been described in individuals with PD with agoraphobia (106). Furthermore, cortisol non-suppression in response to dexamethasone has been described in individuals with agoraphobia and PD (107).

However, studies assessing HPA axis function in these anxiety disorders report mixed results. For instance, in PTSD, basal and diurnal cortisol concentrations have been reported to be either augmented or unchanged compared to controls (108–110). In GAD and PD, CRH concentrations have also been reported to be similar to controls (111,112). The equivocal nature of findings to date regarding the relationship between HPA axis dysregulation and anxiety disorders suggests that other factors may be contributing to HPA dysregulation, such as sex (109), severity of symptoms (113) and altered sympathetic and parasympathetic activity (114).

Regarding autonomic function, studies indicate that individuals with PTSD (115), PD (116,117) and GAD (118) show augmented sympathetic tone. More specifically, PTSD is associated with increased adrenergic activity (115), augmented norepinephrine concentrations at baseline (115,119,120) and in response to a stressor challenge (121,122). Decreased heart rate variability (HRV), a marker of parasympathetic tone, has also been described in PTSD (116,117), PD (116,117), GAD (118), social anxiety (123) and specific phobia (124). Furthermore, a meta-analysis determined that these anxiety disorders are all associated with reduced HRV (125), suggesting another mechanism that may contribute to increased inflammation in individuals with anxiety disorders (Figure 12.1B).

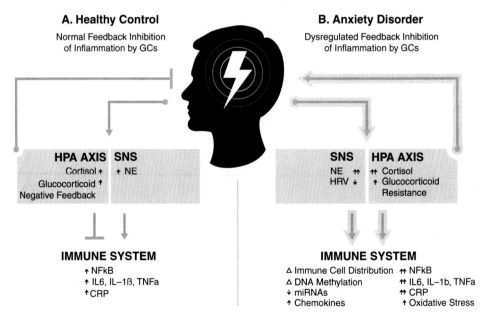

Figure 12.1 (A) Upon stressor exposure, there is an immediate activation of the sympathetic nervous system that facilitates release of NE into the vasculature, which in turn activates the innate immune system to stimulate the synthesis and release of cytokines (IL-6, IL-1β), and TNF-α, which induce CRP release. Activation of the HPA axis upon stressor exposure and subsequent synthesis and release cortisol, act on a slower timeline to attenuate the release of stress-induced cytokines by inhibiting the NFκB pathway. This normal neuroendocrine feedback inhibition of inflammation by glucocorticoids (GCs) functions to maintain immune homeostasis following exposure to threatening stimuli in healthy individuals. (B) Repeated exposures to threatening stimuli in individuals with anxiety disorders results in the dysregulation of the HPA axis, such that this glucocorticoid negative feedback inhibition of the immune system is impaired (GC resistance), facilitating a pro-inflammatory state by driving the NFκB pathway to induce increases in cytokine and CRP levels, as well as increase oxidative stress. Increased inflammation in individuals with anxiety disorders can also arise from augmented sympathetic tone.

12.5 Health Behaviours that Contribute to Inflammation in Anxiety Disorders

Anxiety disorders often disrupt daily functioning and quality of life, and can influence general health by impacting health behaviours, which in turn can contribute to a pro-inflammatory state (126,127). Reductions in the amount and quality of sleep are common in PTSD, GAD and other anxiety disorders, and these disruptions in sleep adversely affect the immune system (128). For example, concentrations of CRP (129) and IL-6 (130) are associated with severe sleep loss, and mild sleep deficits are also associated with increased inflammation (131). Coincident with sleep disturbances in PTSD and other anxiety disorders are changes in eating and exercise behaviours that contribute to obesity, a state also associated with increased CRP and IL-6 concentrations (132). In a recent study, anxiety symptoms were shown to independently contribute to increased CRP concentrations in obese individuals (133). Other physical health conditions, such as diabetes, cardiovascular disease, gastrointestinal disease and autoimmune disorders, such irritable bowel disease, are all highly comorbid with anxiety disorders and PTSD, and are also associated with increased systemic inflammation (5,134,135). Finally, smoking and alcohol dependence are more common in individuals with anxiety disorders and PTSD (127,136,137) and have also been associated with increased inflammation (127,138,139). While the cross-sectional nature of most of the studies reviewed in this chapter limits the ability to address the causality and directionality of the relationship between inflammation and anxiety disorders, a limited number of studies suggest that inflammation contributes to the onset and severity of anxiety symptoms.

12.6 Inflammation Contributes to the Development of Anxiety Disorders

While the majority of studies suggest that the presence of anxiety disorders contributes to increased systemic inflammation in individuals with these psychiatric conditions, significantly fewer studies have assessed whether inflammation contributes to the development of these anxiety disorders. The paucity of such data is likely due to difficulties surrounding implementation of longitudinal, prospective studies of healthy individuals. The limited prospective data that do exist are in the context of PTSD, wherein the onset of the disorder occurs specifically after trauma exposure. Data collected from prospective military cohorts show that greater pre-deployment CRP concentrations and enriched expression of genes involved in the immune system are both associated with increased risk for PTSD for post-deployment, even when accounting for pre-deployment PTSD and trauma exposure (140,141).

It is important to note that similar pre-trauma exposure studies have not been reported in civilian samples. However, studies assessing inflammatory markers in the aftermath of trauma exposure do suggest a link between immune markers and risk for developing PTSD; nonetheless, the results vary by the interval between sample collection and trauma exposure. For instance, higher morning IL-6 levels, greater IL-8 concentrations, and lower levels of low transforming growth factor beta (TFG-beta), all assessed within the first 24 hours from trauma exposure, are associated with PTSD development following trauma exposure (142,143). Contrary to these findings, a recent study that measured pro-inflammatory cytokines on average three hours following trauma exposure found that lower

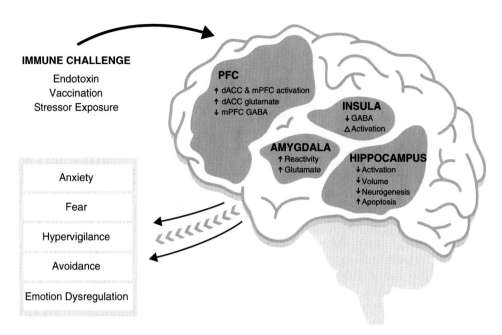

Figure 12.2 Immune challenges arising from experimental procedures (endotoxin or vaccination) or from stressor exposure can induce changes in neurotransmitter systems and impact the function of brain areas (prefrontal cortex, PFC; amygdala; insula; hippocampus) to contribute to emotion dysregulation and symptoms of anxiety, fear, hypervigilance and avoidance.

concentrations of TNF-α and INF-γ were associated with greater risk of chronic PTSD development (144). Overall these data, along with newer literature characterizing the relationship between the immune system and function of brain areas implicated in the aetiology of PTSD and anxiety disorders, suggest that inflammation can contribute to the development and maintenance of anxiety symptoms (Figure 12.2).

One brain area that has been heavily studied in the context of anxiety disorders, including PTSD, is the amygdala, whose activation is increased in response to threatening stimuli in individuals with PTSD, GAD, PD and specific phobia (145–148), and predictive of a greater IL-6 production in response to stressor exposure (149,150). Inducing an inflammatory state via endotoxin administration or vaccination in healthy individuals has also been linked to heightened amygdala activity (149,151) and increased affective and cognitive problems, including greater social disconnection, depressed mood and increased fatigue (150,151). Lipopolysaccharide (LPS) administration in healthy men induces both increased trait anxiety and temporal variance within the amygdala (152). Importantly, increased amygdala activation in anxiety disorders and PTSD is associated with dysfunction of areas of the prefrontal cortex critical for emotion regulation, executive functioning, and responding to threatening stimuli (147,153–161), including the medial prefrontal cortex (mPFC), rostral anterior cingulate cortex (rACC), subgenual ACC (sgACC) and dorsal ACC (dACC).

Activation of the ventral mPFC (vmPFC) is associated with release of IL-1β and TNF receptor II (TNF-RII) in women following a laboratory stress paradigm (162). Similarly, stress-induced increases in IL-6 predict greater functional connectivity between the amygdala and dorsomedial PFC (150). Typhoid vaccination induces mood deterioration while concurrently activating the sgACC and reducing functional connectivity between the sgACC, mPFC, and amygdala in a manner that is predicted by vaccine-induced increases in IL-6 in healthy individuals (163). Typhoid vaccination also elicits increased dACC activation and blood blow during a Stroop task (151,157). Finally, IFN-γ treatment in individuals with hepatitis C is associated with increased dACC activity that is predictive of errors in visuospatial attention (164).

The function of other limbic areas of the brain, including the insula and hippocampus, implicated in the aetiology of anxiety disorders and PTSD (155,165–167) is also impacted by the immune system. Activation of the immune system in healthy humans via typhoid vaccination decreases glucose metabolism in the insula and hippocampus while concurrently compromising spatial memory (168). Similar activation of the immune system by typhoid vaccination and endotoxin administration also results in increased insula activity (151,169) and heightened glucose metabolism in the insula (170). Importantly, increased inflammation is associated with reduced hippocampal volume in PTSD (171), paralleling translational work in rodent models implicated cytokines in the inhibition of neurogenesis and promotion of apoptosis within the hippocampus (172,173). Taken together, these findings indicate that the immune system can impact the function of corticolimbic brain areas critical for affective regulation that is disrupted in anxiety disorders.

It is important to note that the majority of studies discussed above that assess immune effects on the neurobiological pathways underlying anxiety have been conducted in healthy individuals or individuals with depression. Very minimal work has been conducted to characterize the relationships between inflammation and these pathways in individuals with anxiety disorders. A recent study indicates that CRP concentrations correlate negatively with functional connectivity between the amygdala and vmPFC in association with anxiety in individuals with depression (174). While similar studies are lacking in the context of PTSD and other anxiety disorders, there are recent data that suggest a link between increased IL-6 concentrations and decreased amygdala-vmPFC function connectivity in individuals with childhood trauma exposure (physical abuse) (175).

Mechanistically, immune signals can disrupt brain function by altering neurotransmitter pathways in the brain (176), including glutamate, dopamine, serotonin and GABA systems (6). Furthermore, cytokine-induced excitotoxicity from dysregulation of the enzyme that acts to convert tryptophan into kynurenine, indoleamine 2,3 dioxygenase, has been implicated in mood disruption in depression (177,178). Kynurenine can be broken down into quinolinic acid, an N-methyl-D-aspartate (NMDA) receptor agonist that can directly both stimulate and block the reuptake of glutamate (179). Greater CRP concentrations are found in the basal ganglia of depressed individuals (178), and interferon treatment for hepatitis C increases dACC concentrations of glutamate that predict changes in anhedonia and fatigue (180). While there are currently no descriptions of a dysregulated kynurenine pathway in anxiety disorders and PTSD in the literature, animal model work shows that exogenous administration of cytokines, such as IL-6 and TNF-α, into the amygdala of rodents induces glutamate excitotoxicity and impairs fear responses (181,182). However, there are reports of altered neurotransmitter systems in PTSD and anxiety disorders that maybe related to inflammation-induced excitotoxicity (183,184). For examples, PTSD is associated with attenuated insular concentrations of GABA (185), and PD is associated with decreases in prefrontal levels of GABA (186,187).

Cytokines can also induce oxidative stress in the brain by stimulating the release of reactive oxygen species (ROS) in microglia and astrocytes (6). A recent review suggests an association between PTSD and oxidative stress (184). Multiple studies have illustrated increases in ROS and decreases in antioxidant molecules in PTSD (188–190), and show that these changes in ROS occur concomitantly with alterations in GABA levels (188). Furthermore, expression of genes encoding enzymes involved in ROS metabolism, such as glutathione S-transferase mu 1 and 2 (*GSTM1* and *GSTM2*), are altered in chronic PTSD (191), and have been associated with prospective risk for PTSD development (192,193). PTSD has also been associated with augmented expression levels of thioredoxin (*TXNRD1*), a protein critical for responding to oxidative stress (194). Polymorphisms within ROS pathway genes have more recently been associated with PTSD symptom severity (195). Similar studies show that GAD (196) and PD (197) are also associated with oxidative stress.

Preclinical studies in rodents have also highlighted the causal roles of cytokines and other immune signals (e.g., chemokines) in the induction of anxiety behaviour via interaction with other neuropeptide and signalling pathways. For instance, stress-induced increase of central IL-1β or direct infusion of IL-1β into the brain both facilitate anxiogenesis via inhibition of the endocannabinoid system in mice (198). Similarly, intracerebroventricular administration of INF-γ induces anxiety-like behaviour in mice by altering the sensitivity of endocannabinoid receptors (199). Activation of the chemokine CXCL12 (stromal cell-derived factor-1alpha) and its receptor, CXCR4, upon LPS administration in mice induces anxiety-like behaviour (200) and can impact serotonergic neurotransmission that has been implicated in the aetiology of anxiety (201). Expression of brain derived neurotrophic factor (BDNF) within the hippocampus and prefrontal cortex and concentrations of central serotonin and kynurenine are decreased upon a viral challenge that concurrently induces anxiety-like behaviour in mice (202). While the above preclinical data highlight important interactions between immune activation and signalling with other critical pathways implicated in the aetiology of anxiety, further studies are necessary to translate and extend our understanding of mechanisms by which inflammation induces anxiety in people.

- Anxiety disorders are associated with increased systemic inflammation.
- Chronic, unpredictable and repeated exposure to threatening stimuli (stressors) contributes to dysregulation of the HPA axis and drives sympathetic activation that both facilitate systemic inflammation in individuals with anxiety disorders.
- Immune signals can impact the activity of corticolimbic brain regions and signalling systems (e.g., neurotransmitters) to contribute to the aetiology and maintenance of anxiety symptoms.
- Very limited prospective studies indicate a possible role of the immune system in conferring individual risk for the development of PTSD and anxiety disorders.
- Future studies elucidating the mechanisms by which the immune system impacts anxiety will have significant implications for intervention.

Figure 12.3 Key messages.

12.7 Summary and Conclusions

Overall, available data indicate that PTSD, GAD, PD, and phobias are associated with alterations in the immune system that can impact brain regions implicated in anxiety disorders (Figure 12.3). The majority of studies to date conducted in individuals with anxiety disorders have been cross-sectional in nature, limiting our ability to determine whether these disorders are the cause or consequence of increased systemic inflammation. However, the dysregulation of the stress axis and heightened sympathetic activation present in individuals with anxiety disorders likely contribute to augmented systemic inflammation in these individuals. While experimental activation of immune system (either through direct administration of immune activating agents or stress exposure) clearly impacts the neurocircuitry implicated in the aetiology and maintenance of anxiety in healthy individuals, minimal studies address whether similar immune activation is anxiogenic in individuals with anxiety disorders (Figure 12.2). Similarly, there is a general lack of data specifically describing the relationships between inflammation and alterations in structure, function and connectivity of these brain regions in individuals with anxiety disorders; most studies describing these relationships have been conducted in the context of depression. Future clinical and translational studies should focus on conducting similar studies specifically in people with anxiety disorders and on elucidating the biological mechanisms underlying the effects of inflammation on anxiety.

Despite the above-mentioned gaps in knowledge, some have argued that PTSD and these anxiety disorders are immunological disorders themselves, suggesting that targeting inflammation as a therapeutic target may alleviate symptoms in individuals suffering from PTSD and anxiety disorders (203,204). A recent systematic review of prebiotic and probiotic interventions for PTSD revealed only a single pilot study that suggests that these anti-inflammatory interventions may be beneficial for PTSD (205). One pilot study suggests that ingestion of a fermented soy supplement in individuals with PTSD for three months reduces symptoms of anxiety, panic and detachment (206). Diets high in omega-3 polyunsaturated fatty acids (PUFAs) have been associated with decreases in anxiety symptoms and prevention of anxiety in preclinical models (reviewed in (207)). While these limited studies suggest that anti-inflammatory interventions may alleviate symptoms of anxiety, more work needs to be done in the context of these anxiety disorders, similar to what has been done in depression (208,209), where studies have shown that anti-inflammatory interventions only work in people who have significantly elevated levels of inflammation to begin with (209).

Forms of pharmacotherapy and psychotherapy for PTSD and anxiety disorders may also prove efficacious in attenuating augmented inflammation in these disorders. Treatment of PTSD with serotonin reuptake inhibitors (SSRIs) results in decreased peripheral IL-1β concentrations (210), corroborating work showing that SSRIs can prevent stress-induced pro-inflammatory gene expression and attenuate heightened fear responses in a rodent model of PTSD (211). Similarly, treatment of GAD with SSRIs decreases peripheral CRP and IL-6 concentrations in a manner that is predictive of anxiety symptom reduction (212). Psychotherapy has also been associated with reductions in TNF-α in combat-related PTSD that occur concomitantly with reductions in PTSD symptoms (213). Mindfulness-based stress reduction in GAD is associated with a reduction in pro-inflammatory cytokines (IL-6 and TNF-α) following an acute stressor (214). However, studies have also shown no effects of mindfulness and cognitive behavioural therapy for anxiety on inflammatory markers (i.e., IL-6 and CRP) (215). More studies are clearly necessary to assess the effects of the immune system on anxiety symptoms; the need is highlighted by the fact that anxiety disorders and PTSD onset have both been associated with increases in pro-inflammatory markers over time (81,216).

References

1. Kessler RC, Berglund P, Demler O, et al. Lifetime prevalence and age-of-onset distributions of DSM-IV disorders in the National Comorbidity Survey Replication. *Archives of General Psychiatry*. 2005;62 (6):593–602.

2. Gustavsson A, Svensson M, Jacobi F, et al. Cost of disorders of the brain in Europe 2010. *Eur Neuropsychopharmacol*. 2011;21 (10):718–79.

3. American Psychiatric Association. *Diagnostic and Statistical Manual of Mental Disorders*. American Psychiatric Association, Washington; 2013.

4. Singewald N, Schmuckermair C, Whittle N, Holmes A, Ressler KJ. Pharmacology of cognitive enhancers for exposure-based therapy of fear, anxiety and trauma-related disorders. *Pharmacology & Therapeutics*. 2015;149:150–90.

5. Boscarino JA. Posttraumatic stress disorder and physical illness: results from clinical and epidemiologic studies. *Annals of the New York Academy of Sciences*. 2004;1032:141–53.

6. Haroon E, Raison CL, Miller AH. Psychoneuroimmunology meets neuropsychopharmacology: translational implications of the impact of inflammation on behavior. *Neuropsychopharmacology*. 2012;37(1):137–62.

7. Kessler RC, Sonnega A, Bromet E, Hughes M, Nelson CB. Posttraumatic stress disorder in the National Comorbidity Survey. *Archives of General Psychiatry*. 1995;52(12):1048–60.

8. Norrholm SD, Glover EM, Stevens JS, et al. Fear load: the psychophysiological over-expression of fear as an intermediate phenotype associated with trauma reactions. *Int J Psychophysiol*. 2015; 98(2 Pt 2):270–5.

9. Norrholm SD, Jovanovic T, Olin IW, et al. Fear extinction in traumatized civilians with posttraumatic stress disorder: relation to symptom severity. *Biological Psychiatry*. 2011;69(6):556–63.

10. Jovanovic T, Norrholm SD, Blanding NQ, et al. Impaired fear inhibition is a biomarker of PTSD but not depression. *Depress Anxiety*. 2010;27(3):244–51.

11. Michopoulos V, Norrholm SD, Jovanovic T. Diagnostic biomarkers for posttraumatic stress disorder: promising horizons from translational neuroscience research. *Biological Psychiatry*. 2015;78 (5):344–53.

12. Michopoulos V, Rothbaum AO, Jovanovic T, et al. Association of CRP genetic variation and CRP level with elevated PTSD symptoms and physiological responses in a civilian population with high levels of trauma. *The American Journal of Psychiatry*. 2015;172 (4):353–62.

13. O'Donovan A, Ahmadian AJ, Neylan TC, et al. Current posttraumatic stress disorder and exaggerated threat sensitivity associated with elevated inflammation in the Mind Your Heart Study. *Brain Behav Immun*. 2017;60:198–205.

14. Guo M, Liu T, Guo JC, et al. Study on serum cytokine levels in posttraumatic stress disorder patients. *Asian Pac J Trop Med*. 2012;5(4):323–5.

15. Zhou J, Nagarkatti P, Zhong Y, et al. Dysregulation in microRNA expression is associated with alterations in immune functions in combat veterans with post-traumatic stress disorder. *PloS One*. 2014;9(4):e94075.

16. Plantinga L, Bremner JD, Miller AH, et al. Association between posttraumatic stress disorder and inflammation: a twin study. *Brain Behav Immun*. 2013;30:125–32.

17. Sumner JA, Chen Q, Roberts AL, et al. Cross-sectional and longitudinal associations of chronic posttraumatic stress disorder with inflammatory and endothelial function markers in women. *Biological Psychiatry*. 2017;82(12):875–84.

18. von Kanel R, Hepp U, Kraemer B, et al. Evidence for low-grade systemic proinflammatory activity in patients with posttraumatic stress disorder. *Journal of Psychiatric Research*. 2007;41(9):744–52.

19. Oglodek EA, Szota AM, Mos DM, Araszkiewicz A, Szromek AR. Serum concentrations of chemokines (CCL-5 and CXCL-12), chemokine receptors (CCR-5 and CXCR-4), and IL-6 in patients with posttraumatic stress disorder and avoidant personality disorder. *Pharmacol Rep*. 2015;67(6):1251–8.

20. Dalgard C, Eidelman O, Jozwik C, et al. The MCP-4/MCP-1 ratio in plasma is a candidate circadian biomarker for chronic post-traumatic stress disorder. *Transl Psychiatry*. 2017;7(2):e1025.

21. Lindqvist D, Wolkowitz OM, Mellon S, et al. Proinflammatory milieu in combat-related PTSD is independent of depression and early life stress. *Brain Behav Immun*. 2014;42:81–8.

22. Lindqvist D, Dhabhar FS, Mellon SH, et al. Increased pro-inflammatory milieu in combat related PTSD – a new cohort replication study. *Brain Behav Immun*. 2017;59:260–4.

23. Bruenig D, Mehta D, Morris CP, et al. Correlation between interferon gamma and interleukin 6 with PTSD and resilience. *Psychiatry Research*. 2017;260:193–8.

24. Mendoza C, Barreto GE, Avila-Rodriguez M, Echeverria V. Role of neuroinflammation and sex hormones in war-related PTSD. *Molecular and Cellular Endocrinology*. 2016;434:266–77.

25. John-Henderson NA, Marsland AL, Kamarck TW, Muldoon MF, Manuck SB. Childhood socioeconomic status and the occurrence of recent negative life events as predictors of circulating and stimulated levels of interleukin-6. *Psychosom Med*. 2016;78(1):91–101.

26. Devoto C, Arcurio L, Fetta J, et al. Inflammation relates to chronic behavioral and neurological symptoms in military personnel with traumatic brain injuries. *Cell Transplant*. 2017;26(7):1169–77.

27. Tursich M, Neufeld RW, Frewen PA, et al. Association of trauma exposure with proinflammatory activity: a transdiagnostic meta-analysis. *Transl Psychiatry*. 2014;4:e413.

28. Tietjen GE, Khubchandani J, Herial NA, Shah K. Adverse childhood experiences are associated with migraine and vascular biomarkers. *Headache*. 2012;52(6):920–9.

29. Hartwell KJ, Moran-Santa Maria MM, Twal WO, et al. Association of elevated cytokines with childhood adversity in a sample of healthy adults. *Journal of Psychiatric Research*. 2013;47(5):604–10.

30. Smith AK, Conneely KN, Kilaru V, et al. Differential immune system DNA methylation and cytokine regulation in post-traumatic stress disorder. *Am J Med Genet B Neuropsychiatr Genet*. 2011;156B (6):700–8.

31. Gouin JP, Glaser R, Malarkey WB, Beversdorf D, Kiecolt-Glaser JK. Childhood abuse and inflammatory responses to daily stressors. *Ann Behav Med*. 2012;44(2):287–92.

32. Kiecolt-Glaser JK, Gouin JP, Weng NP, et al. Childhood adversity heightens the impact of later-life caregiving stress on telomere length and inflammation. *Psychosom Med*. 2011;73(1):16–22.

33. Danese A, Pariante CM, Caspi A, Taylor A, Poulton R. Childhood maltreatment predicts adult inflammation in a life-course study. *Proceedings of the National Academy of Sciences of the United States of America*. 2007;104(4):1319–24.

34. Rooks C, Veledar E, Goldberg J, Bremner JD, Vaccarino V. Early trauma and inflammation: role of familial factors in a study of twins. *Psychosom Med*. 2012;74(2):146–52.

35. Matthews KA, Chang YF, Thurston RC, Bromberger JT. Child abuse is related to inflammation in mid-life women: role of obesity. *Brain Behav Immun*. 2014;36:29–34.

36. Bertone-Johnson ER, Whitcomb BW, Missmer SA, Karlson EW, Rich-Edwards JW. Inflammation and early-life abuse in

women. *Am J Prev Med.* 2012;43 (6):611–20.

37. Lin JE, Neylan TC, Epel E, O'Donovan A. Associations of childhood adversity and adulthood trauma with C-reactive protein: a cross-sectional population-based study. *Brain Behav Immun.* 2016;53:105–12.

38. Holliday SB, DeSantis A, Germain A, et al. Deployment length, inflammatory markers, and ambulatory blood pressure in military couples. *Mil Med.* 2017;182(7): e1892-e9.

39. Hussein S, Dalton B, Willmund GD, Ibrahim MAA, Himmerich H. A systematic review of tumor necrosis factor-alpha in post-traumatic stress disorder: evidence from human and animal studies. *Psychiatr Danub.* 2017;29 (4):407–20.

40. Waheed A, Dalton B, Wesemann U, Ibrahim MAA, Himmerich H. A systematic review of interleukin-1beta in post-traumatic stress disorder: evidence from human and animal studies. *J Interferon Cytokine Res.* 2018;38(1):1–11.

41. Passos IC, Vasconcelos-Moreno MP, Costa LG, et al. Inflammatory markers in post-traumatic stress disorder: a systematic review, meta-analysis, and meta-regression. *Lancet Psychiatry.* 2015;2 (11):1002–12.

42. Jergovic M, Bendelja K, Savic Mlakar A, et al. Circulating levels of hormones, lipids, and immune mediators in post-traumatic stress disorder – a 3-month follow-up study. *Front Psychiatry.* 2015;6:49.

43. Song Y, Zhou D, Guan Z, Wang X. Disturbance of serum interleukin-2 and interleukin-8 levels in posttraumatic and non-posttraumatic stress disorder earthquake survivors in northern China. *Neuroimmunomodulation.* 2007;14 (5):248–54.

44. Teche SP, Rovaris DL, Aguiar BW, et al. Resilience to traumatic events related to urban violence and increased IL10 serum levels. *Psychiatry Research.* 2017;250:136–40.

45. Jergovic M, Bendelja K, Vidovic A, et al. Patients with posttraumatic stress disorder exhibit an altered phenotype of regulatory T cells. *Allergy Asthma Clin Immunol.* 2014;10(1):43.

46. Altemus M, Cloitre M, Dhabhar FS. Enhanced cellular immune response in women with PTSD related to childhood abuse. *The American Journal of Psychiatry.* 2003;160(9):1705–7.

47. Masoudzadeh A, Modanloo Kordi M, Ajami A, Azizi A. Evaluation of cortisol level and cell-mediated immunity response changes in individuals with post-traumatic stress disorder as a consequence of war. *Med Glas (Zenica).* 2012;9 (2):218–22.

48. Rohleder N, Joksimovic L, Wolf JM, Kirschbaum C. Hypocortisolism and increased glucocorticoid sensitivity of pro-Inflammatory cytokine production in Bosnian war refugees with posttraumatic stress disorder. *Biological Psychiatry.* 2004;55(7):745–51.

49. Gill J, Vythilingam M, Page GG. Low cortisol, high DHEA, and high levels of stimulated TNF-alpha, and IL-6 in women with PTSD. *J Trauma Stress.* 2008;21 (6):530–9.

50. Kawamura N, Kim Y, Asukai N. Suppression of cellular immunity in men with a past history of posttraumatic stress disorder. *American Journal of Psychiatry.* 2001;158(3):484–6.

51. Vidovic A, Gotovac K, Vilibic M, et al. Repeated assessments of endocrine- and immune-related changes in posttraumatic stress disorder. *Neuroimmunomodulation.* 2011;18(4):199–211.

52. Boscarino JA, Chang J. Higher abnormal leukocyte and lymphocyte counts 20 years after exposure to severe stress: research and clinical implications. *Psychosom Med.* 1999;61(3):378–86.

53. Afzali B, Lombardi G, Lechler RI, Lord GM. The role of T helper 17 (Th17) and regulatory T cells (Treg) in human organ transplantation and autoimmune disease. *Clin Exp Immunol.* 2007;148 (1):32–46.

54. Heinzelmann M, Gill J. Epigenetic mechanisms shape the biological response

to trauma and risk for PTSD: a critical review. *Nurs Res Pract.* 2013;2013:417010.

55. Bam M, Yang X, Zumbrun EE, et al. Dysregulated immune system networks in war veterans with PTSD is an outcome of altered miRNA expression and DNA methylation. *Sci Rep.* 2016;6:31209.

56. Kuan PF, Waszczuk MA, Kotov R, et al. An epigenome-wide DNA methylation study of PTSD and depression in World Trade Center responders. *Transl Psychiatry.* 2017;7(6):e1158.

57. Uddin M, Galea S, Chang SC, et al. Gene expression and methylation signatures of MAN2C1 are associated with PTSD. *Dis Markers.* 2011;30(2–3):111–21.

58. Uddin M, Aiello AE, Wildman DE, et al. Epigenetic and immune function profiles associated with posttraumatic stress disorder. *Proceedings of the National Academy of Sciences of the United States of America.* 2010;107(20):9470–5.

59. Miller MW, Maniates H, Wolf EJ, et al. CRP polymorphisms and DNA methylation of the AIM2 gene influence associations between trauma exposure, PTSD, and C-reactive protein. *Brain Behav Immun.* 2018;67:194–202.

60. Pace TW, Wingenfeld K, Schmidt I, et al. Increased peripheral NF-kappaB pathway activity in women with childhood abuse-related posttraumatic stress disorder. *Brain Behav Immun.* 2012;26 (1):13–7.

61. Sarapas C, Cai G, Bierer LM, et al. Genetic markers for PTSD risk and resilience among survivors of the World Trade Center attacks. *Dis Markers.* 2011;30 (2–3):101–10.

62. O'Donovan A, Sun B, Cole S, et al. Transcriptional control of monocyte gene expression in post-traumatic stress disorder. *Dis Markers.* 2011;30 (2–3):123–32.

63. Guardado P, Olivera A, Rusch HL, et al. Altered gene expression of the innate immune, neuroendocrine, and nuclear factor-kappa B (NF-kappaB) systems is associated with posttraumatic stress disorder in military personnel. *J Anxiety Disord.* 2016;38:9–20.

64. Segman RH, Shefi N, Goltser-Dubner T, et al. Peripheral blood mononuclear cell gene expression profiles identify emergent post-traumatic stress disorder among trauma survivors. *Molecular Psychiatry.* 2005;10(5):500–13, 425.

65. Zieker J, Zieker D, Jatzko A, et al. Differential gene expression in peripheral blood of patients suffering from post-traumatic stress disorder. *Molecular Psychiatry.* 2007;12(2):116–8.

66. Yehuda R, Cai G, Golier JA, et al. Gene expression patterns associated with posttraumatic stress disorder following exposure to the World Trade Center attacks. *Biological Psychiatry.* 2009;66 (7):708–11.

67. Mehta D, Gonik M, Klengel T, et al. Using polymorphisms in FKBP5 to define biologically distinct subtypes of posttraumatic stress disorder: evidence from endocrine and gene expression studies. *Archives of General Psychiatry.* 2011;68(9):901–10.

68. Chitrala KN, Nagarkatti P, Nagarkatti M. Prediction of possible biomarkers and novel pathways conferring risk to post-traumatic stress disorder. *PloS One.* 2016;11(12):e0168404.

69. Bam M, Yang X, Zumbrun EE, et al. Decreased AGO2 and DCR1 in PBMCs from War Veterans with PTSD leads to diminished miRNA resulting in elevated inflammation. *Transl Psychiatry.* 2017;7(8): e1222.

70. Wingo AP, Almli LM, Stevens JJ, et al. DICER1 and microRNA regulation in post-traumatic stress disorder with comorbid depression. *Nature Communications.* 2015;6:10106.

71. Bam M, Yang X, Zhou J, et al. Evidence for epigenetic regulation of pro-inflammatory cytokines, interleukin-12 and interferon gamma, in peripheral blood mononuclear cells from PTSD patients. *J Neuroimmune Pharmacol.* 2016;11(1):168–81.

72. Guffanti G, Galea S, Yan L, et al. Genome-wide association study implicates a novel

RNA gene, the lincRNA AC068718.1, as a risk factor for post-traumatic stress disorder in women. *Psychoneuroendocrinology*. 2013;38 (12):3029–38.

73. Bruenig D, Mehta D, Morris CP, et al. Genetic and serum biomarker evidence for a relationship between TNFalpha and PTSD in Vietnam war combat veterans. *Compr Psychiatry*. 2017;74:125–33.

74. Vogelzangs N, Beekman AT, de Jonge P, Penninx BW. Anxiety disorders and inflammation in a large adult cohort. *Transl Psychiatry*. 2013;3:e249.

75. Pitsavos C, Panagiotakos DB, Papageorgiou C, et al. Anxiety in relation to inflammation and coagulation markers, among healthy adults: the ATTICA study. *Atherosclerosis*. 2006;185(2):320–6.

76. Brennan AM, Fargnoli JL, Williams CJ, et al. Phobic anxiety is associated with higher serum concentrations of adipokines and cytokines in women with diabetes. *Diabetes Care*. 2009;32(5):926–31.

77. O'Donovan A, Hughes BM, Slavich GM, et al. Clinical anxiety, cortisol and interleukin-6: evidence for specificity in emotion-biology relationships. *Brain Behav Immun*. 2010;24(7):1074–7.

78. Michopoulos V, Powers A, Gillespie CF, Ressler KJ, Jovanovic T. Inflammation in Fear- and Anxiety-Based Disorders: PTSD, GAD, and Beyond. *Neuropsychopharmacology*. 2017;42 (1):254–70.

79. Belem da Silva CT, Costa MA, Bortoluzzi A, et al. Cytokine levels in panic disorder: evidence for a dose-response relationship. *Psychosom Med*. 2017;79 (2):126–32.

80. Tang Z, Ye G, Chen X, et al. Peripheral proinflammatory cytokines in Chinese patients with generalised anxiety disorder. *Journal of Affective Disorders*. 2018;225:593–8.

81. Glaus J, von Kanel R, Lasserre AM, et al. The bidirectional relationship between anxiety disorders and circulating levels of inflammatory markers: results from a large longitudinal population-based study. *Depress Anxiety*. 2018;35(4):360–71.

82. Vieira MM, Ferreira TB, Pacheco PA, et al. Enhanced Th17 phenotype in individuals with generalized anxiety disorder. *J Neuroimmunol*. 2010;229(1–2):212–8.

83. Hoge EA, Brandstetter K, Moshier S, et al. Broad spectrum of cytokine abnormalities in panic disorder and posttraumatic stress disorder. *Depress Anxiety*. 2009;26 (5):447–55.

84. Rapaport MH, Stein MB. Serum cytokine and soluble interleukin-2 receptors in patients with panic disorder. *Anxiety*. 1994;1(1):22–5.

85. Koh KB, Lee Y. Reduced anxiety level by therapeutic interventions and cell-mediated immunity in panic disorder patients. *Psychother Psychosom*. 2004;73 (5):286–92.

86. Tukel R, Arslan BA, Ertekin BA, et al. Decreased IFN-gamma and IL-12 levels in panic disorder. *Journal of Psychosomatic Research*. 2012;73(1):63–7.

87. Renna ME, O'Toole MS, Spaeth PE, Lekander M, Mennin DS. The association between anxiety, traumatic stress, and obsessive-compulsive disorders and chronic inflammation: A systematic review and meta-analysis. *Depress Anxiety*. 2018;35(11):1081–94.

88. Costello H, Gould RL, Abrol E, Howard R. Systematic review and meta-analysis of the association between peripheral inflammatory cytokines and generalised anxiety disorder. *BMJ Open*. 2019;9(7): e027925.

89. Quagliato LA, Nardi AE. Cytokine alterations in panic disorder: A systematic review. *Journal of Affective Disorders*. 2018;228:91–6.

90. Miller AH, Raison CL. The role of inflammation in depression: from evolutionary imperative to modern treatment target. *Nat Rev Immunol*. 2016;16(1):22–34.

91. Koo JW, Duman RS. IL-1beta is an essential mediator of the antineurogenic and anhedonic effects of stress. *Proceedings*

of the National Academy of Sciences of the United States of America. 2008;105 (2):751–6.

92. Maier SF, Watkins LR. Cytokines for psychologists: implications of bidirectional immune-to-brain communication for understanding behavior, mood, and cognition. *Psychol Rev.* 1998;105(1):83–107.

93. Bierhaus A, Wolf J, Andrassy M, et al. A mechanism converting psychosocial stress into mononuclear cell activation. *Proceedings of the National Academy of Sciences of the United States of America.* 2003;100(4):1920–5.

94. Maslanik T, Mahaffey L, Tannura K, et al. The inflammasome and danger associated molecular patterns (DAMPs) are implicated in cytokine and chemokine responses following stressor exposure. *Brain Behav Immun.* 2013;28:54–62.

95. Iwata M, Ota KT, Duman RS. The inflammasome: pathways linking psychological stress, depression, and systemic illnesses. *Brain Behav Immun.* 2013;31:105–14.

96. Nance DM, Sanders VM. Autonomic innervation and regulation of the immune system (1987–2007). *Brain Behav Immun.* 2007;21(6):736–45.

97. Tan KS, Nackley AG, Satterfield K, et al. Beta2 adrenergic receptor activation stimulates pro-inflammatory cytokine production in macrophages via PKA- and NF-kappaB-independent mechanisms. *Cell Signal.* 2007;19(2):251–60.

98. Rhen T, Cidlowski JA. Antiinflammatory action of glucocorticoids–new mechanisms for old drugs. *The New England Journal of Medicine.* 2005;353(16):1711–23.

99. Yehuda R, Boisoneau D, Lowy MT, Giller EL, Jr. Dose-response changes in plasma cortisol and lymphocyte glucocorticoid receptors following dexamethasone administration in combat veterans with and without posttraumatic stress disorder. *Archives of General Psychiatry.* 1995;52(7):583–93.

100. de Kloet CS, Vermetten E, Geuze E, et al. Elevated plasma corticotrophin-releasing

hormone levels in veterans with posttraumatic stress disorder. *Progress in Brain Research.* 2008;167:287–91.

101. Baker DG, Ekhator NN, Kasckow JW, et al. Higher levels of basal serial CSF cortisol in combat veterans with posttraumatic stress disorder. *The American Journal of Psychiatry.* 2005;162 (5):992–4.

102. Yehuda R, Golier JA, Kaufman S. Circadian rhythm of salivary cortisol in Holocaust survivors with and without PTSD. *The American Journal of Psychiatry.* 2005;162(5):998–1000.

103. Mason JW, Giller EL, Kosten TR, Ostroff RB, Podd L. Urinary free-cortisol levels in posttraumatic stress disorder patients. *J Nerv Ment Dis.* 1986;174 (3):145–9.

104. Staufenbiel SM, Penninx BW, Spijker AT, Elzinga BM, van Rossum EF. Hair cortisol, stress exposure, and mental health in humans: a systematic review. *Psychoneuroendocrinology.* 2013;38 (8):1220–35.

105. Mantella RC, Butters MA, Amico JA, et al. Salivary cortisol is associated with diagnosis and severity of late-life generalized anxiety disorder. *Psychoneuroendocrinology.* 2008;33 (6):773–81.

106. Vreeburg SA, Zitman FG, van Pelt J, et al. Salivary cortisol levels in persons with and without different anxiety disorders. *Psychosom Med.* 2010;72(4):340–7.

107. Coryell W, Noyes R, Jr., Schlechte J. The significance of HPA axis disturbance in panic disorder. *Biological Psychiatry.* 1989;25(8):989–1002.

108. Meewisse ML, Reitsma JB, de Vries GJ, Gersons BP, Olff M. Cortisol and post-traumatic stress disorder in adults: systematic review and meta-analysis. *Br J Psychiatry.* 2007;191:387–92.

109. Freidenberg BM, Gusmano R, Hickling EJ, et al. Women with PTSD have lower basal salivary cortisol levels later in the day than do men with PTSD: a preliminary study. *Physiology & Behavior.* 2010;99(2):234–6.

110. Maes M, Lin A, Bonaccorso S, et al. Increased 24-hour urinary cortisol excretion in patients with post-traumatic stress disorder and patients with major depression, but not in patients with fibromyalgia. *Acta Psychiatr Scand.* 1998;98(4):328–35.

111. Fossey MD, Lydiard RB, Ballenger JC, et al. Cerebrospinal fluid corticotropin-releasing factor concentrations in patients with anxiety disorders and normal comparison subjects. *Biological Psychiatry.* 1996;39 (8):703–7.

112. Jolkkonen J, Lepola U, Bissette G, Nemeroff C, Riekkinen P. CSF corticotropin-releasing factor is not affected in panic disorder. *Biological Psychiatry.* 1993;33(2):136–8.

113. Shea A, Walsh C, Macmillan H, Steiner M. Child maltreatment and HPA axis dysregulation: relationship to major depressive disorder and post traumatic stress disorder in females. *Psychoneuroendocrinology.* 2005;30 (2):162–78.

114. Dieleman GC, Huizink AC, Tulen JH, et al. Alterations in HPA-axis and autonomic nervous system functioning in childhood anxiety disorders point to a chronic stress hypothesis. *Psychoneuroendocrinology.* 2015;51:135–50.

115. Southwick SM, Bremner JD, Rasmusson A, et al. Role of norepinephrine in the pathophysiology and treatment of posttraumatic stress disorder. *Biological Psychiatry.* 1999;46 (9):1192–204.

116. Blechert J, Michael T, Grossman P, Lajtman M, Wilhelm FH. Autonomic and respiratory characteristics of posttraumatic stress disorder and panic disorder. *Psychosom Med.* 2007;69 (9):935–43.

117. Cohen H, Benjamin J, Geva AB, et al. Autonomic dysregulation in panic disorder and in post-traumatic stress disorder: application of power spectrum analysis of heart rate variability at rest and in response to recollection of trauma or panic attacks. *Psychiatry Research.* 2000;96(1):1–13.

118. Thayer JF, Friedman BH, Borkovec TD. Autonomic characteristics of generalized anxiety disorder and worry. *Biological Psychiatry.* 1996;39(4):255–66.

119. Delahanty DL, Nugent NR, Christopher NC, Walsh M. Initial urinary epinephrine and cortisol levels predict acute PTSD symptoms in child trauma victims. *Psychoneuroendocrinology.* 2005;30(2):121–8.

120. Geracioti TD, Jr., Baker DG, Ekhator NN, et al. CSF norepinephrine concentrations in posttraumatic stress disorder. *The American Journal of Psychiatry.* 2001;158 (8):1227–30.

121. Blanchard EB, Kolb LC, Prins A, Gates S, McCoy GC. Changes in plasma norepinephrine to combat-related stimuli among Vietnam veterans with posttraumatic stress disorder. *J Nerv Ment Dis.* 1991;179(6):371–3.

122. Geracioti TD, Jr., Baker DG, Kasckow JW, et al. Effects of trauma-related audiovisual stimulation on cerebrospinal fluid norepinephrine and corticotropin-releasing hormone concentrations in post-traumatic stress disorder. *Psychoneuroendocrinology.* 2008;33(4):416–24.

123. Alvares GA, Quintana DS, Kemp AH, et al. Reduced heart rate variability in social anxiety disorder: associations with gender and symptom severity. *PloS One.* 2013;8(7):e70468.

124. Bornas X, Llabres J, Noguera M, et al. Fear induced complexity loss in the electrocardiogram of flight phobics: a multiscale entropy analysis. *Biological Psychology.* 2006;73(3):272–9.

125. Chalmers JA, Quintana DS, Abbott MJ, Kemp AH. Anxiety disorders are associated with reduced heart rate variability: a meta-analysis. *Front Psychiatry.* 2014;5:80.

126. Gill J, Lee H, Barr T, et al. Lower health related quality of life in U.S. military personnel is associated with service-related disorders and

inflammation. *Psychiatry Research.* 2014;216(1):116–22.

127. Dennis PA, Weinberg JB, Calhoun PS, et al. An investigation of vago-regulatory and health-behavior accounts for increased inflammation in posttraumatic stress disorder. *Journal of Psychosomatic Research.* 2016;83:33–9.

128. Bryant PA, Trinder J, Curtis N. Sick and tired: does sleep have a vital role in the immune system? *Nat Rev Immunol.* 2004;4(6):457–67.

129. Meier-Ewert HK, Ridker PM, Rifai N, et al. Effect of sleep loss on C-reactive protein, an inflammatory marker of cardiovascular risk. *J Am Coll Cardiol.* 2004;43(4):678–83.

130. Vgontzas AN, Papanicolaou DA, Bixler EO, et al. Circadian interleukin-6 secretion and quantity and depth of sleep. *The Journal of Clinical Endocrinology and Metabolism.* 1999;84 (8):2603–7.

131. Vgontzas AN, Zoumakis E, Bixler EO, et al. Adverse effects of modest sleep restriction on sleepiness, performance, and inflammatory cytokines. *The Journal of Clinical Endocrinology and Metabolism.* 2004;89(5):2119–26.

132. Khaodhiar L, Ling PR, Blackburn GL, Bistrian BR. Serum levels of interleukin-6 and C-reactive protein correlate with body mass index across the broad range of obesity. *JPEN J Parenter Enteral Nutr.* 2004;28(6):410–5.

133. Pierce GL, Kalil GZ, Ajibewa T, et al. Anxiety independently contributes to elevated inflammation in humans with obesity. *Obesity (Silver Spring).* 2017;25 (2):286–9.

134. O'Donovan A, Cohen BE, Seal KH, et al. Elevated risk for autoimmune disorders in iraq and afghanistan veterans with posttraumatic stress disorder. *Biological Psychiatry.* 2015;77(4):365–74.

135. Celano CM, Daunis DJ, Lokko HN, Campbell KA, Huffman JC. Anxiety disorders and cardiovascular disease. *Curr Psychiatry Rep.* 2016;18(11):101.

136. Fu SS, McFall M, Saxon AJ, et al. Posttraumatic stress disorder and smoking: a systematic review. *Nicotine Tob Res.* 2007;9(11):1071–84.

137. Morissette SB, Tull MT, Gulliver SB, Kamholz BW, Zimering RT. Anxiety, anxiety disorders, tobacco use, and nicotine: a critical review of interrelationships. *Psychol Bull.* 2007;133 (2):245–72.

138. Frohlich M, Sund M, Lowel H, et al. Independent association of various smoking characteristics with markers of systemic inflammation in men. Results from a representative sample of the general population (MONICA Augsburg Survey 1994/95). *Eur Heart J.* 2003;24 (14):1365–72.

139. Jamal O, Aneni EC, Shaharyar S, et al. Cigarette smoking worsens systemic inflammation in persons with metabolic syndrome. *Diabetol Metab Syndr.* 2014;6:79.

140. Eraly SA, Nievergelt CM, Maihofer AX, et al. Assessment of plasma C-reactive protein as a biomarker of posttraumatic stress disorder risk. *JAMA Psychiatry.* 2014;71(4):423–31.

141. Breen MS, Maihofer AX, Glatt SJ, et al. Gene networks specific for innate immunity define post-traumatic stress disorder. *Molecular Psychiatry.* 2015;20 (12):1538–45.

142. Pervanidou P, Kolaitis G, Charitaki S, et al. Elevated morning serum interleukin (IL)-6 or evening salivary cortisol concentrations predict posttraumatic stress disorder in children and adolescents six months after a motor vehicle accident. *Psychoneuroendocrinology.* 2007;32 (8–10):991–9.

143. Cohen M, Meir T, Klein E, et al. Cytokine levels as potential biomarkers for predicting the development of posttraumatic stress symptoms in casualties of accidents. *International Journal of Psychiatry in Medicine.* 2011;42 (2):117–31.

144. Michopoulos V, Beurel E, Gould F, et al. Association of prospective risk for

chronic PTSD symptoms with low TNFalpha and IFNgamma concentrations in the immediate aftermath of trauma exposure. *The American Journal of Psychiatry*. 2019;177(1):58–65.

145. Fonzo GA, Ramsawh HJ, Flagan TM, et al. Common and disorder-specific neural responses to emotional faces in generalised anxiety, social anxiety and panic disorders. *Br J Psychiatry*. 2015;206 (3):206–15.

146. Killgore WD, Britton JC, Schwab ZJ, et al. Cortico-limbic responses to masked affective faces across ptsd, panic disorder, and specific phobia. *Depress Anxiety*. 2014;31(2):150–9.

147. Monk CS, Telzer EH, Mogg K, et al. Amygdala and ventrolateral prefrontal cortex activation to masked angry faces in children and adolescents with generalized anxiety disorder. *Archives of General Psychiatry*. 2008;65(5):568–76.

148. Stevens JS, Kim YJ, Galatzer-Levy IR, et al. Amygdala reactivity and anterior cingulate habituation predict posttraumatic stress disorder symptom maintenance after acute civilian trauma. *Biological Psychiatry*. 2017;81(12):1023–9.

149. Inagaki TK, Muscatell KA, Irwin MR, Cole SW, Eisenberger NI. Inflammation selectively enhances amygdala activity to socially threatening images. *NeuroImage*. 2012;59(4):3222–6.

150. Muscatell KA, Dedovic K, Slavich GM, et al. Greater amygdala activity and dorsomedial prefrontal-amygdala coupling are associated with enhanced inflammatory responses to stress. *Brain Behav Immun*. 2015;43:46–53.

151. Harrison NA, Brydon L, Walker C, et al. Neural origins of human sickness in interoceptive responses to inflammation. *Biological Psychiatry*. 2009;66(5):415–22.

152. Labrenz F, Ferri F, Wrede K, et al. Altered temporal variance and functional connectivity of BOLD signal is associated with state anxiety during acute systemic inflammation. *NeuroImage*. 2019;184:916–24.

153. Fani N, Jovanovic T, Ely TD, et al. Neural correlates of attention bias to threat in post-traumatic stress disorder. *Biological Psychology*. 2012;90(2):134–42.

154. Banich MT, Mackiewicz KL, Depue BE, et al. Cognitive control mechanisms, emotion and memory: a neural perspective with implications for psychopathology. *Neuroscience and Biobehavioral Reviews*. 2009;33 (5):613–30.

155. Cui H, Zhang J, Liu Y, et al. Differential alterations of resting-state functional connectivity in generalized anxiety disorder and panic disorder. *Hum Brain Mapp*. 2016;37(4):1459–73.

156. Etkin A, Wager TD. Functional neuroimaging of anxiety: a meta-analysis of emotional processing in PTSD, social anxiety disorder, and specific phobia. *The American Journal of Psychiatry*. 2007;164 (10):1476–88.

157. Eisenberger NI, Lieberman MD. Why rejection hurts: a common neural alarm system for physical and social pain. *Trends Cogn Sci*. 2004;8(7):294–300.

158. Shin LM, Bush G, Whalen PJ, et al. Dorsal anterior cingulate function in posttraumatic stress disorder. *J Trauma Stress*. 2007;20(5):701–12.

159. Pannu Hayes J, Labar KS, Petty CM, McCarthy G, Morey RA. Alterations in the neural circuitry for emotion and attention associated with posttraumatic stress symptomatology. *Psychiatry Research*. 2009;172(1):7–15.

160. Felmingham KL, Williams LM, Kemp AH, et al. Anterior cingulate activity to salient stimuli is modulated by autonomic arousal in posttraumatic stress disorder. *Psychiatry Research*. 2009;173 (1):59–62.

161. Eisenberger NI, Lieberman MD, Satpute AB. Personality from a controlled processing perspective: an fMRI study of neuroticism, extraversion, and self-consciousness. *Cogn Affect Behav Neurosci*. 2005;5(2):169–81.

162. O'Connor MF, Irwin MR, Wellisch DK. When grief heats up: pro-inflammatory

cytokines predict regional brain activation. *NeuroImage.* 2009;47 (3):891–6.

163. Harrison NA, Brydon L, Walker C, et al. Inflammation causes mood changes through alterations in subgenual cingulate activity and mesolimbic connectivity. *Biological Psychiatry.* 2009;66(5):407–14.

164. Capuron L, Pagnoni G, Demetrashvili M, et al. Anterior cingulate activation and error processing during interferon-alpha treatment. *Biological Psychiatry.* 2005;58 (3):190–6.

165. Simmons A, Strigo IA, Matthews SC, Paulus MP, Stein MB. Initial evidence of a failure to activate right anterior insula during affective set shifting in posttraumatic stress disorder. *Psychosom Med.* 2009;71(4):373–7.

166. Fani N, King TZ, Jovanovic T, et al. White matter integrity in highly traumatized adults with and without post-traumatic stress disorder. *Neuropsychopharmacology.* 2012;37 (12):2740–6.

167. van Rooij SJH, Stevens JS, Ely TD, et al. The role of the hippocampus in predicting future posttraumatic stress disorder symptoms in recently traumatized civilians. *Biological Psychiatry.* 2017;84 (2):106–15.

168. Harrison NA, Doeller CF, Voon V, Burgess N, Critchley HD. Peripheral inflammation acutely impairs human spatial memory via actions on medial temporal lobe glucose metabolism. *Biological Psychiatry.* 2014;76(7):585–93.

169. Eisenberger NI, Inagaki TK, Rameson LT, Mashal NM, Irwin MR. An fMRI study of cytokine-induced depressed mood and social pain: the role of sex differences. *NeuroImage.* 2009;47(3):881–90.

170. Hannestad J, Subramanyam K, Dellagioia N, et al. Glucose metabolism in the insula and cingulate is affected by systemic inflammation in humans. *J Nucl Med.* 2012;53(4):601–7.

171. O'Donovan A, Chao LL, Paulson J, et al. Altered inflammatory activity associated with reduced hippocampal volume and more severe posttraumatic stress symptoms in Gulf War veterans. *Psychoneuroendocrinology.* 2015;51:557–66.

172. Ekdahl CT, Claasen JH, Bonde S, Kokaia Z, Lindvall O. Inflammation is detrimental for neurogenesis in adult brain. *Proceedings of the National Academy of Sciences of the United States of America.* 2003;100(23):13632–7.

173. Cunningham C, Wilcockson DC, Campion S, Lunnon K, Perry VH. Central and systemic endotoxin challenges exacerbate the local inflammatory response and increase neuronal death during chronic neurodegeneration. *J Neurosci.* 2005;25(40):9275–84.

174. Mehta ND, Haroon E, Xu X, et al. Inflammation negatively correlates with amygdala-ventromedial prefrontal functional connectivity in association with anxiety in patients with depression: preliminary results. *Brain Behav Immun.* 2018;73:725–30.

175. Kraynak TE, Marsland AL, Hanson JL, Gianaros PJ. Retrospectively reported childhood physical abuse, systemic inflammation, and resting corticolimbic connectivity in midlife adults. *Brain Behav Immun.* 2019;82:203–13.

176. Dunn AJ, Wang J, Ando T. Effects of cytokines on cerebral neurotransmission. Comparison with the effects of stress. *Advances in Experimental Medicine and Biology.* 1999;461:117–27.

177. Schwarcz R. The kynurenine pathway of tryptophan degradation as a drug target. *Curr Opin Pharmacol.* 2004;4(1):12–7.

178. Haroon E, Fleischer CC, Felger JC, et al. Conceptual convergence: increased inflammation is associated with increased basal ganglia glutamate in patients with major depression. *Molecular Psychiatry.* 2016;21(10):1351–7.

179. Tavares RG, Tasca CI, Santos CE, et al. Quinolinic acid stimulates synaptosomal glutamate release and inhibits glutamate uptake into astrocytes. *Neurochem Int.* 2002;40(7):621–7.

180. Haroon E, Woolwine BJ, Chen X, et al. IFN-alpha-induced cortical and subcortical glutamate changes assessed by magnetic resonance spectroscopy. *Neuropsychopharmacology*. 2014;39 (7):1777–85.

181. Jing H, Hao Y, Bi Q, Zhang J, Yang P. Intra-amygdala microinjection of TNF-alpha impairs the auditory fear conditioning of rats via glutamate toxicity. *Neurosci Res*. 2015;91:34–40.

182. Hao Y, Jing H, Bi Q, et al. Intra-amygdala microinfusion of IL-6 impairs the auditory fear conditioning of rats via JAK/ STAT activation. *Behavioural Brain Research*. 2014;275:88–95.

183. Crowley T, Cryan JF, Downer EJ, O'Leary OF. Inhibiting neuroinflammation: the role and therapeutic potential of GABA in neuro-immune interactions. *Brain Behav Immun*. 2016;54:260–77.

184. Miller MW, Lin AP, Wolf EJ, Miller DR. Oxidative stress, inflammation, and neuroprogression in chronic PTSD. *Harv Rev Psychiatry*. 2018;26(2):57–69.

185. Rosso IM, Weiner MR, Crowley DJ, et al. Insula and anterior cingulate GABA levels in posttraumatic stress disorder: preliminary findings using magnetic resonance spectroscopy. *Depress Anxiety*. 2014;31(2):115–23.

186. Long Z, Medlock C, Dzemidzic M, et al. Decreased GABA levels in anterior cingulate cortex/medial prefrontal cortex in panic disorder. *Prog Neuropsychopharmacol Biol Psychiatry*. 2013;44:131–5.

187. Goddard AW, Mason GF, Almai A, et al. Reductions in occipital cortex GABA levels in panic disorder detected with 1h-magnetic resonance spectroscopy. *Archives of General Psychiatry*. 2001;58 (6):556–61.

188. Michels L, Schulte-Vels T, Schick M, et al. Prefrontal GABA and glutathione imbalance in posttraumatic stress disorder: preliminary findings. *Psychiatry Research*. 2014;224(3):288–95.

189. Borovac Stefanovic L, Kalinic D, Mimica N, et al. Oxidative status and the severity of clinical symptoms in patients with post-traumatic stress disorder. *Ann Clin Biochem*. 2015;52(Pt 1):95–104.

190. Atli A, Bulut M, Bez Y, et al. Altered lipid peroxidation markers are related to post-traumatic stress disorder (PTSD) and not trauma itself in earthquake survivors. *Eur Arch Psychiatry Clin Neurosci*. 2016;266(4):329–36.

191. Neylan TC, Sun B, Rempel H, et al. Suppressed monocyte gene expression profile in men versus women with PTSD. *Brain Behav Immun*. 2011;25(3):524–31.

192. Glatt SJ, Tylee DS, Chandler SD, et al. Blood-based gene-expression predictors of PTSD risk and resilience among deployed marines: a pilot study. *Am J Med Genet B Neuropsychiatr Genet*. 2013;162B (4):313–26.

193. Tylee DS, Chandler SD, Nievergelt CM, et al. Blood-based gene-expression biomarkers of post-traumatic stress disorder among deployed marines: a pilot study. *Psychoneuroendocrinology*. 2015;51:472–94.

194. Logue MW, Smith AK, Baldwin C, et al. An analysis of gene expression in PTSD implicates genes involved in the glucocorticoid receptor pathway and neural responses to stress. *Psychoneuroendocrinology*. 2015;57:1–13.

195. Bruenig D, Morris CP, Mehta D, et al. Nitric oxide pathway genes (NOS1AP and NOS1) are involved in PTSD severity, depression, anxiety, stress and resilience. *Gene*. 2017;625:42–8.

196. Bulut M, Selek S, Bez Y, et al. Reduced PON1 enzymatic activity and increased lipid hydroperoxide levels that point out oxidative stress in generalized anxiety disorder. *Journal of Affective Disorders*. 2013;150(3):829–33.

197. Ozdemir O, Selvi Y, Ozkol H, et al. Comparison of superoxide dismutase, glutathione peroxidase and adenosine deaminase activities between respiratory and nocturnal subtypes of patients with

panic disorder. *Neuropsychobiology.* 2012;66(4):244–51.

198. Rossi S, Sacchetti L, Napolitano F, et al. Interleukin-1beta causes anxiety by interacting with the endocannabinoid system. *J Neurosci.* 2012;32 (40):13896–905.

199. Mandolesi G, Bullitta S, Fresegna D, et al. Interferon-gamma causes mood abnormalities by altering cannabinoid CB1 receptor function in the mouse striatum. *Neurobiol Dis.* 2017;108:45–53.

200. Yang L, Wang M, Guo YY, et al. Systemic inflammation induces anxiety disorder through CXCL12/CXCR4 pathway. *Brain Behav Immun.* 2016;56:352–62.

201. Heinisch S, Kirby LG. SDF-1alpha/ CXCL12 enhances GABA and glutamate synaptic activity at serotonin neurons in the rat dorsal raphe nucleus. *Neuropharmacology.* 2010;58(2):501–14.

202. Gibney SM, McGuinness B, Prendergast C, Harkin A, Connor TJ. Poly I:C-induced activation of the immune response is accompanied by depression and anxiety-like behaviours, kynurenine pathway activation and reduced BDNF expression. *Brain Behav Immun.* 2013;28:170–81.

203. Wang Z, Caughron B, Young MRI. Posttraumatic stress disorder: an immunological disorder? *Front Psychiatry.* 2017;8:222.

204. Michopoulos V, Jovanovic T. Chronic inflammation: a new therapeutic target for post-traumatic stress disorder? *Lancet Psychiatry.* 2015;2(11):954–5.

205. Brenner LA, Stearns-Yoder KA, Hoffberg AS, et al. Growing literature but limited evidence: a systematic review regarding prebiotic and probiotic interventions for those with traumatic brain injury and/or posttraumatic stress disorder. *Brain Behav Immun.* 2017;65:57–67.

206. Gocan AG, Bachg D, Schindler AE, Rohr UD. Balancing steroidal hormone cascade in treatment-resistant veteran soldiers with PTSD using a fermented soy product (FSWW08): a pilot study.

Horm Mol Biol Clin Investig. 2012;10 (3):301–14.

207. Su KP, Matsuoka Y, Pae CU. Omega-3 Polyunsaturated Fatty Acids in Prevention of Mood and Anxiety Disorders. *Clin Psychopharmacol Neurosci.* 2015;13(2):129–37.

208. Uher R, Tansey KE, Dew T, et al. An inflammatory biomarker as a differential predictor of outcome of depression treatment with escitalopram and nortriptyline. *The American Journal of Psychiatry.* 2014;171(12):1278–86.

209. Raison CL, Rutherford RE, Woolwine BJ, et al. A randomized controlled trial of the tumor necrosis factor antagonist infliximab for treatment-resistant depression: the role of baseline inflammatory biomarkers. *JAMA Psychiatry.* 2013;70(1):31–41.

210. Tucker P, Ruwe WD, Masters B, et al. Neuroimmune and cortisol changes in selective serotonin reuptake inhibitor and placebo treatment of chronic posttraumatic stress disorder. *Biological Psychiatry.* 2004;56(2):121–8.

211. Kao CY, He Z, Zannas AS, et al. Fluoxetine treatment prevents the inflammatory response in a mouse model of posttraumatic stress disorder. *Journal of Psychiatric Research.* 2016;76:74–83.

212. Hou R, Ye G, Liu Y, et al. Effects of SSRIs on peripheral inflammatory cytokines in patients with Generalized Anxiety Disorder. *Brain Behav Immun.* 2019;81:105–10.

213. Himmerich H, Willmund GD, Zimmermann P, et al. Serum concentrations of TNF-alpha and its soluble receptors during psychotherapy in German soldiers suffering from combat-related PTSD. *Psychiatr Danub.* 2016;28(3):293–8.

214. Hoge EA, Bui E, Palitz SA, et al. The effect of mindfulness meditation training on biological acute stress responses in generalized anxiety disorder. *Psychiatry Research.* 2018;262:328–32.

215. Memon AA, Sundquist K, Ahmad A, et al. Role of IL-8, CRP and epidermal growth

factor in depression and anxiety patients treated with mindfulness-based therapy or cognitive behavioral therapy in primary health care. *Psychiatry Research.* 2017;254:311–6.

216. Sumner JA, Chen Q, Roberts AL, et al. Posttraumatic stress disorder onset and inflammatory and endothelial function biomarkers in women. *Brain Behav Immun.* 2018;69:203–9.

217. Heath NM, Chesney SA, Gerhart JI, et al. Interpersonal violence, PTSD, and inflammation: potential psychogenic pathways to higher C-reactive protein levels. *Cytokine.* 2013;63(2):172–8.

218. Miller RJ, Sutherland AG, Hutchison JD, Alexander DA. C-reactive protein and interleukin 6 receptor in post-traumatic stress disorder: a pilot study. *Cytokine.* 2001;13(4):253–5.

219. Bersani FS, Wolkowitz OM, Lindqvist D, et al. Global arginine bioavailability, a marker of nitric oxide synthetic capacity, is decreased in PTSD and correlated with symptom severity and markers of inflammation. *Brain Behav Immun.* 2016;52:153–60.

220. Miller K, Driscoll D, Smith LM, Ramaswamy S. The role of inflammation in late-life post-traumatic stress disorder. *Mil Med.* 2017;182(11):e1815-e8.

221. Rosen RL, Levy-Carrick N, Reibman J, et al. Elevated C-reactive protein and posttraumatic stress pathology among survivors of the 9/11 World Trade Center attacks. *Journal of Psychiatric Research.* 2017;89:14–21.

222. Sondergaard HP, Hansson LO, Theorell T. The inflammatory markers C-reactive protein and serum amyloid A in refugees with and without posttraumatic stress disorder. *Clinica Chimica Acta: International Journal of Clinical Chemistry.* 2004;342(1–2): 93–8.

223. McCanlies EC, Araia SK, Joseph PN, et al. C-reactive protein, interleukin-6, and posttraumatic stress disorder symptomology in urban police officers. *Cytokine.* 2011;55(1):74–8.

224. Muhtz C, Godemann K, von Alm C, et al. Effects of chronic posttraumatic stress disorder on metabolic risk, quality of life, and stress hormones in aging former refugee children. *J Nerv Ment Dis.* 2011;199(9):646–52.

225. Maes M, Lin AH, Delmeire L, et al. Elevated serum interleukin-6 (IL-6) and IL-6 receptor concentrations in posttraumatic stress disorder following accidental man-made traumatic events. *Biological Psychiatry.* 1999;45(7):833–9.

226. Newton TL, Fernandez-Botran R, Miller JJ, Burns VE. Interleukin-6 and soluble interleukin-6 receptor levels in posttraumatic stress disorder: associations with lifetime diagnostic status and psychological context. *Biological Psychology.* 2014;99:150–9.

227. Oganesyan LP, Mkrtchyan GM, Sukiasyan SH, Boyajyan AS. Classic and alternative complement cascades in post-traumatic stress disorder. *Bull Exp Biol Med.* 2009;148(6):859–61.

228. Spivak B, Shohat B, Mester R, et al. Elevated levels of serum interleukin-1 beta in combat-related posttraumatic stress disorder. *Biological Psychiatry.* 1997;42(5):345–8.

229. Naude PJW, Roest AM, Stein DJ, de Jonge P, Doornbos B. Anxiety disorders and CRP in a population cohort study with 54,326 participants: The LifeLines study. *World J Biol Psychiatry.* 2018;6:1–10.

230. Copeland WE, Shanahan L, Worthman C, Angold A, Costello EJ. Generalized anxiety and C-reactive protein levels: a prospective, longitudinal analysis. *Psychol Med.* 2012;42(12):2641–50.

231. Khandaker GM, Zammit S, Lewis G, Jones PB. Association between serum C-reactive protein and DSM-IV generalized anxiety disorder in adolescence: findings from the ALSPAC cohort. *Neurobiol Stress.* 2016;4:55–61.

232. Bankier B, Barajas J, Martinez-Rumayor A, Januzzi JL. Association between C-reactive protein and generalized

anxiety disorder in stable coronary heart disease patients. *Eur Heart J.* 2008;29 (18):2212–7.

233. Wagner EY, Wagner JT, Glaus J, et al. Evidence for chronic low-grade systemic inflammation in individuals with agoraphobia from a population-based prospective study. *PloS One.* 2015;10(4): e0123757.

234. Brambilla F, Bellodi L, Perna G, et al. Plasma interleukin-1 beta concentrations in panic disorder. *Psychiatry Research.* 1994;54(2):135–42.

235. Brambilla F, Bellodi L, Perna G. Plasma levels of tumor necrosis factor-alpha in patients with panic disorder: effect of alprazolam therapy. *Psychiatry Research.* 1999;89(1):21–7.

Chapter 13

Microbiome-Gut-Brain Interactions in Neurodevelopmental Disorders: Focus on Autism and Schizophrenia

Kiran V. Sandhu, Eoin Sherwin, Ted G. Dinan and John F. Cryan

13.1 Introduction

Human brain development is a complex process. For instance, in the third week of gestation, many of the ~ 86 billion neurons observed in the adult brain are being produced (1). Subsequently, there is a constant refining and fine-tuning of these connections that continues after birth until late adolescence. This process of circuit remodelling is critical for normal brain function and behaviour (2) and factors that interfere with these processes can result in brain miswiring and associated behavioural manifestations. Genetic and environmental factors have long been recognized to modulate this complex process of brain development (2). However, there is a growing appreciation of the role that bacterial commensals of the gastrointestinal (GI) system (collectively referred to as gut microbiota which also includes viruses, fungi and protozoans) have in shaping host health and behaviour following birth (3,4). The gut microbiota plays a critical role in the maturation of the immune system especially in the early stages of life. The colonization and development of gut microbiota in early life has been associated with disease later in life (5). The gut microbiota comprises trillions of bacteria, which play a key role in morphological and neurological processes such as brain development, neurotransmission, neuroinflammation, neurogenesis and modulation of behaviour (6–9). Deleterious alterations to the gut microbiota through various factors such as diet, age, stress, mode of delivery and antibiotic administration can disrupt brain physiology and behaviour. Administration of antibiotics is one such example, where ablation of the gut microbiota composition can result in cognitive impairments (10), metabolic alterations (11) and disrupted immune function (12). Cumulative data from both preclinical and clinical studies suggest a key role for the gut microbiota in the onset of various psychiatric and neurological conditions including depression (13,14), anxiety (15), stroke (16), autism (17) and schizophrenia (18).

In this chapter we will explore the supporting evidence demonstrating importance of the microbiota-gut-brain axis in the regulation of brain development at critical windows and its implications in the manifestation of various neurodevelopmental disorders.

13.2 The Gut-Brain Axis

The gut-brain axis is a bidirectional pathway, amalgamating immune and endocrine systems along with efferent, and afferent neuronal signals between the GI tract and the brain (Figure 13.1) (19). Cumulative evidence demonstrates the microbiota to be a key player in the modulation of this gut-brain axis. This complex network of communication between the gut microbiota and central nervous system (CNS) is mediated through the interplay of the autonomic nervous system (ANS), visceral afferent fibres travelling in autonomic nerves, the enteric nervous system (ENS), the hypothalamic–pituitary–adrenal axis (HPA) and bacterial metabolites (20). Visceral afferent fibres travelling within the sympathetic and parasympathetic divisions of the autonomic system signal from the gut lumen to the CNS through enteric, spinal and vagal pathways (21). While efferent autonomic signals from CNS traverse the intestinal wall (21–23). Here, we focus on the bidirectional communication between the gut microbiota and the host in terms of effects of commensal microbiota on the HPA axis response, modulation of neurotransmitter release, and the role of the neural networks in mediating this communication. We also discuss effects of various metabolites released by the commensal microbiota on the host immune system.

13.2.1 Hormones

The HPA axis is the core stress efferent axis that processes stressors to mediate adaptive fight or flight responses (24). For instance, environmental stress conditions or elevated systemic pro-inflammatory cytokines can result in activation of this axis stimulating secretion of corticotrophin-releasing factor (CRF) from the hypothalamus, which triggers adrenocorticotropic hormone (ACTH) secretion from pituitary gland, culminating in the release of cortisol from the adrenal glands. Cortisol is a major stress hormone known to act on many tissues and organs including the brain. Similarly, the microbiota is sensitive to levels of cortisol/corticosterone, with the relative abundance of certain bacteria reduced in the presence of elevated levels of the stress hormone. For example, a recent study showed that exposure to a stressor (e.g., a male aggressor) for a period of ten days decreased the relative levels of bacteria within the Firmicutes and Verrucomicrobia phyla in the gut microbiota (25). On the other hand, some probiotic strains have been shown to modulate levels of stress-induced corticosterone release in rodents. *Lactobacillus rhamnosus,* for instance, has been shown to reduce stress-induced corticosterone levels in mice (26). Conversely, healthy male volunteers who consumed the probiotic strain, *Bifidobacterium longum* 1714, reported improved levels of perceived psychological stress in addition to a reduction in levels of salivary cortisol (27). Together, this demonstrates that the ability of the microbiota to modulate activation of the HPA axis is a trait that is evolutionarily conserved across species from mice to humans.

Perhaps the most pronounced effects of the microbiota on the activation of the HPA axis were observed in germ-free mouse (have no microbiota) studies. Indeed, exposure of germ-free mice to restraint stress resulted in exaggerated levels of circulating ACTH and corticosterone relative to conventionally colonized animals (28). This exaggerated stress response in germ-free mice is attenuated following treatment with either a *Bifidobacterium* strain or reconstitution with a normal microbiota, further reaffirming the influence that the gut bacteria has upon HPA axis activation (28). However, corticosterone is not the only hormone in the mammalian body under the influence of the microbiota. For example, gut

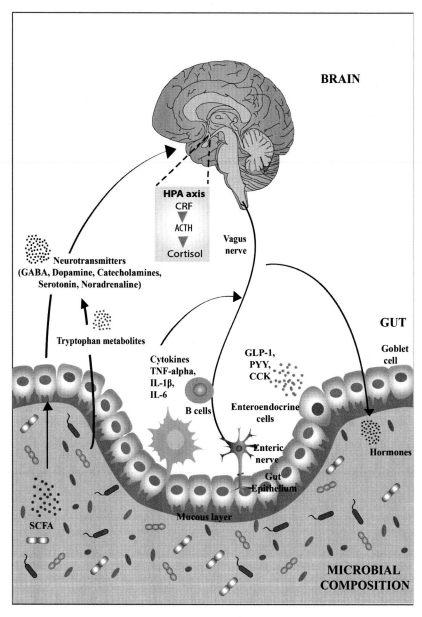

Figure 13.1 Key communicating pathways of the microbiome-gut-brain axis. There are different mechanisms via which the bacteria commensals in our gut signal to the brain. These include activation of the vagus nerve, production of microbial metabolites (short chain fatty acids: SCFA), immune mediators and endocrine cell signalling. Alteration in the gut microbiota subsequently results in the disruption in central processes. Numerous studies have shown alteration in the gut microbiota in neuropsychiatric conditions, which may account for the behaviour abnormalities. Normalization of the gut composition with microbial therapy (prebiotics or probiotics) may offer a viable treatment for neuropsychiatric conditions. ACTH Adrenocorticotropic hormone; CCK cholecystokinin; CRF Corticotropin-releasing factor; GABA γ-aminobutyric acid; GLP glucagon-like peptide; IL interleukin; PYY peptide YY; TNF tumour necrosis factor. (A black and white version of this figure will appear in some formats. For the colour version, please refer to the plate section.)

bacteria have been shown to influence the expression of the 'prosocial' hormone, oxytocin. Poutahidis and colleagues demonstrated that the probiotic strain, *Lactobacillus reuteri*, was capable of increasing the release of oxytocin from the pituitary gland in a manner that was dependent upon the vagus nerve, given that this effect of the bacterium was lost following vagotomy (29). In a separate study, *Lactobacillus reuteri* was also shown to increase oxytocin immunoreactivity within the paraventricular nucleus of the hypothalamus and its signalling to the dorsolateral periaqueductal grey (30). This effect of *Lactobacillus reuteri* corresponded with an improvement in social behaviour, indicating that this probiotic could be a potential therapeutic strategy to improve deficits in sociability e.g., autism.

13.2.2 Neurotransmitters

The microbiota also plays a role in modulation of several neurotransmitters including the serotonergic and GABAergic systems (Figure 13.1) (31). Studies on germ-free mice have been instrumental in highlighting the impact that the gut microbiota has upon central neurotransmitter turnover. Germ-free mice show a significant increase in the hippocampal concentration of serotonin (5-hydroxytryptamine; 5-HT) and its primary metabolite, 5-hydroxyindoleacetic acid (5-HIAA). Moreover, plasma levels of the dietary amino acid and serotonin precursor, tryptophan, were elevated in germ-free mice relative to conventionally colonized mice which may explain the increased concentration of the neurotransmitter in the brain (32). Further corroborating the effect of the microbiota on tryptophan and serotonin metabolism, recolonization of germ-free mice with microbiota resulted in the normalization of tryptophan concentrations (32). This study demonstrated the crucial role of gut microbiota in the regulation of brain function and neurotransmitter synthesis (32).

The impact of the gut microbiota on neurotransmitter turnover is further supported by studies that modulate the microbiota using prebiotics (indigestible dietary components metabolized by gut bacteria) and probiotics (commensal bacteria with beneficial effects on the host) (33). For instance, chronic treatment of mice with the probiotic bacterium, *Lactobacillus rhamnosus* JB-1, induced region-specific changes in the expression of GABA receptor subunits in the brain. More specifically, treatment with this probiotic increased expression of the GABA B1b subunit in the cingulate cortex and prelimbic cortical regions, but reduced it in the hippocampus, amygdala and locus coeruleus (26). In contrast, the same probiotic reduced expression of mRNA for the GABA Aα2 subunit in the prefrontal cortex and amygdala, but increased it in the hippocampus. Administration of *this probiotic* also attenuated the stress-induced release of corticosterone and ameliorated anxiety- and depression-related behaviours (26).

More recently, a combination of two prebiotics, fructo-oligosaccharide and galacto-oligosaccharide, were found to increase the expression of the GABA B1 and B2 receptors in the hippocampus of mice and simultaneously improve depression and anxiety-related behaviours following exposure to chronic stress using the chronic social defeat model (34). Thus, the GABAergic and serotonergic systems appear to be under close regulation by the gut microbiota and may be one potential mechanism through which gut commensals influence behaviours such as anxiety.

Interestingly, several strains of gut bacteria possess the enzymatic potential to produce GABA itself through the metabolism of monosodium glutamate (35). However, GABA is not the only neurotransmitter that gut bacteria are capable of synthesizing. There is considerable evidence to demonstrate that certain bacterial strains are also capable of synthesizing catecholamines such as noradrenaline. Whether these locally produced neuro-transmitters in the gut are capable of reaching the brain to influence behaviour in any capacity is currently unknown (23). Other neurotransmitters produced by the gut micro-biota act locally to regulate vital physiological functions such as gut motility. *Lactobacilli*, for instance, are capable of metabolizing nitrate and nitrite to generate the gaseous neurotrans-mitters nitric oxide and hydrogen sulphide. These atypical neurotransmitters can bind to the vanilloid receptor expressed on pain (capsaicin)-sensitive nerve fibres to mediate gut motility (36,37).

13.2.3 Neural

Visceral afferent fibres travelling in the vagus nerve, are another route through which the gut can communicate with the brain. These fibres converge near the intestinal mucosa, mediating information from the intestine to the brainstem via nuclei such as the nucleus tractus solitarius and the nodose ganglion (38). While these fibres do not project directly into the lumen of the gut, their activation is mediated through the secretion of various peptide hormones including glucagon-like peptide1 (GLP-1), peptide hormones YY (PYY) and cholecystokinin (CCK) from enteroendocrine cells acting upon receptors expressed on the nerve (Figure 13.1) (39). The binding of these gut hormones to their cognate receptors on sensory vagus nerve fibres mediates different behaviours. For example, PYY has been associated with the modulation of food intake and, in part, mediates its effect by binding to the hypothalamic neuropeptide YY2 receptor (40). However, vagotomy blocks this inter-action resulting in the attenuation of PYY-induced hypophagia and the associated activa-tion of neurons in the hypothalamic arcuate nucleus (41). Numerous studies have further established the critical role of vagus nerve fibres in mediating the bidirectional communi-cation between the gut microbiota and the brain. For instance, the bacterium *Lactobacillus rhamnosus* was shown to improve anxiety-related behaviour in mice. However, the benefi-cial effect of this probiotic strain on behaviour was absent in mice that underwent vagotomy (26) Similarly, in a mouse model of chronic colitis, administration of *Bifidobacterium longum* (another probiotic) attenuated anxiety-like behaviour, which was also blocked in mice that underwent vagotomy before the induction of colitis (42). Moreover, the probiotic *Lactobacillus reuteri* increased the secretion of the prosocial hormone, oxytocin, from the pituitary gland in a manner that was dependent upon the integrity of the vagus nerve (29). Collectively these studies demonstrate that sensory fibres travelling within the vagus nerve are a crucial conduit through which the gut and its associated microbiota mediates its effects upon the brain. Modulation of afferent sensory nerves by the microbiota is another potential mechanism through which microbiota influences the gut-brain axis. For example, adminis-tration of *Lactobacillus reuteri* increased neuronal excitability and action potential fre-quency, accompanied by a decrease in calcium-dependent potassium channel opening, modulation of gut motility and pain perception (43).

13.2.4 Immune System

The immune system forms a close relationship with the host microbiota; with the highest number of immune cells in the body resident at sites colonized by commensals such as the GI tract. One strategy utilized by the host to maintain its homeostatic relationship with the microbiota is to minimize contact between the commensal bacterial and the epithelial cells surface, thereby limiting microbial translocation and tissue inflammation (44). The mucus produced by goblet cells represents the first line of defence limiting contact between the microbiota and the host tissue (45). In addition to the production of mucus by goblet cells, intestinal epithelial cells produce anti-microbial peptides that play a significant role in limiting exposure to the commensal microbiota (46). These proteins have been shown to exert their anti-microbial functions through the disruption of the bacterial inner membrane or through the enzymatic degradation of the bacterial cell wall (46). Reg-IIIγ constitutes one of the best characterized mucosal anti-microbial peptides and its expression appears to be under the control of the microbiota. Germ-free mice (which do not have a microbiota), display profound immunological deficits, along with reduced levels of the anti-microbial peptide Reg-IIIγ in the intestinal epithelium (47). Colonization of these germ-free mice with the gram-negative bacterium, *Bacteroides thetaiotaomicron,* restored expression of Reg-IIIγ in the intestines, indicating that the gut microbiota can influence the expression of a host anti-microbial peptide. However, colonization with Gram-positive bacteria reduced Reg-IIIγ expression in germ-free mice suggesting that this immunomodulatory role of the gut microbiota is dependent upon the ratio of gram-negative to gram-positive bacteria in the gut (46–48).

The immune system is not only associated with establishing homeostasis between the intestinal microbiota and the gut, but also functions as an intermediary between the gut microbiota and the brain (49). For example, the gut microbiota can elicit an immune response through the secretion of certain pathogen associated molecular patterns (PAMPs), such as lipopolysaccharide (LPS), which is a key component of the cell wall of gram-negative bacteria. In conditions where the integrity of the intestinal mucosal barrier is compromised, gram-negative bacteria expressing LPS are capable of translocating from the gut into the circulatory system leading to peripheral immune activation through LPS binding to Toll-like receptor 4 (TLR4) on immune cells. There is considerable clinical and preclinical evidence to demonstrate that peripheral and central immune activation can affect behaviours related to depression (50,51). Indeed, depressed patients were found to display increased serum IgM antibodies raised against the gram-negative bacterium, *Enterobacteriaceae,* suggestive of bacterial translocation (52). Aside from LPS, bacterial peptidoglycan also appears to be an important intermediary in mediating the gut microbiota's influence on brain and behaviour. In the absence of a microbiota, germ-free mice display alterations in the central expression of peptidoglycan-sensing molecules, a class of pathogen recognition receptor (21). Moreover, knock-down of one of these peptidoglycan-sensing molecules, Pglyrp2, resulted in alterations to social behaviour in mice, highlighting the importance of bacterial-immune signalling in the development of critical behaviours such as sociability (21).

In addition to influencing behaviour via the modulation of immune signalling to the CNS, the neuroinflammatory status of the brain is also under the control of the gut bacteria. Germ-free mice display deficits in microglia morphology, with altered cell proportions and an immature phenotype (53). Moreover, microglial activation in response to LPS exposure is reduced in germ-free mice, indicating that microglia require signals from the gut microbiota to elicit a proper neuroinflammatory response. These findings in germ-free mice were corroborated in antibiotic treated animals thereby ruling out any developmental defect in germ-free mice that may give rise to this deficit in microglial physiology (53).

13.2.5 Microbial Metabolites

The microbiota may also partly mediate its effect on the brain through the production of bacterial metabolites (Figure 13.1). Short chain fatty acids (SCFA) are one of the main bacterial metabolites produced by gut bacteria and include molecules such as butyric acid, valeric acid, propionic acid and acetic acid. SCFAs are predominately found in the colon and the small intestine through bacterial fermentation (54). Bacteria belonging to the phyla Bacteroidetes mainly produce acetate and propionate, whereas Firmicutes mediate the production of butyrate. SCFAs account for 2–10% of the total energy consumption in humans and are the main energy source for large intestinal epithelial cells that mediate the production of mucins (mucus). At the level of the GI system, SCFAs mediate several important physiological functions such as influencing blood flow to the colonic mucosal membrane, the absorption of fluids and electrolytes, and the secretion of gut hormones (55). SCFAs regulate such a vast array of physiological functions through their epigenetic and signalling properties. For instance, acetate possesses epigenetic modulatory properties through its ability to inhibit histone deacetylases (56). In contrast, butyrate offers as a major source of energy for colonic epithelial cells (57). Propionic acid mediates its beneficial effects through the modulation of glucose metabolism and body weight control by activating free fatty acid receptor (FFAR) 3 on nerve fibre endings of the portal vein (58). SCFAs also possess neuroactive properties and can influence brain and behaviour through a variety of ways (59). For instance, some SCFAs may be able to influence monoaminergic neurotransmission in the brain through regulating the expression of enzymes involved in their biosynthesis. Butyric and propionic acid have both been shown in vitro to increase expression of tyrosine hydroxylase, the rate-limiting enzyme in dopamine and noradrenaline synthesis. Moreover, these SCFAs attenuated the expression of dopamine-β-hydroxylase, the enzyme responsible for converting dopamine into noradrenaline (60).

While these effects were observed in vitro, exposure to propionic acid attenuated the levels of γ-aminobutyric acid (GABA), adrenaline and dopamine in the rat brain (9,61). This ability of SCFAs to modulate neurotransmitters such as GABA, noradrenaline and dopamine is likely to have some bearing upon anxiety and depression-related behaviours (59). SCFAs can also mediate the secretion of satiety hormones such as PYY, GLP-1 and CCK (59). Through binding and activating FFAR2 and FFAR3 receptors present on intestinal epithelial cells, SCFAs can facilitate the secretion of satiety peptides thereby influencing feeding behaviour (62). SCFAs also appear to be the main intermediary in the microbiota modulation of the brain's neuroinflammatory status. Germ-free mice display alterations in microglial morphology and function, with increased numbers and a blunted activation in response to stimulation with LPS (53). However, supplementation of germ-free mice with a cocktail of SCFAs (propionic acid, acetic acid and butyric acid) was capable of restoring microglial density, morphology and function to levels observed in conventional animals (53). While the mechanisms through which SCFAs modulate microglial morphology and activation are currently unknown, these seminal experiments shed some light on how gut bacteria are capable of influencing a physiological process as crucial as neuroinflammation.

13.3 Impact of Microbiota Manipulation on Brain and Behaviour

13.3.1 Germ-Free Mice

Preclinical work with germ-free mice (devoid of any microbiota) has provided considerable insight into how the gut microbiota can influence brain function and behaviour (63). For instance, germ-free mice display elevated levels of the stress hormone corticosterone in comparison to conventionally colonized mice raised with a normal gut microbiota (28). Moreover, levels of brain derived neurotrophic factor (BDNF), a key protein involved in plasticity and learning and memory (64), were reduced in both the cortex and hippocampus of germ-free mice (31). Administration of a single strain of bacterium, *Bifidobacterium infantis*, attenuated the enhanced HPA axis response in germ-free mice. Further, these data showed that there is a critical period during development in which the microbiota is capable of regulating this effect upon the HPA axis as it was ineffective in adult animals (28). Moreover, germ-free mice also display reduced anxiety-like behaviour along with increased locomotor activity which could be reversed by colonization with gut microbiota at a younger age compared to at a later time point, further suggesting that there is a critical period for the effect of gut microbes on neuronal circuitry and behaviour (2).

Profiling of gene expression changes from the hippocampus, frontal cortex and striatum of germ-free mice revealed that there are significantly different changes in the transcriptome compared to conventionally colonized mice (31). For example, synaptophysin, a protein important for synaptic vesicle endocytosis and synaptogenesis (65,66), and PSD 95, involved in excitatory synapse maturation and plasticity, were reduced in the striatum of germ-free mice (31,67,68). Another study reported downregulation of the N-methyl-D-aspartate receptor subunit 2B (NR2B) subunit of the N-methyl-D-aspartate (NMDA) receptor, which is crucial for synaptic plasticity and memory processes, in the amygdala of germ-free mice (69). With changes in the expression of crucial genes linked to synaptic plasticity, perhaps it is no surprise that there are considerable morphological changes of neurons along with volumetric enlargement of the hippocampus and amygdala in germ-free mice. Germ-free mice demonstrate region-specific alterations in dendritic spine density and morphology along with dendritic length. One may argue that these alterations in the morphology of neurons and the structure of brain regions provide a neurobiological correlate for the observed behaviour phenotype of germ-free mice (63).

The influence of the microbiota upon neurons is not limited to its morphology and function as it has also been shown that myelination is also under the control of gut bacteria (70). Germ-free mice display increased myelination in brain regions such as the prefrontal cortex relative to conventionally colonized animals, which likely influences the rate of neurotransmission between individual neurons in the germ-free brain (70). This ability of the microbiota to influence the level of myelination in the brain has important implications for diseases in which myelination is affected (i.e., multiple sclerosis).

The influence of gut microbiota on the brain is not only limited to structure and morphology but also extends to neurochemical release. Serotonin, a neurotransmitter associated with a wide range of physiological functions and involved in the modulation of anxiety, sociability, fear responses and reward behaviour (71,72), is under the influence of commensal gut bacteria. For instance, germ-free mice display reduced expression of the 5-HT1A receptor in the hippocampus compared with conventionally colonized animals (69). Moreover, germ-free mice display elevated levels of both serotonin and its metabolite, 5-HIAA, in the hippocampus which corresponded with elevated circulating plasma levels of tryptophan (32). It is likely that in the absence of a gut microbiota, there is a greater availability of circulating tryptophan that can reach the brain and be metabolized to serotonin. This is supported by the fact that germ-free mice display reduced colonic expression of the rate-limiting enzyme in serotonin synthesis, tryptophan hydroxylase 1 (73).

Interestingly, this effect of the microbiota upon serotonin metabolism is apparent in male but not in female germ-free mice (32). Consequently, it is likely that there exists a sexual dimorphism in the regulation of the microbiota upon central serotonergic neurotransmission. Restoration of germ-free mice with microbiota reverted to anxiety-like behaviour to control levels, while also normalizing plasma tryptophan concentrations. However, this was independent of any alterations to the elevated levels of hippocampal 5-HT (32).

13.3.2 Antibiotic Treatments

Germ-free mice are a widely used model to study causality in gut microbiota and brain physiology (63). However, there are certain limitations with using germ-free mice to investigate the microbiome-gut-brain axis. For example, these mice display numerous physiological abnormalities such as deficits in the integrity of the blood-brain-barrier (BBB) and alterations in brain structure. An alternative approach is to use antibiotics to diminish the intestinal microbiota (12). Dysregulation of the gut microbiota composition following antibiotic administration has been shown to have a profound effect on brain chemistry and behaviour (74). Another advantage of antibiotics over germ-free animals is that they offer a greater degree of temporal manipulation of the microbiome-gut-brain axis and allow us to assess the impact of microbiota depletion at different stages of life. For instance, depletion of the gut microbiota from weaning onwards produces an anxiolytic-like effect while also impairing cognitive behaviour. It also alters tryptophan metabolism and attenuates hippocampal BDNF expression (74).

Even in adulthood this effect of, administration of an antibiotic cocktail (ampicillin, bacitracin, meropenem, neomycin, vancomycin) induces cognitive deficits, along with reducing expression of BDNF, the serotonin transporter (SERT), neuropeptide Y (NPY), and NR2B (8). Interestingly, similar to what is observed with germ-free mice, the ablation of the gut microbiota through antibiotic treatment is also associated with an increase in circulating corticosterone despite the apparent anxiolytic-like profile of these animals (10,28,32). This disparity is difficult to explain, especially considering the complex intricacies behind each experimental study; however, this disagreement highlights the complex relationship between the gut microbiota and the brain. Future experiments should aim to investigate this complex interaction.

Antibiotic studies have also been incredibly beneficial in elucidating a role for the gut microbiota in modulating neurogenesis. For example, chronic antibiotic treatment of adult mice resulted in the reduction of hippocampal neurogenesis, although it could be completely restored following probiotic administration or exercise (2). Ablation of the gut microbiota following antibiotic administration resulted in a reduction in neurogenesis which was associated with decreased infiltration of a particular type of Ly6Chi monocytes. Furthermore, administration of probiotics or exercise were able to promote neurogenesis while also restoring Ly6Chi cells to control levels which suggests that the gut microbiota may mediate its regulation of neurogenesis via the immune system (75).

13.4 Gut Microbiota and Brain Development

The development of the brain is a complex process starting from the third week of gestation and continuing after birth through to late adolescence. This process is mediated through the interaction of genes and the environmental factors that play a fundamental role in refining neuronal networks (76). Disruption of these interactions are known to alter normal developmental trajectories and result in neuropsychiatric outcomes in later life (2). During the last few years, several studies have indicated that the gut microbiota influences fine maturation of the brain while having long-lasting effects on brain physiology.

13.4.1 Prenatal Neurodevelopment

Neuronal development begins early in embryonic development with numerous stages occurring before birth (77). During this period, the brain is highly vulnerable to various factors such as maternal immunity and metabolism, which can impact upon neurodevelopment and behaviour (78). Perturbations to maternal homeostasis through infection, diet or stress, have been reported as risk factors for the development of neuropsychiatric disorders such as anxiety, autism, attention deficit hyperactive disorder, depression and schizophrenia in offspring (72,79). Interestingly, recent data suggest a potential role for the *maternal* microbiome in offspring neurodevelopment. For example, pregnant mice colonized with segmented filamentous bacteria were more likely to produce offspring that displayed an autistic-like phenotype (80). Moreover, female mice fed a high fat diet (HFD) during pregnancy, led to the development of social and anxiety-related behavioural disturbances in offspring which was attributed to the absence of specific *Lactobacillus* species from the gut microbiota of these animals (30,81).

The interaction between the maternal microbiome and the HPA axis can influence both fetal brain development and maturation, and infant cognitive functioning (82,83). Stress-induced activation of the HPA axis can lead to changes in maternal gut microbiome composition (84). These changes in the gut microbiota can then feedback to influence HPA axis dysfunction through modulating tryptophan metabolism, pro-inflammatory immune responses and triggering other pathways linked to the stress axis (77). Through changes in the dynamics between the gut microbiota and the HPA axis, alterations in the level of cortisol reaching the fetal brain from the maternal bloodstream can subsequently affect neurodevelopment. In addition, there is some evidence supporting the role of the gut microbiome in regulating placental function of the placenta through the HPA axis, which will subsequently influence fetal exposure to potentially toxic compounds *in utero* (85,86).

Another possible mechanism via which the maternal gut microbiota can influence fetal neurodevelopment is through the modulation of circulating 5-HT. Maternal plasma serotonin is important for fetal neuronal development, with embryos depending more on maternal plasma serotonin than their own during *in utero* development (87). The gut microbiome regulates 5-HT biosynthesis from enterochromaffin (EC) cells and in turn, 5-HT has been shown to regulate fetal neuronal cell division, synaptogenesis and differentiation. Moreover, transient disruptions to maternal-offspring 5-HT signalling during development has been shown to result in offspring behavioural abnormalities (88). Furthermore, the maternal gut microbiota is essential for offspring BBB formation. Analysis of the germ-free mouse embryos revealed that the integrity of the developing BBB is compromised relative to conventional animals (89). Consequently, any increase in the permeability of the BBB would leave the developing fetal brain far more vulnerable to exposure of exogenous chemical signals with potentially maladaptive consequences. These studies collectively highlight the fundamental role that the maternal microbiota in mediating *in utero* neurodevelopment.

13.4.2 Postnatal Neurodevelopment

The postnatal period is another critical period of brain development, which is characterized by profound remodelling of cortical and subcortical structures (88). Synaptogenesis begins soon after birth and culminates at two years of age, whereas remodelling continues until the third decade of life, providing a lengthy window of vulnerability to external insults that could affect development and behaviour (79). Evidence has shown that this crucial period of neurodevelopment runs parallel to the establishment and maturation of the gut microbiota, a process critical for normal immune function, establishment of neuroendocrine system and for metabolic regulations (2). Consequently, early-life changes in the gut microbiota composition has the potential to affect neurodevelopment, give rise to behaviour abnormalities and increase the risk of psychiatric conditions (91).

Microbiota colonization is influenced by mode of delivery and feeding patterns (91–93). Clinical data of children born by Caesarean section report a lower abundance of species assigned to the Actinobacteria and Bacteroidetes phyla, with a higher abundance of species within the Firmicute phylum (93). At the genus level, the relative abundance of *Bifidobacterium* and *Bacteroides* appear to be significantly reduced in children born by caesarean section when compared to naturally born infants (93). Given, that *Bifidobacteria* are largely considered to be beneficial for host health, their reduction in children born via Caesarean section may provide insight as to why birth via this delivery method is associated with an increase susceptibility to autoimmune and metabolic disorders (90). Preclinical models of Caesarean sections allows further investigation of the impact that this mode of delivery has on offspring development and behaviour. Indeed, offspring mice born via Caesarean section exhibit an altered gut microbiota while also displaying increased anxiety, and deficits in social and stereotypical behaviours compared to vaginally delivered mice (90). One suggestive mechanism is the interaction between the emerging gut microbial ecology and the developing mucosal immune system. In the absence of key bacterial genera, such as *Bifidobacteria*, which possess potent immunoregulatory properties, the development of the GI immune response is likely to be affected by caesarean section. Future studies are aimed at dissecting the interaction between the developing immune system and the intestinal microbiota and the influence of delivery mode on these phenomena (94).

Diet is another critical factor in regulating the composition of the gut microbiota and neurodevelopment during early life. Human milk is the gold standard for nourishment of early infants because it includes numerous bioactive components, such as human milk oligosaccharides (HMOs). HMOs are a group of complex and diverse glycans, resistant to GI digestion and are the first prebiotics to reach the infant colon (95). They are known to modulate epithelial and immune cell responses, reduce excessive mucosal leukocyte infiltration and activation, lower the risk for necrotizing enterocolitis and provide the infant with sialic acid as a potential nutrient for brain development and cognition (96,97). HMOs offer a selective growth substrate for intestinal *Bifidobacteria*, which represent the dominant microbiota of breast-fed infants. Numerous studies have shown that breast-fed infants have a higher count of *Bifidobacteria* and stable gut colonization patterns compared to formula-fed infants (98). Through influencing the gut microbiota, these early-life dietary lifestyle choices influence offspring neurodevelopment. For instance, breast-fed infants demonstrate better neurodevelopmental outcomes and higher scores on intelligence tests compared to infants that were formula-fed infants (97). Corroborating these clinical observations,

Stanton and colleagues showed that feeding mice with *Bifidobacterial* isolates from infant faeces beneficially affected brain fatty acid composition (99).

The gut microbiota also synthesizes vitamins such as vitamins K2 and B12 that are essential for normal brain functioning and nervous system development. For example, the probiotic strain *Lactobacillus reuteri* has been shown to be crucial in facilitating the production of vitamin B12, or cobalamin (100). In addition to neonatal dietary intake, maternal diet is also a crucial factor for healthy brain development in the offspring (101). Studies have shown that diet-induced alterations to maternal metabolism and microbiota affects early-life neurodevelopment through altering milk composition. For example, offspring of mice fed an HFD during lactation show developmental and neurobehavioural changes, with disruption of sensory-motor and physical maturation, and increased susceptibility to depressive and aggressive-like behaviour (102). These observations suggest a crucial role of diet during early-life brain development.

After the postnatal stage, the brain undergoes a process of synaptic refinement and elimination which results in the reduction of the number of synapses in a region-specific manner to adult levels by mid-adolescence. This refinement of the synapses, also known as 'synaptic pruning', is facilitated by microglia and is crucial for the development of cognitive abilities and behavioural transition from developmental stage to adulthood. This process of synaptic pruning is vulnerable to various environmental factors and has been suggested to increase the onset of neurodevelopmental disorders like autism (103) and schizophrenia (104). Remarkably, the gut microbiota is important for the maturation and function of microglial cells. Erny and colleagues demonstrated that depletion of the gut microbiota dramatically interferes with microglia development and function in adult mice. Microglia from germ-free mice displayed prominent morphological alterations and were unable to respond to inflammatory insults compared to microglia isolated from conventionally colonized mice. Interestingly, administration of SCFAs to germ-free mice was able to completely reverse this impairment, indicating the essential role of gut microbial metabolites in regulating microglial function (53).

13.5 Neurodevelopmental Disorders and Microbiota

13.5.1 Autism Spectrum Disorder (ASD)

ASD is a heterogeneous neurodevelopmental disorder with a prevalence of 1 in 68 children (105). It is characterized by deficits in social communication, repetitive/stereotypic behaviour patterns and cognitive impairments. For instance, the processing of emotional stimuli, facial expression or language is altered in individuals with ASD (106,107). While ASD is aetiologically heterogenous, it is believed that both genetic and environmental factors influence the onset and development of this neurodevelopmental disorder (108,109). Individuals with ASD often report comorbid GI symptoms such as abdominal pain, gaseousness, diarrhoea, flatulence and constipation (110). Interestingly, there is some evidence to suggest that comorbid GI symptoms can be linked with the severity of ASD (110,111). ASD individuals with GI symptoms display significant behavioural hallmarks, including anxiety, self-injury and aggression (112). In a clinical study of 2,973 children with ASD, 24% of the subjects experienced at least one type of GI problem. Excessive sensory responsiveness and anxiety were highly associated with GI problems, and each could serve as a predictor for chronic GI problems in ASD (113).

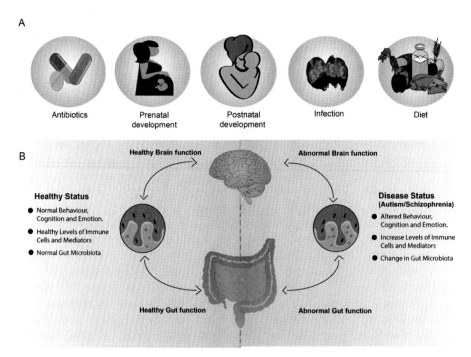

Figure 13.2 A. Different factors associated with neuropsychiatric onset (Autism and Schizophrenia) via targeting the gut-brain axis: antibiotics, prenatal neurodevelopment, postnatal neurodevelopment, infection by *Toxoplasma gondii*, diet. B. The gut microbiota axis in healthy and disease state.

Alterations in gut bacterial composition in individuals with ASD provide further evidence for the role of the microbiota in this neurodevelopmental disorder (Figure 13.2 A, B) (Table 13.1). Data from clinical studies sequencing analysis of the faecal microbiota from autistic children indicate reduced bacterial diversity, namely within the Actinobacteria and Firmicutes phyla such as *Lactobacilli*, *Clostridia*, *Desulfovibrio* and *Sarcina* (111,114–116). In a separate clinical study, a reduced abundance in the *Prevotella*, *Coprococcus* and unclassified *Veillonellaceae* genera were associated with GI symptoms in children with ASD (117). Consequently, the loss of some key bacterial genera may negatively affect GI homeostasis and give rise to symptoms such as constipation and diarrhoea. Indeed, one such potentially harmful bacterial genus contributing towards the neurodevelopmental disorder is *Clostridium*. Analysis of the faecal microbiota of autistic children revealed an increase in the relative abundance of the clostridium genus when compared to non-autistic controls, with nine species of *Clostridia* present in the microbiota of autistic children that were not found to be present in control microbiota (114). Other clinical studies have identified and isolated clostridial strains such as *Clostridium perfringens*, *Clostridium histoyticum* and *Clostridium bolteae* that were found to be elevated in the microbiota of autistic children (118–120). Interestingly, gene expression analysis of the *Clostridium perfringens* genome revealed the presence of the β2 toxin gene only in strains isolated from autistic children with gastrointestinal symptoms (120). Moreover, levels of the clostridial-derived metabolite, 3-(3-hydroxy phenyl)-3-hydroxypropionic acid (HPHPA), were found to be higher in the urine of children with ASD relative to controls, supporting the premise of increased

Table 13.1 Role of microbiota in ASD reported in clinical studies

Experimental layout	Study information	Quantification criteria	Results	References
FMT – 18 weeks in total; 10 week open label and 8 week follow-up	ASD (n = 18) Age (7–16 years) Controls (n = 20) Age and Gender matched	Gastrointestinal Symptom Rating Scale Parent Global Impressions-III (PGI-II) Childhood Autism Rating Scale (CARS) Aberrant Behaviour Checklist (ABC) Social Responsiveness Scale (SRS) Vineland Adaptive Behaviour Scale II (VABS-II)	ASD-related behaviour improved (PGI-II) (CARS) (SRS) (ABC) 80% reduction of GI symptoms (persisted for 8 weeks post-FMT) *Bifidobacterium, Prevotella,* and *Desulfovibrio* increased post-FMT (persisted for 8 weeks post-FMT)	(172)
Antibiotic – 12-week trial of open label oral vancomycin	ASD, regressive-onset autism (n = 11) Age (43–84 months) No control group	CARS Developmental Profile II Coded, paired videotapes scored by a clinical psychologist blinded to treatment status	Short-term improvement was noted using multiple pre- and post-therapy evaluations	(173)
Cross-sectional	ASD (n = 20) Age (6.7 ± 2.7 years) 20 neurotypical children Age (8.3 ± 4.4 years)	Faecal samples Autism Diagnostics Interview – Revised (ADI-Revised) Autism Diagnostics Observation Schedule (ADOS) Autism Treatment Evaluation Checklist (ATEC) Pervasive Developmental Disorder Behaviour Inventory (PDD-BI) Limited dietary data Most ASD had GI symptom	ASD – less diverse gut microbial compositions with lower levels of *Prevotella, Coprococcus,* and unclassified *Veillonellaceae* autistic symptoms, rather than the severity of GI symptoms, was associated with less diverse gut microbiota	(117)

Table 13.1 (cont.)

Experimental layout	Study information	Quantification criteria	Results	References
Cross-sectional	ASD, regressive-onset autism (n = 13) Controls (n = 8)	All ASD had GI symptoms (diarrhoea and constipation) Gastric and small-bowel specimens (7 ASD, 4 controls) Limited dietary data: patients were on a gluten-free (GF), casein-free (CF) diet	Total absence of non-spore-forming anaerobes (clostridia) and microaerophilic bacteria from control children and significant numbers of such bacteria from children with autism	(114)
Cross-sectional	ASD patients (n = 58) Age (3–16 years) Two control groups (n = 22); Non-autistic sibling group (n = 12) Age (2–10 years) Unrelated healthy group (n = 10) Age (3–12 years of age)	91.4% of ASD had GI Symptoms Limited dietary data; Most of the children were on GF/CF diets and many were taking probiotics/prebiotics/antibiotics	ASD – higher *Clostridium histolyticum* group compared to controls Non-autistic sibling group had an intermediate level of the *C. histolyticum* group – not significantly different from ASD or controls	(118)
Cross-sectional	ASD (n = 40) Age (11.1 ± 6.8 years) Neurotypical controls (n = 40) Age (9.2 ± 7.9 years)	CARS Autism Diagnostic Observation Schedule and Autism Behaviour Checklist Constipation defined according to Rome III criteria All subjects of in this study were on a Mediterranean-based diet, and no antibiotics, probiotics, or prebiotics taken in the 3 months prior to the sample collection	ASD – increase in the Firmicutes/Bacteroidetes ratio due to a reduction of the Bacteroidetes relative abundance ASD – at the genus level – decrease in *Alistipes, Bilophila, Dialister, Parabacteroides,* and *Veillonella,* while *Collinsella, Corynebacterium, Dorea,* and *Lactobacillus* were significantly increased in	(174)

			constipated ASD – high levels of bacterial taxa belonging to *Escherichia/Shigella* and *Clostridium* cluster XVIII ASD – fungal genus Candida increased	
Cross-sectional	ASD (n = 23) Age (123 ± 9 months) Controls (n = 31) Age (136 ± 9 months)	SCFAs Dietary intake of macro-nutrients	ASD – faecal acetic, butyric, isobutyric, valeric, and isovaleric acid were all significantly higher compared with controls	(123)
Cross-sectional	ASD (n = 58, GI symptoms) Age (6.91 ± 3.4 years) Controls (n = 39) Age (7.7 ± 4.4 years)	GI symptoms (assessed by the six-item GI Severity Index (6-GSI) questionnaire) Autism Treatment Evaluation Checklist (ATEC) Diet not recorded, ASD on probiotics	ASD – decreased faecal SCFAs, acetate, propionate, and valerate ASD – lower levels of Bifidobacterium and higher levels of Lactobacillus GI symptoms were strongly correlated with the severity of autism	(111)
Cross-sectional	ASD (n = 23, without GI symptoms) ASD (n = 28, with GI symptoms) Age range (2–12 years) Neurotypical siblings (n = 53) Age range (2–12 years)	CARS Limited dietary data; Probiotics not excluded	No significant change in microbiota between the groups	(175)
Cross-sectional	ASD (n = 33, varying GI symptoms) Controls (n = 15); 7 sibling controls 8 non-sibling controls Age (all ASD	No information regarding diet	Bacteroidetes was found at high levels in the severely autistic group Firmicutes were more predominant in	(115)

Table 13.1 (cont.)

Experimental layout	Study information	Quantification criteria	Results	References
	and controls between 2 and 13 years)		the control group Smaller, but significant, differences also in the Actinobacterium and Proteobacterium phyla *Desulfovibrio* species and *Bacteroides vulgatus* present in significantly higher numbers in stools of severally in autistic children compared to control	
Cross-sectional	ASD children (n = 23) Age (123 ± 9 months) Controls (n = 31); Typically developing siblings (n = 22) Community controls (n = 9) Age (136 ± 9 months)	Macronutrient intake determined from dietary records kept by caregivers, did not differ significantly between study groups	ASD – elevated faecal acetic, butyric, isobutyric, valeric, isovaleric, and caproic acids, ammonia	(122)
Meta-analysis of 15 cross-sectional studies			11 studies (n = 562) reported significant gut microbiota differences between ASD children and controls, particularly in the Firmicutes, Bacteroidetes and Proteobacteria phyla Substantial heterogeneity in methodology and the often, contradictory results of different studies – not possible to pool the results into a meta-analysis	(176)

Cross-sectional	Healthy children (n = 77) Age (18–27 months)	Early Childhood Behaviour Questionnaire (ECBQ) (18 dimensions of temperament, three composite scales: Negative Affectivity, Surgency/Extraversion, Effortful Control)	Greater surgery/extraversion was associated greater phylogenetic diversity Boys only – subscales loading on this composite scale were associated with differences in phylogenetic diversity, the Shannon Diversity index (SDI), beta diversity, and differences in abundances of *Dialister, Rikenellaceae, Ruminococcaceae,* and *Parabacteroides* Higher effortful control was associated with a lower SDI score and differences in both beta diversity and *Rikenellaceae* were observed in relation to Fear Associations between temperament and dietary patterns were observed	(177)
Probiotic Intervention – "Children Dophilus" oral capsule containing 3 strains of *Lactobacillus* (60%), 2 strains of *Bifidumbacteria* (25%) and one strain of	ASD (n = 10) Age (2–9 years) Siblings (n = 9) Age (5–17 years) Controls (n = 10) Age (2–11 years)	Autism Diagnostic Interview (ADI) CARS	ASD – decrease of the Bacteroidetes/Firmicutes ratio and elevation of the amount of *Lactobacillus Desulfovibrio* decreased postprobiotic *Desulfovibrio spp.* associated with the	(178)

Table 13.1 (cont.)

Experimental layout	Study information	Quantification criteria	Results	References
Streptococcus (15%), times a day for 4 months			severity of autism (ADI) restricted/repetitive behaviour subscale score Probiotic significantly decreased faecal TNF-α levels in ASD. No correlation between plasma levels of oxytocin, testosterone, DHEA-S and faecal microbiota	
Cross-sectional	ASD probands (n = 66) Neurotypical (NT) siblings (n = 37) Age (7–14 years)	Parent-completed ROME III questionnaire for paediatric Functional gastrointestinal disorders (FGIDs) Child Behaviour Check List (CBCL) Targeted quantitative polymerase chain reaction (qPCR) assays were conducted on selected taxa implicated in ASD, including *Sutterella spp*, *Bacteroidetes spp*, and *Prevotella spp*.	No significant difference in macronutrient intake between ASD and NT siblings There was no significant difference in ASD severity scores between ASD children with and without FGID No significant difference in diversity or overall microbial composition was detected between ASD children with NT siblings	(126)

clostridial abundance and its associated metabolism in the microbiota of autistic individuals (121). Therefore, microbial transplant therapy (MTT) has shown to be promising in autistic individuals because recent study has shown long-lasting effects with improvement both in behavioural and gastrointestinal symptoms. The autistic individuals post MTT showed increased gut microbiota diversity and an increase in *Bifidobacteria* and *Prevotella* (122). This suggests targeting the gut microbiota as a potential therapy to abate autistic phenotype.

Accompanying the reported alterations in gut bacteria composition in ASD, are changes in bacterial metabolite concentrations. Analysis of faecal SCFA levels from autistic children reveals marked increase in the concentrations of acetic acid, isobutyric acid, butyric acid, valeric acid and propionic acid (123). Given that SCFAs possess neuroactive properties, the reported alterations in the levels of these metabolites in ASD may have some bearing upon the observed behavioural deficits (59). In addition to altered microbiota composition, increased GI tract permeability has also been reported in individuals with ASD (124). Increased intestinal permeability can facilitate translocation of bacteria or bacterial components (i.e., LPS) into systemic circulation whereby they can elicit an inflammatory response. Indeed, elevated levels of circulating inflammatory cytokines such as (interleukin) IL-1β, IL-6 and IL-8 have been documented in children with ASD lending support to the premise of a 'leaky gut' and bacterial-mediated inflammation (125). While these clinical studies have provided the field with an insight into how the microbiome-gut-brain axis may be involved in ASD, there are certain considerations that we must be cautious of when interpreting the data. For instance, several clinical studies that have profiled the gut microbiota of autistic children did not account for diet as an important covariable. Diet is well known to have a fundamental impact in shaping the gut microbiota (20), and its documentation is vital when performing clinical studies in ASD individuals. Indeed, one clinical study reported an increase in the low occurring cyanobacterium/chloroplast genus in children with ASD (126). The authors cautioned, however, that the presence of this genus may have been due to participants in the study consuming large quantities of chia seeds (126). Consequently, future clinical studies will need to appropriately control for such influential covariates such as diet as many autistic children adopt stereotyped eating patterns.

Evidence from preclinical studies provide us with an insight into how the gut microbiota may influence autism-related behaviours. Prenatal exposure to propionic acid significantly impairs cognition and social behaviour of neonatal and adolescent offspring, as well as increasing the neuroinflammatory response (127,128). Data from the widely used maternal immune activation (MIA) model for autism demonstrated microbial shifts within the gut (129). This was associated with changes in serum metabolites and the development of autistic-like behaviours. Moreover, GI barrier defects were observed in these mice, further underscoring the crucial role of microbiota and their ligands in maintaining the cell-cell junctions critical to barrier integrity (129). Interestingly the behavioural, physiological and GI deficits observed in MIA mice were ameliorated following administration of *Bacteroides fragilis*, (129). In a separate animal model of autism, offspring born to mothers fed an HFD, the deficits in social behaviour and anxiety were partly attributed to the absence of specific *Lactobacillus* species. Supplementation of these autistic-like mice with *Lactobacillus reuteri* improved social behaviour and anxiety while also increasing the central expression of the prosocial hormone, oxytocin, (30).

The BTBR inbred mouse displays an inherent autistic-like phenotype including dysregulation of social communication (130,131), occurrence of repetitive behaviours (132,133), reduction of neurogenesis (134) and an aberrant immune state (135). Consequently, it

Table 13.2 Role of microbiota in schizophrenia demonstrated in preclincial studies

Experimental layout	Study information	Quantification criteria	Results	References
Cross-sectional	Schizophrenia (n = 16) Years (34.7 ± 4.8) Controls (n = 16) Years (34.3 ± 10.1) Differences in smoking and BMI between groups	Shotgun metagenomic analysis of the oropharyngeal microbiome	SCZ – higher proportions of Firmicutes, Ascomycota, Bifidobacterium and *Lactobacilli* (largest effect was observed in *Lactobacillus gasseri*) SCZ – increase Candida and Eubacterium and reduction of *Neisseria, Haemophilus* and *Capnocytophaga* SCZ – increased number of metabolic pathways related to metabolite transport systems including siderophores, glutamate and vitamin B12 Carbohydrate and lipid pathways and energy metabolism were abundant in controls	(161)
Cross-sectional	Schizophrenia (n = 41) Years (39.2 ± 9.9) Controls (n = 33) Years (30.9 ± 8.8) Differences in smoking, BMI and age	Metagenomic analysis to characterize bacteriophage genomes in oral pharynx	SCZ – increased *Lactobacillus* phage phiadh (controlling for age, gender, race, socioeconomic status, or smoking)	(162)
Two case-control cohorts (n = 947)	Schizophrenia (n = 261), including; First-episode schizophrenia (n = 139, 78	Repeatable Battery for the Assessment of	No differences in C. albicans exposures were found until diagnostic groups stratified by	(179)

Intervention/Population	Measure	Outcome	Ref
antipsychotic naïve) Years (37.71 ± 13.69) Bipolar (n = 270) Years (34.08 ± 13.15) Controls (n = 277) Years (32.02 ± 11.31)	Neuropsychological Status (RBANS)	sex SCZ – in males, C. albicans seropositivity conferred increased odds (OR 2.04–9.53) for a SCZ diagnosis SCZ – in females, C. albicans seropositivity conferred increased odds (OR 1.12) for lower cognitive scores on RBANS with significant decreases on memory modules C. albicans IgG levels were not impacted by antipsychotic medications gastrointestinal (GI) disturbances were associated with elevated C. albicans in males with SCZ and females with bipolar	
14 week double-blind, placebo controlled. Lactobacillus rhamnosus strain GG and Bifidobacterium animalis subsp. lactis Bb12 (10⁹ cfu) Schizophrenia (n = 56) Probiotic (n = 30) Placebo (n = 26) Years (44.66 + 11.4)	Biweekly Positive and Negative Syndrome Scale (PANSS) Self-reported – bowel score (scale of 1–4)	SCZ – in males – reduced C. albicans antibodies S. cerevisiae were not altered. Trends toward improvement in positive psychiatric symptoms in males treated with probiotics who were seen to be negative for C. albicans	(180)

represents an appropriate and popular animal model for addressing the underlying neuro-biology of autism. In addition to their profound autistic-like behavioural phenotype, BTBR mice demonstrate alterations in gut physiology, with an increase in gut permeability and a decrease in intestinal motility. These GI deficits are also associated with alterations to the composition of the gut microbiota. Indeed, the relative abundance of *Blautia*, *Bifidobacteria* and *Rikenella* genera all reduced in the microbiota of the BTBR mouse (136). Given that *Bifidobacteria* have been shown to have a beneficial effect on brain physiology and behaviour, its absence in the microbiota of the BTBR mouse may contribute towards the behavioural deficits observed in these animals. Moreover, both *Bifidobacteria* and *Blautia* carry out a vital role in the de-conjugation of primary and secondary bile acids in the GI tract. Their absence from the microbiota of the BTBR mouse may provide some insight into the gastrointestinal abnormalities reported in this strain (136,137).

13.5.2 Schizophrenia

Schizophrenia is a heterogenous neurodevelopmental disorder with a prevalence of approximately 0.87% worldwide with a higher prevalence in males compared to females, and onset of psychotic symptoms typically occurring during adolescence (138). This disorder is associated with a detrimental impact on normal day-to-day functioning, and it is associated with a reduced life expectancy and a suicide rate of 5% (139). Schizophrenia is classically characterized with positive (delusion, hallucinations), negative (affective flattening, alogia and avolition) and cognitive symptoms (140,141). Deficits in social interaction and communication are normally manifested during the adolescent period (142).

One of the suggested underlying mechanisms in schizophrenia is a disruption of immune processes in the CNS and various lines of evidence support this hypothesis. For instance, genes linked to B-lymphocyte lineages associated with acquired immunity (CD19 and CD20 lines), and the major histocompatibility complex locus, are known to be associated with schizophrenia (143). Studies have shown elevated levels of peripheral cytokines in patients with schizophrenia (144–147). Moreover, data from national cohort studies found that schizophrenia patients display an increased risk for autoimmune diseases further indicating dysfunction to immune homeostasis (148). There is also considerable evidence to suggest that the immune status of the brain is affected in this neurodevelopmental disorder. Patients with schizophrenia show a significant increase in the density of microglial cells in the brain compared to control subjects (149). Furthermore, schizophrenia patients' plasma showed an increase in pro-inflammatory genes on the transcript and protein level compared to control groups, suggesting that an aberrant central immune response may be contributing towards the neurodevelopmental conditions (150).

Studies on host-parasitic infections have provided the field with an insight into how microorganisms such as the gut microbiota may contribute to schizophrenia (Table 13.2). Infection with the protozoan, *Toxoplasma gondii*, for example, establishes latent infection within the CNS of immune-competent hosts. A meta-analysis of 16 studies demonstrated increased *T. gondii* IgM levels in patients with acute psychosis. While the precise mechanism is not clear, a putative role for ablated CD8 T-cells response in individuals with *T. gondii* infection has been suggested to precipitate psychosis. *T. gondii* infection has also been shown to lead to an increase in the central production of cytokines through microglia activation, astrocytes and neurons (151). Infection with *T. gondii* can also influence dopaminergic neurotransmission, which may be one possible mechanism as to how the protozoan can induce psychosis (152,153).

Interestingly, acute infection of mice with *T. gondii* can also lead to alterations to the gut microbiota, indicating that the microorganism may influence its psychotomimetic effects through modulating gut bacteria (Figure 13.2 A, B) (154). It is noteworthy that other infections, such as *Chlamydophila pneumoniae*, *Chlamydophila psittaci* and *Retrovirus W* are also associated with schizophrenia in humans (155). This raises the question regarding the role of microbes and their influence on schizophrenia.

A growing number of studies have shown alterations to the gut microbiota in schizophrenia (Table 13.2). A recent study showed that the relative abundances of *Succinivibrio*, *Megasphaera*, *Collinsella*, *Clostridia*, *Klebsiella* and *Methanobrevibacter* genera were all significantly higher whereas levels of *Blautia*, *Coprococcus*, *Roseburia* were all decreased relative to healthy controls (156). A recent study profiled the gut microbiota composition in first-episode psychosis (FEP) patients (157). The data showed significance difference between patients and healthy controls at the family levels: Lactobacillaceae, Halothiobacillaceae, Brucellaceae, and Micrococcineae were increased, whereas Veillonellaceae were reduced in FEP patients. At the genus level, there was an increase in *Lactobacillus*, *Tropheryma*, *Halothiobacillus*, *Saccharophagus*, *Ochrobactrum*, *Deferribacter* and *Halorubrum*, whereas *Anabaena*, *Nitrosospira* and *Gallionella* were decreased in FEP (157). It is noteworthy that the vast majority of FEP patients were prescribed antipsychotic medication, which can impact gut microbiota composition (158–160). Interestingly, an oropharyngeal microbiome analysis in schizophrenia patients showed an increased abundance of *Lactobacillus*, in addition to *Bifidobacterium* and *Ascomycota*, when compared to heathy individuals (161). Another study of the oropharyngeal microbiota revealed an increase in the abundance of a bacteriophage specific for *lactobacilli*, *lactobacillus* phage phiadh (162).

Whether these alterations to the oropharyngeal microbiota have any bearing upon the behavioural disturbances of patients with schizophrenia is unknown. However, these studies highlight that various microbiomes are affected in this neurodevelopmental disorder (72). Preclinical and clinical data have documented the beneficial effects of the antibiotic minocycline on the behavioural and physiological symptoms of schizophrenia (Figure 13.2 A, B) (163,164). Minocycline has been shown to improve sensorimotor deficits and visual-spatial memory in animal models of schizophrenia in a manner comparable to the classical antipsychotic, haloperidol (165, 166). Moreover, treatment with minocycline improved both the negative symptoms and cognitive deficits in patients with schizophrenia (165,167,168). Minocycline mediated its effect through suppressing microglia activation and modulation of excitatory neurotransmission. In contrast, a recent study showed administration of minocycline failed to abate negative symptoms in patients with recent-onset of psychosis (169). The absence of a minocycline effect may be because the active neuroinflammation involving microglial activation and neuropathology is not prevalent during the first years of schizophrenia (169). The gut microbiome holds a promising future as a potential therapy for schizophrenia, but there may be a need to have a more personalized approach compared to a one glove fits all. Therefore, more studies are required to understand different targets to better understand role of gut microbiome in schizophrenia.

13.6 Conclusion

Human brain development is a highly complex process and it is becoming increasingly recognized that the gut microbiome influences it. Recent developments in the field of neurodevelopmental disorders such as ASD and schizophrenia has further supported the importance of this mutual coordination. Preclinical studies have started to elucidate the underlying mechanisms for how the gut microbiota participates in the regulation of social, cognitive and emotional behaviours, all of which are hallmarks of neurodevelopment disorders. Evidence has shown that restoration of the gut microbiota can result in the improvement of the behavioural symptoms of neurodevelopmental disorders, including ASD and schizophrenia. These findings have led to the concept of psychobiotics, (live bacteria, probiotics which when ingested confer mental health benefits through interaction with commensal gut bacteria) that may offer improvements in the therapeutic index of autism and schizophrenia pharmacology (170,171). Indeed, more robust clinical studies are required to delineate the efficacy of potential psychobiotics. Nonetheless, the preclinical and clinical data generated thus far provide a promising glimpse into the future treatments of these neurodevelopmental disorders.

References

1. Azevedo FA, Carvalho LR, Grinberg LT, et al. Equal numbers of neuronal and nonneuronal cells make the human brain an isometrically scaled-up primate brain. *J. Comp. Neurol.* 2009; 513: 532–541.

2. Tognini P. Gut microbiota: a potential regulator of neurodevelopment. *Front Cell Neurosci.* 2017;11:25.

3. Sekirov I, Russell SL, Antunes LC, Finlay BB. Gut microbiota in health and disease. *Physiol Rev.* 2010;90:859–904.

4. Derrien M, Alvarez AS, de Vos WM. The gut microbiota in the first decade of life. *Trends Microbiol.* 2019;27:997–1010.

5. Zhuang L, Chen H, Zhang S, Zhuang J, Li Q, Feng Z. Intestinal microbiota in early life and its implications on childhood health. *Genomics Proteomics Bioinformatics.* 2019;17:13–25.

6. Qin J, Li R, Raes J, et al. A human gut microbial gene catalogue established by metagenomic sequencing. *Nature.* 2010;464:59–65.

7. Dinan TG, Cryan JF. The microbiome-gut-brain axis in health and disease. *Gastroenterol Clin North Am.* 2017;46:77–89.

8. Sampson TR, Debelius JW, Thron T, et al. Gut microbiota regulate motor deficits and neuroinflammation in a model of Parkinson's disease. *Cell.* 2016;167:1469–80 e12.

9. Sherwin E, Sandhu KV, Dinan TG, Cryan JF. May the force be with you: the light and dark sides of the microbiota-gut-brain axis in neuropsychiatry. *CNS Drugs.* 2016;30:1019–41.

10. Frohlich EE, Farzi A, Mayerhofer R, et al. Cognitive impairment by antibiotic-induced gut dysbiosis: analysis of gut microbiota-brain communication. *Brain Behav Immun.* 2016;56:140–55.

11. Yang JH, Bhargava P, McCloskey D, et al. Antibiotic-induced changes to the host metabolic environment inhibit drug efficacy and alter immune function. *Cell Host Microbe.* 2017;22:757–65 e3.

12. Becattini S, Taur Y, Pamer EG. Antibiotic-induced changes in the intestinal microbiota and disease. *Trends Mol Med.* 2016;22:458–78.

13. Kelly JR, Borre Y, O'Brien C, et al. Transferring the blues: depression-associated gut microbiota induces neurobehavioural changes in the rat. *J Psychiatr Res.* 2016;82:109–18.

14. Jiang H, Ling Z, Zhang Y, et al. Altered fecal microbiota composition in patients with major depressive disorder. *Brain Behav Immun.* 2015;48:186–94.

15. Clapp M, Aurora N, Herrera L, et al. Gut microbiota's effect on mental health: The gut-brain axis. *Clin Pract.* 2017;7:987.

16. 1Ridler C. Gut microbiota: gut bacteria affect post-ischaemic inflammation in stroke by modulating intestinal T cells. *Nat Rev Gastroenterol Hepatol.* 2016;13:250.

17. Mulle JG, Sharp WG, Cubells JF. The gut microbiome: a new frontier in autism research. *Curr Psychiatry Rep.* 2013;15:337.

18. Dinan TG, Borre YE, Cryan JF. Genomics of schizophrenia: time to consider the gut microbiome? *Mol Psychiatry.* 2014;19:1252–7.

19. Sandhu KV, Sherwin E, Schellekens H, et al. Feeding the microbiota-gut-brain axis: diet, microbiome, and neuropsychiatry. *Transl Res.* 2017;179:223–44.

20. Arentsen T, Qian Y, Gkotzis S, et al. The bacterial peptidoglycan-sensing molecule Pglyrp2 modulates brain development and behavior. *Mol Psychiatry.* 2017;22:257–66.

21. Critchley HD, Harrison NA. Visceral influences on brain and behavior. *Neuron.* 2013;77(4):624–38.

22. Carabotti M. SAM, Maselli AM, Severia C. The gut-brain axis: interactions between enteric microbiota, central and enteric nervous systems. *Annals of Gastroenterology.* 2015;28:203–9.

23. Lyte M. Microbial endocrinology in the microbiome-gut-brain axis: how bacterial production and utilization of neurochemicals influence behavior. *PLoS Pathog.* 2013;9:e1003726.

24. Foster JA, Rinaman L, Cryan JF. Stress & the gut-brain axis: regulation by the microbiome. *Neurobiol Stress.* 2017;7:124–36.

25. Gautam A, Kumar R, Chakraborty N, et al. Altered fecal microbiota composition in all male aggressor-exposed rodent model simulating features of post-traumatic stress disorder. *J Neurosci Res.* 2018;96:1311–23.

26. Bravo JA, Forsythe P, Chew MV, et al. Ingestion of Lactobacillus strain regulates emotional behavior and central GABA receptor expression in a mouse via the vagus nerve. *Proc Natl Acad Sci USA.* 2011;108:16050–5.

27. Allen AP, Hutch W, Borre YE, et al. Bifidobacterium longum 1714 as a translational psychobiotic: modulation of stress, electrophysiology and neurocognition in healthy volunteers. *Transl Psychiatry.* 2016; 6:e939.

28. Sudo N, Chida Y, Aiba Y, et al. Postnatal microbial colonization programs the hypothalamic-pituitary-adrenal system for stress response in mice. *J Physiol.* 2004;558:263–75.

29. Poutahidis T, Kearney SM, Levkovich T, et al. Microbial symbionts accelerate wound healing via the neuropeptide hormone oxytocin. *PLoS One.* 2013 Oct 30;8(10):e78898.

30. Buffington SA, Di Prisco GV, Auchtung TA, et al. Microbial Reconstitution Reverses Maternal Diet-Induced Social and Synaptic Deficits in Offspring. *Cell.* 2016;165:1762–75.

31. Diaz Heijtz R, Wang S, Anuar F, et al. Normal gut microbiota modulates brain development and behavior. *Proc Natl Acad Sci USA.* 2011;108:3047–52.

32. Clarke G, Grenham S, Scully P, et al. The microbiome-gut-brain axis during early life regulates the hippocampal serotonergic system in a sex-dependent manner. *Mol Psychiatry.* 2013;18:666–73.

33. Saulnier DM, Ringel Y, Heyman MB, et al. The intestinal microbiome, probiotics and prebiotics in neurogastroenterology. *Gut Microbes.* 2013;4:17–27.

34. Burokas A, Arboleya S, Moloney RD, et al. Targeting the microbiota-gut-brain axis: prebiotics have anxiolytic and antidepressant-like effects and reverse the impact of chronic stress in mice. *Biol Psychiatry.* 2017;82:472–87.

35. Marques TM, Patterson E, Wall R, et al. Influence of GABA and GABA-producing Lactobacillus brevis DPC 6108 on the development of diabetes in a streptozotocin rat model. *Benef Microbes.* 2016;7:409–20.

36. Sobko T. Influence of the microflors on gastrointestinal nitric oxide generation.

Unpublished Ph.D. thesis, Karolinska Institutet, Sweden, 2006.

37. Schicho R, Krueger D, Zeller F, et al. Hydrogen sulfide is a novel prosecretory neuromodulator in the Guinea-pig and human colon. *Gastroenterology.* 2006;131:1542–52.

38. Latorre R, Sternini C, De Giorgio R, Greenwood-Van Meerveld B. Enteroendocrine cells: a review of their role in brain-gut communication. *Neurogastroenterol Motil.* 2016;28:620–30.

39. Berthoud HR. The vagus nerve, food intake and obesity. *Regul Pept.* 2008;149:15–25.

40. Batterham RL, Cowley MA, Small CJ, et al. Gut hormone PYY3-36 physiologically inhibits food intake. *Nature.* 2002;418:650–4.

41. Koda S, Date Y, Murakami N, et al. The role of the vagal nerve in peripheral PYY3-36-induced feeding reduction in rats. *Endocrinology.* 2005;146:2369–75.

42. Bercik P, Denou E, Collins J, et al. The intestinal microbiota affect central levels of brain-derived neurotropic factor and behavior in mice. *Gastroenterology.* 2011;141:599–609, e1-3.

43. Kunze WA, Mao YK, Wang B, et al. Lactobacillus reuteri enhances excitability of colonic AH neurons by inhibiting calcium-dependent potassium channel opening. *J Cell Mol Med.* 2009;13:2261–70.

44. Macpherson AJ, Slack E, Geuking MB, McCoy KD. The mucosal firewalls against commensal intestinal microbes. *Semin Immunopathol.* 2009;31:145–9.

45. McGuckin MA, Linden SK, Sutton P, Florin TH. Mucin dynamics and enteric pathogens. *Nat Rev Microbiol.* 2011;9:265–78.

46. Hooper LV, Macpherson AJ. Immune adaptations that maintain homeostasis with the intestinal microbiota. *Nat Rev Immunol.* 2010;10:159–69.

47. Pamer EG. Immune responses to commensal and environmental microbes. *Nat Immunol.* 2007;8:1173–8.

48. Cash HL, Whitham CV, Behrendt CL, Hooper LV. Symbiotic bacteria direct expression of an intestinal bactericidal lectin. *Science.* 2006;313:1126–30.

49. Bengmark S. Gut microbiota, immune development and function. *Pharmacol Res.* 2013;69:87–113.

50. Dantzer R, O'Connor JC, Freund GG, Johnson RW, Kelley KW. From inflammation to sickness and depression: when the immune system subjugates the brain. *Nat Rev Neurosci.* 2008;9:46–56.

51. Steer T, Carpenter H, Tuohy K, Gibson GR. Perspectives on the role of the human gut microbiota and its modulation by pro- and prebiotics. *Nutr Res Rev.* 2000;13:229–54.

52. Maes M, Kubera M, Leunis J-C, Berk M. Increased IgA and IgM responses against gut commensals in chronic depression: further evidence for increased bacterial translocation or leaky gut. *J Affect Disord.* 2012;141:55–62.

53. Erny D, Hrabe de Angelis AL, Jaitin D, et al. Host microbiota constantly control maturation and function of microglia in the CNS. *Nat Neurosci.* 2015;18: 965–77.

54. Kau AL, Ahern PP, Griffin NW, Goodman AL, Gordon JI. Human nutrition, the gut microbiome and the immune system. *Nature.* 2011;474:327–36.

55. Koh A, De Vadder F, Kovatcheva-Datchary P, Backhed F. From dietary fiber to host physiology: short-chain fatty acids as key bacterial metabolites. *Cell.* 2016;165:1332–45.

56. Stilling RM, Dinan TG, Cryan JF. Microbial genes, brain & behaviour – epigenetic regulation of the gut-brain axis. *Genes Brain Behav.* 2014;13:69–86.

57. Hullar MA, Fu BC. Diet, the gut microbiome, and epigenetics. *Cancer J.* 2014;20:170–5.

58. den Besten G, van Eunen K, Groen AK, et al. The role of short-chain fatty acids in the interplay between diet, gut microbiota, and host energy metabolism. *J Lipid Res.* 2013;54:2325–40.

59. Stilling RM, van de Wouw M, Clarke G, et al. The neuropharmacology of butyrate: The bread and butter of the

microbiota-gut-brain axis? *Neurochem Int.* 2016;99:110–32.

60. Nankova BB AR, MacFabe DF, La Gamma EF. Enteric bacterial metabolites propionic and butyric acid modulate gene expression, including CREB-dependent catecholaminergic neurotransmission, in PC12 cells – possible relevance to autism spectrum disorders. *PLOS One.* 2014;9(8): e103740.

61. El-Ansary AK, Ben Bacha A, Kotb M. Etiology of autistic features: the persisting neurotoxic effects of propionic acid. *J Neuroinflammation.* 2012;9:74.

62. Bourassa MW, Alim I, Bultman SJ, Ratan RR. Butyrate, neuroepigenetics and the gut microbiome: Can a high fiber diet improve brain health? *Neurosci Lett.* 2016;625:56–63.

63. Luczynski P, Whelan SO, O'Sullivan C, et al. Adult microbiota-deficient mice have distinct dendritic morphological changes: differential effects in the amygdala and hippocampus. *Eur J Neurosci.* 2016;44:2654–66.

64. Park H, Poo MM. Neurotrophin regulation of neural circuit development and function. *Nat Rev Neurosci.* 2013;14:7–23.

65. Tarsa L, Goda Y. Synaptophysin regulates activity-dependent synapse formation in cultured hippocampal neurons. *Proc Natl Acad Sci USA.* 2002;99:1012–6.

66. Kwon SE, Chapman ER. Synaptophysin regulates the kinetics of synaptic vesicle endocytosis in central neurons. *Neuron.* 2011;70:847–54.

67. El-Husseini AE SE, Chetkovich DM, Nicoll RA, Bredt DS. PSD-95 involvement in maturation of excitatory synapses. *SCIENCE.* 2000;290:1364–8.

68. Béïque J-C, Andrade R. PSD-95 regulates synaptic transmission and plasticity in rat cerebral cortex. *The Journal of Physiology.* 2003;546:859–67.

69. Neufeld KM, Kang N, Bienenstock J, Foster JA. Reduced anxiety-like behavior and central neurochemical change in germ-free mice. *Neurogastroenterol Motil.* 2011;23:255–64, e119.

70. Hoban AE, Stilling RM, Ryan FJ, et al. Regulation of prefrontal cortex myelination by the microbiota. *Transl Psychiatry.* 2016;6:e774.

71. Asan E, Steinke M, Lesch KP. Serotonergic innervation of the amygdala: targets, receptors, and implications for stress and anxiety. *Histochem Cell Biol.* 2013;139:785–813.

72. Kelly JR, Minuto C, Cryan JF, Clarke G, Dinan TG. Cross talk: the microbiota and neurodevelopmental disorders. *Front Neurosci.* 2017; 11:490.

73. Reigstad CS, Salmonson CE, Rainey JF, 3rd, et al. Gut microbes promote colonic serotonin production through an effect of short-chain fatty acids on enterochromaffin cells. *FASEB J.* 2015;29:1395–403.

74. Desbonnet L, Clarke G, Traplin A, et al. Gut microbiota depletion from early adolescence in mice: Implications for brain and behaviour. *Brain Behav Immun.* 2015;48:165–73.

75. Mohle L, Mattei D, Heimesaat MM, et al. Ly6C(hi) monocytes provide a link between antibiotic-induced changes in gut microbiota and adult hippocampal neurogenesis. *Cell Rep.* 2016;15: 1945–56.

76. Stiles J, Jernigan TL. The basics of brain development. *Neuropsychol Rev.* 2010;20:327–48.

77. O'Mahony SM, Clarke G, Borre YE, Dinan TG, Cryan JF. Serotonin, tryptophan metabolism and the brain-gut-microbiome axis. *Behav Brain Res.* 2015;277:32–48.

78. Jasarevic E, Rodgers AB, Bale TL. A novel role for maternal stress and microbial transmission in early life programming and neurodevelopment. *Neurobiol Stress.* 2015;1:81–8.

79. Rogers GB, Keating DJ, Young RL, et al. From gut dysbiosis to altered brain function and mental illness: mechanisms and pathways. *Mol Psychiatry.* 2016;21:738–48.

80. Kim S, Kim H, Yim YS, et al. Maternal gut bacteria promote neurodevelopmental abnormalities in mouse offspring. *Nature*. 2017;549:528–32.

81. Sasaki A, de Vega W, Sivanathan S, St-Cyr S, McGowan PO. Maternal high-fat diet alters anxiety behavior and glucocorticoid signaling in adolescent offspring. *Neuroscience*. 2014;272:92–101.

82. Davis EP, Sandman CA. The timing of prenatal exposure to maternal cortisol and psychosocial stress is associated with human infant cognitive development. *Child Dev*. 2010;81:131–48.

83. Sandman CA, Davis EP, Buss C, Glynn LM. Exposure to prenatal psychobiological stress exerts programming influences on the mother and her fetus. *Neuroendocrinology*. 2012;95:7–21.

84. Golubeva AV, Crampton S, Desbonnet L, et al. Prenatal stress-induced alterations in major physiological systems correlate with gut microbiota composition in adulthood. *Psychoneuroendocrinology*. 2015;60:58–74.

85. Jansson T, Powell TL. Role of the placenta in fetal programming: underlying mechanisms and potential interventional approaches. *Clin Sci (Lond)*. 2007;113:1–13.

86. Glover V, Bergman K, Sarkar P, O'Connor TG. Association between maternal and amniotic fluid cortisol is moderated by maternal anxiety. *Psychoneuroendocrinology*. 2009;34:430–5.

87. Côté F FC, Bayard E, Launay JM, et al. Maternal serotonin is crucial for murine embryonic development. *Proc Natl Acad Sci USA*. 2007;104:329–34.

88. Bonnin A, Levitt P. Placental source for 5-HT that tunes fetal brain development. *Neuropsychopharmacology*. 2012;37:299–300.

89. Braniste V, Al-Asmakh M, Kowal C, et al. The gut microbiota influences blood-brain barrier permeability in mice. *Sci Transl Med*. 2014;6:263ra158.

90. Borre YE, O'Keeffe GW, Clarke G, et al. Microbiota and neurodevelopmental windows: implications for brain disorders. *Trends Mol Med*. 2014;20:509–18.

91. O'Mahony SM, Clarke G, Dinan TG, Cryan JF. Early-life adversity and brain development: Is the microbiome a missing piece of the puzzle? *Neuroscience*. 2017;342:37–54.

92. Timmerman HM, Rutten N, Boekhorst J, et al. Intestinal colonisation patterns in breastfed and formula-fed infants during the first 12 weeks of life reveal sequential microbiota signatures. *Sci Rep*. 2017;7:8327.

93. Rutayisire E, Huang K, Liu Y, Tao F. The mode of delivery affects the diversity and colonization pattern of the gut microbiota during the first year of infants' life: a systematic review. *BMC Gastroenterol*. 2016;16:86.

94. Neu J, Rushing J. Cesarean versus vaginal delivery: long-term infant outcomes and the hygiene hypothesis. *Clin Perinatol*. 2011;38:321–31.

95. Musilova S, Rada V, Vlkova E, Bunesova V. Beneficial effects of human milk oligosaccharides on gut microbiota. *Benef Microbes*. 2014;5:273–83.

96. Bode L. Human milk oligosaccharides: every baby needs a sugar mama. *Glycobiology*. 2012;22:1147–62.

97. Toscano M, De Grandi R, Grossi E, Drago L. Role of the human breast milk-associated microbiota on the newborns' immune system: a mini review. *Front Microbiol*. 2017;8:2100.

98. Andreas NJ, Kampmann B, Mehring Le-Doare K. Human breast milk: a review on its composition and bioactivity. *Early Hum Dev*. 2015;91:629–35.

99. Wall R, Marques TM, O'Sullivan O, et al. Contrasting effects of Bifidobacterium breve NCIMB 702258 and Bifidobacterium breve DPC 6330 on the composition of murine brain fatty acids and gut microbiota. *Am J Clin Nutr*. 2012;95:1278–87.

100. Santos F, Spinler JK, Saulnier DM, et al. Functional identification in Lactobacillus reuteri of a PocR-like transcription factor regulating glycerol utilization and vitamin

B12 synthesis. *Microb Cell Fact.* 2011;10:55.

101. Innis SM. Impact of maternal diet on human milk composition and neurological development of infants. *Am J Clin Nutr.* 2014;99:734S-41S.

102. Edlow AG. Maternal obesity and neurodevelopmental and psychiatric disorders in offspring. *Prenat Diagn.* 2017;37:95-110.

103. Kim HJ, Cho MH, Shim WH, et al. Deficient autophagy in microglia impairs synaptic pruning and causes social behavioral defects. *Mol Psychiatry.* 2017;22:1576-84.

104. Boksa P. Abnormal synaptic pruning in schizophrenia: Urban myth or reality? *J Psychiatry Neurosci.* 2012;37:75-7.

105. Christensen DL, Baio J, Van Naarden Braun K, et al. Prevalence and characteristics of autism spectrum disorder among children aged 8 years – autism and developmental disabilities monitoring network, 11 Sites, United States, 2012. *Surveillance Summaries.* 2016;65(3):1-23.

106. Lartseva A, Dijkstra T, Buitelaar JK. Emotional language processing in autism spectrum disorders: a systematic review. *Front Hum Neurosci.* 2014;8:991.

107. Wang S, Adolphs R. Reduced specificity in emotion judgment in people with autism spectrum disorder. *Neuropsychologia.* 2017;99:286-95.

108. Li Q, Zhou JM. The microbiota-gut-brain axis and its potential therapeutic role in autism spectrum disorder. *Neuroscience.* 2016;324:131-9.

109. De Rubeis S, He X, Goldberg AP, et al. Synaptic, transcriptional and chromatin genes disrupted in autism. *Nature.* 2014;515:209-15.

110. Gorrindo P, Williams KC, Lee EB, et al. Gastrointestinal dysfunction in autism: parental report, clinical evaluation, and associated factors. *Autism Res.* 2012;5:101-8.

111. Adams JB, Johansen LJ, Powell LD, Quig D, Rubin RA. Gastrointestinal flora and gastrointestinal status in children with autism–comparisons to typical children and correlation with autism severity. *BMC Gastroenterol.* 2011;11:22.

112. Buie T, Fuchs GJ, 3rd, Furuta GT, et al. Recommendations for evaluation and treatment of common gastrointestinal problems in children with ASDs. *Pediatrics.* 2010;125(Suppl 1):S19-29.

113. Mazurek MO, Vasa RA, Kalb LG, et al. Anxiety, sensory over-responsivity, and gastrointestinal problems in children with autism spectrum disorders. *J Abnorm Child Psychol.* 2013;41:165-76.

114. Finegold SM MD, Song Y, Liu C, et al. Gastrointestinal microflora studies in late-onset autism. *Clin Infect Dis.* 2002;35:S6-S16.

115. Finegold SM, Dowd SE, Gontcharova V, et al. Pyrosequencing study of fecal microflora of autistic and control children. *Anaerobe.* 2010;16:444-53.

116. De Angelis M, Piccolo M, Vannini L, et al. Fecal microbiota and metabolome of children with autism and pervasive developmental disorder not otherwise specified. *PLoS One.* 2013;8:e76993.

117. Kang DW, Park JG, Ilhan ZE, et al. Reduced incidence of Prevotella and other fermenters in intestinal microflora of autistic children. *PLoS One.* 2013;8:e68322.

118. Parracho HM, Bingham MO, Gibson GR, McCartney AL. Differences between the gut microflora of children with autistic spectrum disorders and that of healthy children. *J Med Microbiol.* 2005;54:987-91.

119. Pequegnat B, Sagermann M, Valliani M, et al. A vaccine and diagnostic target for Clostridium bolteae, an autism-associated bacterium. *Vaccine.* 2013;31:2787-90.

120. Finegold SM, Summanen PH, Downes J, Corbett K, Komoriya T. Detection of Clostridium perfringens toxin genes in the gut microbiota of autistic children. *Anaerobe.* 2017;45:133-7.

121. Shaw W. Increased urinary excretion of a 3-(3-hydroxyphenyl)-

3-hydroxypropionic acid (HPHPA), an abnormal phenylalanine metabolite of Clostridia spp. in the gastrointestinal tract, in urine samples from patients with autism and schizophrenia. *Nutr Neurosci* 2010;13:135–43.

122. Kang DW, Adams JB, Coleman DM, et al. Long-term benefit of Microbiota Transfer Therapy on autism symptoms and gut microbiota. *Sci Rep.* 2019;9:5821.

123. Wang L, Christophersen CT, Sorich MJ, et al. Elevated fecal short chain fatty acid and ammonia concentrations in children with autism spectrum disorder. *Dig Dis Sci.* 2012;57:2096–102.

124. de Magistris L, Familiari V, Pascotto A, et al. Alterations of the intestinal barrier in patients with autism spectrum disorders and in their first-degree relatives. *J Pediatr Gastroenterol Nutr.* 2010;51:418–24.

125. Ashwood P, Krakowiak P, Hertz-Picciotto I, et al.Elevated plasma cytokines in autism spectrum disorders provide evidence of immune dysfunction and are associated with impaired behavioral outcome. *Brain Behav Immun.* 2011;25:40–5.

126. Son JS, Zheng LJ, Rowehl LM, et al. Comparison of fecal microbiota in children with autism spectrum disorders and neurotypical siblings in the Simons Simplex Collection. *PLoS One.* 2015;10: e0137725.

127. Shultz SR, Macfabe DF, Martin S, et al. Intracerebroventricular injections of the enteric bacterial metabolic product propionic acid impair cognition and sensorimotor ability in the Long-Evans rat: further development of a rodent model of autism. *Behav Brain Res.* 2009;200:33–41.

128. Shultz SR, MacFabe DF, Ossenkopp KP, et al. Intracerebroventricular injection of propionic acid, an enteric bacterial metabolic end-product, impairs social behavior in the rat: implications for an animal model of autism. *Neuropharmacology.* 2008;54:901–11.

129. Hsiao EY, McBride SW, Hsien S, et al. Microbiota modulate behavioral and physiological abnormalities associated with neurodevelopmental disorders. *Cell.* 2013;155:1451–63.

130. Pobbe RL, Pearson BL, Defensor EB, et al. Expression of social behaviors of C57BL/6J versus BTBR inbred mouse strains in the visible burrow system. *Behav Brain Res.* 2010;214:443–9.

131. Weissbrod A, Shapiro A, Vasserman G, et al. Automated long-term tracking and social behavioural phenotyping of animal colonies within a semi-natural environment. *Nat Commun.* 2013;4:2018.

132. Pearson BL, Pobbe RL, Defensor EB, et al. Motor and cognitive stereotypies in the BTBR T+tf/J mouse model of autism. *Genes Brain Behav.* 2011;10:228–35.

133. Karvat G, Kimchi T. Systematic autistic-like behavioral phenotyping of 4 mouse strains using a novel wheel-running assay. *Behav Brain Res.* 2012;233:405–14.

134. Stephenson DT, O'Neill SM, Narayan S, et al. Histopathologic characterization of the BTBR mouse model of autistic-like behavior reveals selective changes in neurodevelopmental proteins and adult hippocampal neurogenesis. *Mol Autism.* 2011;2:7.

135. Heo Y, Zhang Y, Gao D, Miller VM, Lawrence DA. Aberrant immune responses in a mouse with behavioral disorders. *PLoS One.* 2011;6: e20912.

136. Golubeva AV, Joyce SA, Moloney G, et al. Microbiota-related changes in bile acid & tryptophan metabolism are associated with gastrointestinal dysfunction in a mouse model of autism. *EBioMedicine.* 2017;24:166–78.

137. Coretti L, Cristiano C, Florio E, et al. Sex-related alterations of gut microbiota composition in the BTBR mouse model of autism spectrum disorder. *Sci Rep.* 2017;7:45356.

138. Perälä J SJ, Saarni SI, Kuoppasalmi K, et al. Lifetime prevalence of psychotic and

bipolar I disorders in a general population. *Arch Gen Psychiatry.* 2007;64:19–28.

139. Hor K, Taylor M. Suicide and schizophrenia: a systematic review of rates and risk factors. *J Psychopharmacol.* 2010;24:81–90.

140. JH G. Understanding what causes schizophrenia: a developmental perspective. *AM J Psychiatry.* 2008;167:8–10.

141. Kahn RS, Keefe RS. Schizophrenia is a cognitive illness: time for a change in focus. *JAMA Psychiatry.* 2013;70:1107–12.

142. Hommer RE, Swedo SE. Schizophrenia and autism-related disorders. *Schizophr Bull.* 2015;41:313–4.

143. Corvin A, Morris DW. Genome-wide association studies: findings at the major histocompatibility complex locus in psychosis. *Biol Psychiatry.* 2014;75:276–83.

144. Miller BJ, Buckley P, Seabolt W, Mellor A, Kirkpatrick B. Meta-analysis of cytokine alterations in schizophrenia: clinical status and antipsychotic effects. *Biol Psychiatry.* 2011;70:663–71.

145. Di Nicola M, Cattaneo A, Hepgul N, et al. Serum and gene expression profile of cytokines in first-episode psychosis. *Brain Behav Immun.* 2013;31:90–5.

146. de Witte L, Tomasik J, Schwarz E, et al. Cytokine alterations in first-episode schizophrenia patients before and after antipsychotic treatment. *Schizophr Res.* 2014;154:23–9.

147. Upthegrove R, Manzanares-Teson N, Barnes NM. Cytokine function in medication-naive first episode psychosis: a systematic review and meta-analysis. *Schizophr Res.* 2014;155:101–8.

148. Cremaschi L, Kardell M, Johansson V, et al. Prevalences of autoimmune diseases in schizophrenia, bipolar I and II disorder, and controls. *Psychiatry Res.* 2017;258:9–14.

149. Notter T, Meyer U. Microglia and schizophrenia: where next? *Mol Psychiatry.* 2017;22:788–9.

150. van Kesteren CF, Gremmels H, de Witte LD, et al. Immune involvement in the pathogenesis of schizophrenia: a meta-analysis on postmortem brain studies. *Transl Psychiatry.* 2017;7:e1075.

151. Schwarcz R, Hunter CA. Toxoplasma gondii and schizophrenia: linkage through astrocyte-derived kynurenic acid? *Schizophr Bull.* 2007;33:652–3.

152. Prandovszky E, Gaskell E, Martin H, et al. The neurotropic parasite Toxoplasma gondii increases dopamine metabolism. *PLoS One.* 2011;6:e23866.

153. Havlícek J, Gasová ZG, Smith AP, et al. Decrease of psychomotor performance in subjects with latent 'asymptomatic' toxoplasmosis. *Parasitology.* 2001 May;122(Pt 5):515–20.

154. Molloy MJ, Grainger JR, Bouladoux N, et al. Intraluminal containment of commensal outgrowth in the gut during infection-induced dysbiosis. *Cell Host Microbe.* 2013;14:318–28.

155. Arias I, Sorlozano A, Villegas E, et al. Infectious agents associated with schizophrenia: a meta-analysis. *Schizophr Res.* 2012;136:128–36.

156. Shen Y, Xu J, Li Z, et al. Analysis of gut microbiota diversity and auxiliary diagnosis as a biomarker in patients with schizophrenia: a cross-sectional study. *Schizophr Res.* 2018;197:470–77.

157. Schwarz E, Maukonen J, Hyytiainen T, Kieseppa T, Oresic M, Sabunciyan S, et al. Analysis of microbiota in first episode psychosis identifies preliminary associations with symptom severity and treatment response. *Schizophr Res.* 2018;192:398–403.

158. Davey KJ, Cotter PD, O'Sullivan O, et al. Antipsychotics and the gut microbiome: olanzapine-induced metabolic dysfunction is attenuated by antibiotic administration in the rat. *Transl Psychiatry.* 2013;3:e309.

159. Davey KJ, O'Mahony SM, Schellekens H, et al. Gender-dependent consequences of chronic olanzapine in the rat: effects on body weight, inflammatory, metabolic

and microbiota parameters.
Psychopharmacology (Berl).
2012;221:155–69.

160. Bahr SM, Tyler BC, Wooldridge N, et al.
Use of the second-generation
antipsychotic, risperidone, and secondary
weight gain are associated with an altered
gut microbiota in children. *Transl
Psychiatry.* 2015;5:e652.

161. Castro-Nallar E, Bendall ML, Perez-
Losada M, et al. Composition, taxonomy
and functional diversity of the
oropharynx microbiome in individuals
with schizophrenia and controls. *PeerJ.*
2015;3:e1140.

162. Yolken RH, Severance EG, Sabunciyan S,
et al. Metagenomic sequencing indicates
that the oropharyngeal phageome of
individuals with schizophrenia differs
from that of controls. *Schizophr Bull.*
2015;41:1153–61.

163. Chaves C, Marque CR, Trzesniak C, et al.
Glutamate-N-methyl-D-aspartate
receptor modulation and minocycline for
the treatment of patients with
schizophrenia: an update. *Braz J Med Biol
Res.* 2009;42(11):1002–14.

164. Solmi M, Veronese N, Thapa N, et al.
Systematic review and meta-analysis of
the efficacy and safety of minocycline in
schizophrenia. *CNS Spectr.*
2017;22:415–26.

165. Levkovitz Y, Levi U, Braw Y, Cohen H.
247 – Minocycline, a second-generation
tetracycline, as a neuroprotective agent in
an animal model of schizophrenia.
Schizophrenia Research. 2008;98:135.

166. Zhang L, Zhao J. Profile of minocycline
and its potential in the treatment of
schizophrenia. *Neuropsychiatr Dis Treat.*
2014;10:1103–11.

167. Chaudhry IB, Hallak J, Husain N, et al.
Minocycline benefits negative symptoms
in early schizophrenia: a randomised
double-blind placebo-controlled clinical
trial in patients on standard treatment.
J Psychopharmacol. 2012;26:
1185–93.

168. Liu F, Guo X, Wu R, et al. Minocycline
supplementation for treatment of

negative symptoms in early-phase
schizophrenia: a double blind,
randomized, controlled trial. *Schizophr
Res.* 2014;153:169–76.

169. Deakin B, Suckling J, Barnes TRE, et al.
The benefit of minocycline on negative
symptoms of schizophrenia in patients
with recent-onset psychosis (BeneMin):
a randomised, double-blind,
placebo-controlled trial. *Lancet
Psychiatry.* 2018;5:885–94.

170. Dinan TG, Stanton C, Cryan JF.
Psychobiotics: a novel class of
psychotropic. *Biol Psychiatry.*
2013;74:720–6.

171. Sarkar A, Lehto SM, Harty S, et al.
Psychobiotics and the manipulation of
bacteria-gut-brain signals. *Trends
Neurosci.* 2016;39:763–81.

172. Kang DW, Adams JB, Gregory AC, et al.
Microbiota transfer therapy alters gut
ecosystem and improves gastrointestinal
and autism symptoms: an
open-label study. *Microbiome.*
2017;5:10.

173. Sandler RH, Finegold SM, Bolte ER, et al.
Short-term benefit from oral vancomycin
treatment of regressive-onset autism.
J Child Neurol. 2000;15(7):429–35.

174. Strati F, Cavalieri D, Albanese D, et al.
New evidences on the altered gut
microbiota in autism spectrum
disorders. *Microbiome.*
2017;5:24.

175. Gondalia SV, Palombo EA, Knowles SR,
et al. Molecular characterisation of
gastrointestinal microbiota of children
with autism (with and without
gastrointestinal dysfunction) and their
neurotypical siblings. *Autism Res.*
2012;5:419–27.

176. Cao X, Lin P, Jiang P, Li C. Characteristics
of the gastrointestinal microbiome in
children with autism spectrum
disorder: a systematic review.
Shanghai Arch Psychiatry.
2013;25:342–53.

177. Christian LM, Galley JD, Hade EM, et al.
Gut microbiome composition is

associated with temperament during early childhood. *Brain Behav Immun.* 2015;45:118–27.

178. Tomova A, Husarova V, Lakatosova S, et al. Gastrointestinal microbiota in children with autism in Slovakia. *Physiol Behav.* 2015;138:179–87.

179. Severance EG, Yolken RH, Eaton WW. Autoimmune diseases, gastrointestinal disorders and the microbiome in schizophrenia: more than a gut feeling. *Schizophr Res.* 2016;176: 23–35.

180. Severance EG, Gressitt KL, Stallings CR, et al. Probiotic normalization of Candida albicans in schizophrenia: a randomized, placebo-controlled, longitudinal pilot study. *Brain Behav Immun.* 2017;62: 41–5.

Depression and the Adaptive Immune System

Robert Dantzer

14.1 Introduction

In the context of immunopsychiatry it is important to know whether the association between psychiatric disorders and the immune system that is reported in more and more scientific publications is a real one or just another manifestation of the many comorbid physical conditions that are affecting psychiatric patients. In the case this association is real, the next question is whether the reported alterations in immunity are causal to the psychiatric disorder or just one of its consequences, in the form for instance of the impact of unhealthy lifestyles on the microbiota. Causality, when it exists, provides a unique opportunity to identify new mechanistic targets for drug development. The observation of consistent immune alterations in psychiatric patients also leads to the important interrogation of their functional outcome on the organism resistance to infection or the progression of somatic diseases such as cancer and autoimmunity.

The answers to all these questions are relatively straightforward when examining the relationship between major depressive disorder and inflammation. Several reviews and books have been published on the inflammatory component of major depressive disorder (1–5). As discussed in other chapters of the present book, there is plenty of clinical and preclinical evidence for a causal effect of activation of the innate immune system in the development of symptoms of depression. It is therefore not surprising that anti-inflammatory cytokine treatment can have antidepressant activity both in chronic inflammatory conditions (6) and in depressed individuals who have no sign of physical illness (7) even if the conditions in which such an effect can occur remain to be better defined.

The situation is much less clear when it comes to the adaptive immune system as we will discuss in the present chapter. It is generally believed that the adaptive immune system and the innate immune system vary in opposite directions in depressed subjects. For instance, a recent genome-wide differential gene expression analysis of microarray data collected on whole blood from two independent case-control studies of patients with major depressive disorder compared with healthy control subjects revealed an overexpression of several genes associated with activation of the immune system and a decreased expression of genes associated with the adaptive immune response (8). These findings match the results obtained from smaller-scale studies that showed a positive association between depressive symptoms and inflammation (9–12) and a negative association between these symptoms and lymphocyte proliferation in response to mitogens and other markers of adaptive immunity, ranging from lymphopenia to decreased natural killer cell cytotoxicity (13–16).

Whether such results are generalizable to all cellular components of the adaptive immune system and the relative immunodepression that is apparent in depressed subjects has adverse functional consequences on the physical health of depressed patients is not always clear. A Danish prospective population-based study appears at first face to support this last possibility. This study included more than 970,000 individuals, of whom 14% had a history of depression. It revealed an increased risk for a wide range of infections, with an incidence-rate ratio of 1.64 subsequent to the onset of depression (17). This risk remained elevated for the 11 years of follow up and was higher after several depressive episodes (increasing to 1.84) than after a single event. However, as the immune status of the population under study was not examined, this study provides no evidence in favour of an increased risk of infection in depressed subjects with reduced immunity compared to depressed subjects whose immunity was not affected. It is therefore not possible to determine whether this type of observation is nothing else than another example of the depression-associated higher risk for morbidity or mortality in many medical conditions that do not always involve the adaptive immune system (18).

The objective of the present chapter is not just to examine in details what has been learned on the association between major depressive disorder (MDD) and the adaptive immune system but mainly to discuss whether certain immune cell subsets can play a role in the pathophysiology of depression.

14.2 Clinical Data

14.2.1 Lymphocyte Proliferation Studies

The earliest studies of immunity in depressive disorders took place in the 1980s. The clinical immunology techniques that were available at the time consisted of assessing lymphocyte function by measuring proliferation of peripheral blood mononuclear cells in vitro in response to concavalin A (ConA), phytohemagglutin (PHA), pokeweed mitogen (PWM) and lipopolysaccharide (LPS). The lymphocyte proliferation induced by mitogens is not antigen specific and therefore not very informative for assessing the functional capacity of lymphocytes. PHA and ConA are assumed to preferentially activate T cells, PWM both T cells and B cells, and LPS only B cells. Cell proliferation in these in vitro assays is measured by the amount of ^{3}H-thymidine incorporated into the DNA of rapidly dividing cells.

Melancholic patients were found to have lower lymphocyte responses to mitogens than did non-melancholic patients, who did not differ from normal controls. While studying lymphocyte function in bereaved individuals, Schleifer and colleagues observed that the decreased lymphocyte function that was apparent in the first two months after the bereavement did not recover in a small subset of study participants (20). On the basis of the high prevalence of depressive disorders in bereaved persons and the reported association between melancholic depression and decreased lymphocyte function (21), they initiated a series of systematic studies on the relationship between depressive disorders and lymphocyte function. Depressed hospitalized patients were found to have low counts of T cells and B cells and reduced lymphocyte response to mitogens (Figure 14.1) (22). This was not related solely to hospitalization in a psychiatric unit, as hospitalized patients with schizophrenia did not differ from controls (23). These results were also specific to depressed hospitalized patients, as ambulatory patients with major depressive disorders were not affected (23). Despite their innovative aspect and their importance for the still nascent field of psychoneuroimmunology, these data were met with some scepticism by other physicians, given the absence of an obvious relationship between lymphocyte proliferation

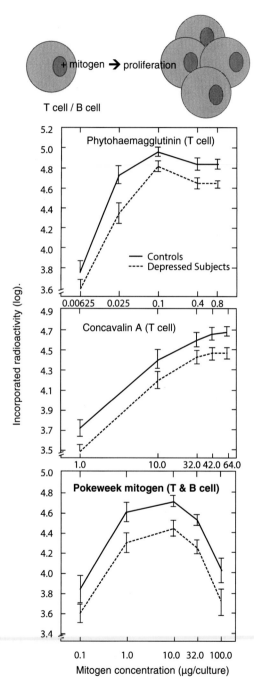

Figure 14.1 A typical example of the decreased lymphocyte proliferation in depressed subjects compared to controls reported in early studies of depression and immunity. The results were obtained in 18 inpatients and 18 non-hospitalized controls. Purified blood lymphocytes were stimulated by various concentrations of phytohaemagglutinin (PHA), concanavalin A (ConA) and pokeweed mitogen. Cell proliferation was measured by incorporation of ^{3}H-thymidine. Modified from Schleifer SJ, et al. *Arch Gen Psychiat.* 1984;41:484–8.

responses and relevant host defences and the lack of consideration of important factors such as treatment, diet, and lifestyle (24).

However, these issues did not prevent this field of research from moving forward. For instance, a study carried out with a limited number of inpatients with a DSM-III diagnosis of major depression who were carefully selected for physical health and lack of psychotropic medication (other than low-dose benzodiazepines) confirmed the occurrence of a decreased mitogen responsiveness to ConA compared with that found in controls (hospital staff members) and in other forms of depression (atypical, dysthymic or atypical bipolar) (25). A meta-analytic review published by Herbert and Cohen in 1993 confirmed that clinical depression is associated with several alterations in cellular immunity. In a total of 35 studies, the effect size for decreased proliferative responses to PHA, ConA, and PWM reached 0.25 to 0.45, and alterations in several white blood cell populations reached 0.11 to 0.77 (26). In general, the immune alterations associated with depression were more pronounced in both older and hospitalized patients. Once more, the authors noted the limitations related to existing published studies, due to the lack of relevance of the measurements of immune function to disease resistance or susceptibility.

14.2.2 T-Cell Subsets and T-Cell Cytokines

The introduction of fluorescence-activated cell-sorting analysis for separating and characterizing subsets of T cells and enzyme-linked immunosorbent assay measurement of cytokines produced by activated immune cells in clinical immunology helped the field of research on depression and immunity to move forward. However, these improvements in clinical immunology did not really change the general approach to the study of the relationship between depression and immunity but allowed a more elaborate description of immune alterations associated with depression. Under the influence of various cytokines, naïve T cells can be differentiated into pro-inflammatory T helper (Th)-1 cells that are involved in protecting the host against intracellular and viral pathogens, and anti-inflammatory Th-2 cells that dampen the inflammatory response and are necessary for induction of humoral immunity, B-cell activation, and production of immunoglobulin E and G. Regulatory T (Treg) cells, previously known as T suppressor cells, downregulate inflammation and control immunotolerance. They are characterized by expression of the fork head box P3 transcription factor (FOXP3) and the alpha chain of the interleukin-2 (IL-2) receptor (CD25). Tissue-resident Treg cells have trophic actions, with those in the brain promoting in particular oligodendrocyte differentiation and remyelination. A number of studies on T cells in depressed individuals refer to the CD4/CD8 ratio that has mainly been used in the context of human immunodeficiency virus infection to predict the likely course of the disease. CD4 is a marker of T helper cells while CD8 is a marker of cytotoxic T cells. CD4$^+$ T cells include both T helper cells and Treg cells. The CD4/CD8 ratio is normally around 2 and a decreased ratio either due to a decrease in CD4$^+$ T cells, an increase in CD8$^+$ T cells or a combination of both phenomena. This decrease is usually interpreted as indicative of a reduced resistance to infection. Naïve T cells and Treg cells can differentiate intoTh-17 cells under the influence of IL-6 and transforming growth factor (TGF)-β. Th-17 cells produce IL-17. They promote inflammation and are involved in the pathogenesis of several autoimmune conditions including rheumatoid arthritis, multiple sclerosis and lupus erythematosus.

A non-exhaustive description of the dysregulation of Th-1/Th-2 cytokines in depressive disorders is given by Hughes and colleagues in a review published in 2016 (27). The general pattern that emerges is suggestive of a predominance of Th-1 activity over Th-2 activity, although this varies according to factors such as depression subtypes, comorbid disorders (including obesity and drug abuse), and medications.

A series of studies carried out in the 1990s on $CD4^+$ and $CD8^+$ T cells in depressed patients revealed a pattern of what was called at the time T cell activation characterized by a higher percentage of $CD4^+$ T cells with or without a lower number of $CD8^+$ T cells, leading to a higher CD4/CD8 ratio (28–30). This pattern was described as being characteristic of melancholic/endogenous depression and treatment-resistant depression (31). There was even description of a highly positive correlation between the CD4/CD8 ratio and the Hamilton Anxiety Score in depressed patients whose dexamethasone suppression test is negative (32), showing once more the necessity of avoiding generalization between different subtypes of depression. It is therefore not necessarily surprising that negative results have also been reported (33–36). However, more questionable is the specificity of the relationship between the increase in CD4/C8 ratio and depression as the same pattern could be observed also in schizophrenic patients (37).

More recent studies have focused on other T-cell subsets. There has been some specula- tion on the wealth of preclinical and clinical evidence in favour of a Treg insufficiency in major depressive disorder (38). As a decreased Treg cell phenotype is associated with a pattern of inflammatory monocyte activation (13) it is tempting to claim that Treg insufficiency could play a causal role in inflammatory depression (38). The Treg deficiency would be secondary to an increase in soluble IL-2 receptor concentrations (39) which would decrease the bioavailability of IL-2 for Treg survival and expansion. Based on this reasoning it should be possible to treat inflammatory depression by low-dose IL-2, which would become the first example of an immune-based treatment for treatment-resistant depression (38). The problem is that there are once more divergent findings in the literature concerning both soluble IL-2 receptor and Treg cells. For instance, treatment-resistant depression was found to be associated with decreased rather than increased soluble IL-2 receptor (40). This finding cannot be due to a deficit in enzymatic processes responsible for shedding of receptors from the cell membrane as soluble receptors of TNF and IL-6 were simultaneously increased. In the same manner, Treg were found to be increased in at least two studies in untreated depressed patients (41,42).

A possible involvement of Th-17 cells in the pathophysiology of MDD has also been proposed based on the role of IL-17 in neuroinflammation in autoimmune disorders (43,44). However, only one of five clinical studies that examined the association between IL-17 levels and depression reported some evidence of increased IL-17 levels and Th-17 cells associated with decreased Treg cells (45). In addition, the percentage of circulating Th-17 cells was found to correlate positively to the structural and functional integrity of the brain in both bipolar depression and healthy controls (46). In view of the role of Th-17 cells in pregnancy morbidities, the possibility that Th-17 cells mediate perinatal mood and anxiety disorders in this condition has been proposed recently (47) but is still awaiting confirmation.

14.2.3 B Cells

Relatively little work has been done on B cells and depression. As too often the case in the field contradictory data on the number and percent of B cells in depressed subjects compared to controls can be found in the literature, with decreases as well as increases and even no difference being reported (22,48–50). As B cells are highly heterogeneous and are involved not only in the production of antibodies but also in the regulation of the inflammatory response, more recent studies have investigated the relationship between depression and specific subsets of B cells. A recent study focused on regulatory B cells, also known as $CD5^+CD1d^+B$ cells, that suppress immune responses through IL-10, TGF-β and IL-35 (51). Although there was no difference in the overall frequency of B cells in depressed subjects compared to controls, transitional B cells that normally mature into B cells were lower in MDD possibly because of a switch to production of myeloid cells. In addition, B cells with a regulatory phenotype were decreased in MDD, which could promote an inflammatory phenotype.

14.2.4 Depression as an Autoimmune Disease

Several studies have attempted to relate the alterations in B and T lymphocytes in MDD with a possible autoimmune condition that would be responsible for the production of anti-brain autoantibodies. This aspect of the relationship between depression and immunity dates back to the origin of this field in the 1970s, when evidence for higher anti-nuclear antibodies was reported in patients with depression (52–54). However, a subsequent semi-systematic review concluded that there are more negative than positive studies and that once more confounding factors were not controlled, casting some doubt on the role of anti-nuclear antibodies (55); even so, attempts at resuscitating this hypothesis persist (45,56).

As noted in (56), most studies that have examined a possible relationship between autoantibodies and depressive symptoms have done this in a cross-sectional manner, therefore failing to establish a temporal association. In one of the rare prospective studies in this field, a wide range of anti-nuclear autoantibodies was measured at baseline in a population-based cohort of 2,049 Australians aged 55–85 years. Autoantibodies were not rare in the population, but they were not predictive markers for the development of depressive symptoms measured at baseline and five years later (57). In the same manner, no evidence was found for an association between depression and thyroid autoimmunity in a general population study carried out in 8,214 Danish subjects (58). A meta-analysis of the association between N-methyl-D-aspartate (NMDA) receptor antibodies and MDD showed an odds ratio of 3 for higher NMDA receptor antibody titres in depressed participants compared with healthy controls (59). However, this association was not specific to depression, as it was also found for schizophrenia, schizo-affective disorder and bipolar disorder. In addition, it was based on a small number of studies that were inadequately powered and lacked a prospective dimension.

In the context of the neuroinflammatory theory of depression, it has been suggested that activation of oxidative and nitrosative stress pathways leads to the switch of autoepitopes to neoantigens which have immunogenicity and could cause autoimmune responses (60). In accordance with this hypothesis, patients with chronic depression were found to have higher rates of IgM antibodies directed against membrane fatty acids, by-products of oxidative damage to fatty acids, and nitrosylated amino acids (61). However, this immune signature is not necessarily specific of depression as it can be found also in other conditions, including in chronic fatigue (62).

14.2.5 Depressive Symptoms and Immunity

In view of the heterogeneity of symptoms in MDD, attempts have been made to determine whether markers of the adaptive immune system are more commonly associated with some symptoms than with others. In particular, epidemiological studies reveal a stronger association of inflammatory markers with somatic symptoms (e.g., fatigue, reduced appetite, sleep disorders) than with cognitive and affective symptoms of depression (63,64). In general, increased CD4$^+$ percentages and CD4$^+$/CD8$^+$ ratios are more apparent in severe depression than in moderate depression (31,65). However, their relation to specific symptoms has not been investigated. More recently, some attention has been paid to sleep disturbance, a core symptom of MDD, in the alterations in lymphocyte distributions that are associated with depression (42). Depressed patients showed increased CD127^{low}/CCR4$^+$ Treg cells and memory Treg cells and a trend for lower CD56$^+$/CD16$^-$ natural killer cells and higher effector memory CD8$^+$ cell counts. Effector memory CD8$^+$ counts were positively correlated with self-reported sleep disturbance. Despite anhedonia being one of the core symptoms of depression, not much has been done on its immune correlates. Circulating levels of IL-17 were found to be associated with greater severity of anhedonia but this association was apparent only in males, not in females (66). There is clearly a need for further studies on the immune phenotype associated with different dimensions of depressive disorders.

14.2.6 Factors of Variation in the Relationship Between Depression and Immunity

There has not been much interest in the influence of the many factors that are related to the clinical presentation of depression including lifestyle factors on the relationship between depression and adaptive immunity. We have already mentioned possible differences between melancholic/endogenous depression and reactive depression and between treatment-resistant depression and other subtypes of depression. We have also presented the possible influence of age on differences in findings between studies based on lymphocyte proliferation measures. These factors certainly contribute to the variability between studies but it is difficult at this stage to predict in which way as they are usually not systemically investigated in available studies. Just to take one example of their importance, the age factor has been considered as one possible explanation for the existence of contradictory findings for the role of T cells in depression. We have seen that there are two sets of data, one in favour of immune suppression, in the form of reduced proliferation in response to mitogens and reduced function of NK cells, and another one in favour of immune hyperactivation, in the form of enhanced proliferation and increased production of pro-inflammatory cytokines. Depressed patients older than 28 years of age were found to have increased monocyte gene expression while patients younger than 28 years had a reverse immune response. Examination of lymphocyte subsets in these two populations revealed that older patients had decreased percentage of CD4$^+$CD25$^+$Foxp3$^+$ Treg inversely associated with activation of the monocyte system whereas younger patients had impaired maturation of Th-2 and Th-17 cells and decreased serum levels of IL-7 and soluble CD25 (13).

14.2.7 Impact of Immune Alterations Associated with Depression on Physical Health

As emphasized by the authors of this last study, these findings indicate that signs of immune suppression and activation can coexist in the same patients therefore making any generalization premature. This does not facilitate the resolution of a lingering issue in the study of the relationship between depression and immunity, that is whether the immune changes that are reported in depressed patients can negatively impact health and promote diseases. A series of studies carried out by Michael Irwin and colleagues shows that the occurrence of major depression in older adults lowers varicella zoster virus cell-mediated immunity in vaccinated individuals (67–69). These effects are a function of the severity of depressive symptoms and increasing age and are abrogated by antidepressant treatment. Because higher levels of antibody titres to the vaccine correlate with lower risk and severity of herpes zoster, the authors propose that untreated depression might increase the risk and severity of the disease and reduce the effectiveness of vaccination. No similar study has been conducted on other forms of vaccination, including the commonly administered influenza vaccine.

In terms of disease outcomes, depressed individuals are well known to have a worse prognosis in chronic medical conditions. In a Danish population-based cohort study, individuals with depression were found to have a significantly shorter life expectancy, and this effect was more pronounced for men than for women (70). Independently of mortality due to unnatural causes (e.g., suicide), comorbid physical illness partially mediated the association between depression and mortality, which is consistent with depression as a risk factor for a variety of diseases including cancer, stroke, cardiovascular diseases and metabolic syndrome. Of course, many factors other than alterations in immunity can explain this association, including deficient compliance with medical prevention and treatment, poor hygiene and substance abuse. The difficulty of controlling for all these factors plus the issue of reverse causality explain why it is difficult to isolate possible biological causal factors in studies on depression as a risk factor for morbidity and mortality.

14.2.8 Influence of Treatment

The association between depression and immune alterations has stimulated the search for biomarkers of subtypes of depression and predictors of response to antidepressant treatment. Investigation into the possible relationships between antidepressant treatment outcomes and immune markers of depression has yielded mixed results. In a systematic review of the modulatory effects of different classes of antidepressants on the innate and adaptive immune system in depression, Bernhard Baune and colleagues concluded that antidepressants in general appear to reduce pro-inflammatory cytokine levels (71). However, their effect on the adaptive immune system is much more difficult to capture because available studies have substantial methodological heterogeneity and very small sample sizes. Despite this rather bleak context, some attempt has been made to use immune factors as predictive markers of the effects of antidepressants. In one study comparing imipramine and venlafaxine in melancholic patients who had lower percentages of Treg, imipramine increased Treg cells more than venlafaxine did, but this effect was independent of the treatment outcome (72). In contrast, response to treatment was associated with different lymphocyte subsets. Those who did not respond to the antidepressants showed increased CD8$^+$ cytotoxic T cell percentages and decreased natural killer cell percentages at inception of treatment compared with responders, but these differences did not vary according to treatment. In another study investigating a range of cytokines in depressed patients treated with different combinations of antidepressants, higher baseline IL-17 levels were found to be associated with greater reduction in severity of depression in response to bupropion plus escitalopram but not to escitalopram alone or venlafaxine plus mirtazapine (73). These findings provide some encouraging support for the use of immune biomarkers as predictors of treatment outcomes in MDD.

14.2.9 Mechanisms

In terms of mechanisms, the impairments in the adaptive immune system that are observed in depressive disorders are hypothesized to be mediated by activation of the classic neurohormonal stress pathways involving glucocorticoid and adrenergic signalling (74). However, most studies on depression and immunity do not assess the functionality of these pathways. In addition, it is difficult to relate the relative invariability of the stress response to the diversity of the findings in the immune status of depressed subjects. A role for inflammation-driven activation of the kynurenine pathway that leads to the formation of cytotoxic kynurenine metabolites has been proposed to cause T cell apoptosis and therefore reduced T cell counts (75). The intriguing observation that suppressed T cells in depressed patients could be due to an expansion of myeloid derived suppressor cells (76) is still waiting for confirmation as this monocytic subset is mainly studied in immuno-oncology but has received little attention elsewhere.

14.3 Preclinical Data

The first preclinical studies on the influence of the adaptive immune system on brain functions have compared immune-deficient mice to normal mice. Most of these studies have been carried out by Michal Schwartz's group at the Weissman Institute in Rehovot, Israel. On the basis of her earlier work showing that autoreactive T cells contribute to the formation of the brain-derived neurotrophic factor (BDNF) and the development of hippocampal neurogenesis, Schwartz proposed that T cells recognizing brain antigens could help to treat depression by promoting neurogenesis and increasing BDNF. To test this hypothesis, she produced weakly self-reactive T cells in rats immunized with a modified fragment of myelin basic protein and showed that naïve rats were protected when exposed to a chronic mild stress that induces depression-like behaviour in non-immunized rats (77). The possibility that self-reactive T cells can participate in the protection or repair of the central nervous system is obviously in contrast with the literature on the association between autoantibodies and depression that we examined in Section 14.2.4, even if this literature is largely inconclusive. More recent attempts have searched for a role of the adaptive immune system in mood regulation. In particular, the clinical evidence for the occurrence of comorbid symptoms of depression in autoimmune disorders has been confirmed experimentally by the demonstration that animal models of autoimmune disorders are associated with behavioural signs of depression (78–81). Whether this is due to the cytokines that are released during the autoimmune process (81) or primarily driven by brain-intrinsic factors the nature of which remains to be discovered (80) remains controversial. Whatever the case, it is clear that adaptive immunity has potent effects on brain functions even if they have been less well studied than those of innate immunity.

An innovative series of studies has been carried out on the influence of Th-17 cells on depression-like behaviour by Eleonore Beurel at the University of Miami. In a mouse model of depression induced by exposure to inescapable electric shock, mice that developed depression-like behaviour characterized by the inability to learn to escape further electric shocks when exposed to them later on had higher levels of Th-17 cells but normal levels of Treg cells trafficking into their brains, compared with mice which recovered and learned to escape later on (82). Because Th-17 cells are mainly present in the lamina propria of the small intestine where their expression is dependent on the gut microbiome it has been proposed that this is the site from which they traffic into the brain in response to stress (Figure 14.2) (83).

This hypothesis opens a number of possibilities to abrogate Th-17-dependent depression from modification of the microbiome to prevention of increased permeability of the blood-brain-barrier (BBB) under the influence of TNF (84). Administration of Th-17 cells to naïve mice increased the number of mice that subsequently failed to learn to escape after exposure to inescapable electric shocks, and this effect generalized to other tests of depression-like behaviour. Depletion of the transcription factor that drives the differentiation of

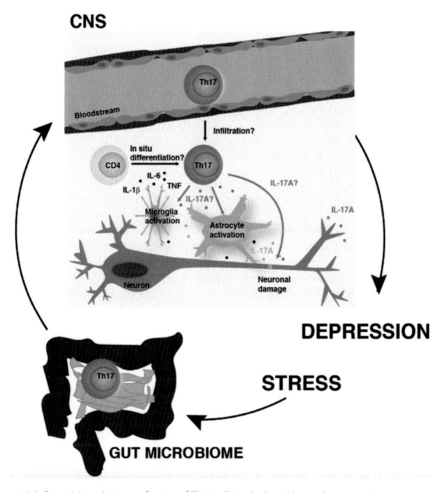

Figure 14.2 Potential mechanisms of action of Th17 cells in the brain during depression. In response to stress, peripheral Th17 cells (possibly released from the lamina propria of the small intestine) may infiltrate the brain parenchyma, or surveying CD4+T cells may differentiate into Th17 cells *in situ* after receiving signals from pro-inflammatory cytokines (e.g., IL-6, IL-1α, TNF) generated during the neuroinflammatory response to stress. Once in the brain parenchyma, Th17 cells may exert direct or indirect effects on the brain via production of IL-17A or other cytokines or factors produced by Th17 cells by either inducing activation of astrocytes and microglia, and/or by inducing neuronal damage, enhancing the neuroinflammatory response (including the production of IL-17A by CNS resident cells) and leading to increased susceptibility to depressive-like behaviours. Reproduced from Beurel E, Lowell JA. *Brain Behav Immun.* 2018; 69:28–34.

CD4$^+$ T cells in Th-17 cells made mice resistant to the effects of exposure to inescapable electric shocks.

Activation of the adaptive immune system can promote depression or protect from it. The protection effect does not need self-reactive T cells. In a series of different experiments, adoptive transfer of lymphocytes from socially defeated mice to naïve T-cell-deficient mice conferred resistance to the development of anxiety- and depression-like behaviour induced by chronic exposure to stress (85). The same treatment was also able to treat anxiety and depression-like behaviour in T-cell-deficient mice that had been chronically exposed to restraint stress (86). The exact nature of the T-cell population that is required for these effects has not yet been identified.

T-cell-deficient mice are actually characterized by their propensity to develop chronic pain as well as long lasting depression-like behaviour when exposed to various stressors. Adoptive transfer of CD8$^+$ T cells normalize their recovery, indicating that activation of the adaptive immune system is necessary for repair and recovery (87). This influence of CD8$^+$ T cells on recovery is mediated by the production of the anti-inflammatory cytokine IL-10 by macrophages residing in the meninges and the brain parenchyma as it is abrogated by inhibition of IL-10 signalling by intranasal administration of a neutralizing anti-IL-10 antibody. How the adaptive immune system is mobilized to act in the brain, and in particular whether it needs to enter the brain parenchyma or can act in the meninges and the choroid plexus, and how it promotes repair, are all questions that require further research.

14.4 Conclusions

The clinical and preclinical evidence presented in this chapter converge on the notion that depression is associated with alterations in the adaptive immune system that add to those already described in the innate immune system. Vice versa, activation of the adaptive immune system can precipitate the development of depression as we have seen with Th-17 cells and, in some conditions, facilitate its recovery and even prevent its occurrence in response to stressors as we have seen with CD8$^+$ T cells.

Despite its clinical importance, it is still uncertain whether the association between depression and altered immune function is sufficient to explain morbidity and mortality associated with depression, knowing that the medical conditions that are worsened by depression involve immune processes that can by themselves increase the risk of depression.

How can the conflicting evidence of a relationship between depression and the adaptive immune system be improved? It should be clear at the end of this review that in contrast to the advances in our understanding on the relationship between depression and inflammation the research investment in the relationship between depression and the adaptive immune system has not paid off. It is still much too early to describe a T cell or a B cell immune-based phenotype of depression that can either serve as a biomarker or help for selection of more appropriate treatments. Not surprisingly, two recent meta-analyses of cytokine levels in MDD and their response to treatment reveal a hardly more than average quality of the available studies and a high heterogeneity across them (11,88). Part of this is due to the high number of cross-sectional studies and the very small numbers of subjects in most published studies which much too often present preliminary findings without any follow up in larger populations. In such a situation it is always tempting to believe that the solution is to refine the methodology and assess immune function based on advances in post-genomic biology. As a typical example of this move, recent application of high-content, single-cell screening of ligand receptor interactions and downstream signalling mechanisms to explore differences in cell signalling dynamics across the neuropsychiatric spectrum using PBMCs ex vivo revealed that MDD was characterized by alterations in T cell nuclear factor-kappaB p65 (one of the effector of Toll-like receptor activation), S6 phosphorylation (a key mediator of neuronal activity-dependent protein synthesis that is downstream of mTORC1) and STAT3 (an effector of JAK/STAT signalling) (89). However, in striking contrast with the technological advances these results illustrate, it is important to note that the corresponding study was carried out in only 25 patients per disease condition and without any indication of their clinical and medication status. This means that the results of this study represent more a demonstration of the feasibility of the approach than real progress in characterization of the immune profiling of depression.

Ultimately it is clear that like in other domains of biological psychiatry advances in immunopsychiatry will not come from more sophisticated studies based on traditional research paradigms comparing depressed to healthy individuals, but on different conceptual approaches to psychiatric disorders.

14.5 Acknowledgements

Robert Dantzer's research work is funded by a Brain and Behavior Distinguished Research Award, grants from the National Institutes of Health (R01 CA193522 and R01 NS073939), and a MD Anderson Cancer Support Grant (P30 CA016672).

References

1. Raison CL, Miller AH. Role of inflammation in depression: implications for phenomenology, pathophysiology and treatment. *Mod Trends Pharmacopsychiatry.* 2013;28:33–48.

2. Miller AH, Raison CL. The role of inflammation in depression: from evolutionary imperative to modern treatment target. *Nat Rev Immunol.* 2016;16 (1):22–34.

3. Dantzer R, O'Connor JC, Freund GG, Johnson RW, Kelley KW. From inflammation to sickness and depression: when the immune system subjugates the brain. *Nat Rev Neurosci.* 2008;9(1):46–56.

4. Dantzer R, O'Connor JC, Lawson MA, Kelley KW. Inflammation-associated depression: from serotonin to kynurenine. *Psychoneuroendocrinology.* 2011;36 (3):426–36.

5. Dantzer R, Capuron L. *Inflammation-Associated Depression: Evidence, Mechanisms, and Implicaiton.* Geyer MA, Ellenbroek BA, Marsden CA, Barnes TRE, eds. Springer. Switzerland; 2017.

6. Kappelmann N, Lewis G, Dantzer R, Jones PB, Khandaker GM. Antidepressant activity of anti-cytokine treatment: a systematic review and meta-analysis of clinical trials of chronic inflammatory conditions. *Mol Psychiatry.* 2018 Feb;23 (2):335–43. doi:10.1038/mp.2016.167. Epub 2016 Oct 18.

7. Raison CL, Rutherford RE, Woolwine BJ, et al. A randomized controlled trial of the tumor necrosis factor antagonist infliximab for treatment-resistant depression: the role of baseline inflammatory biomarkers. *JAMA Psychiatry.* 2013;70(1):31–41.

8. Leday GGR, Vertes PE, Richardson S, et al. Replicable and coupled changes in innate and adaptive immune gene expression in two case-control studies of blood microarrays in major depressive disorder. *Biol Psychiatry.* 2018 Jan;83(1):70–80. doi:10.1016/j.biopsych.2017.01.021. Epub 2017 Jul 6.

9. Haapakoski R, Mathieu J, Ebmeier KP, Alenius H, Kivimaki M. Cumulative meta-analysis of interleukins 6 and 1beta, tumour necrosis factor alpha and C-reactive protein in patients with major depressive

disorder. *Brain Behav Immun.* 2015;49:206–15.

10. Howren MB, Lamkin DM, Suls J. Associations of depression with C-reactive protein, IL-1, and IL-6: a meta-analysis. *Psychosom Med.* 2009;71(2):171–86.

11. Kohler CA, Freitas TH, Stubbs B, et al. Peripheral alterations in cytokine and chemokine levels after antidepressant drug treatment for major depressive disorder: systematic review and meta-analysis. *Mol Neurobiol.* 2018 May;55(5):4195–206. doi:10.1007/s12035-017-0632-1. Epub 2017 Jun 13.

12. Valkanova V, Ebmeier KP, Allan CL. CRP, IL-6 and depression: a systematic review and meta-analysis of longitudinal studies. *J Affect Disord.* 2013;150(3):736–44.

13. Grosse L, Hoogenboezem T, Ambree O, et al. Deficiencies of the T and natural killer cell system in major depressive disorder: T regulatory cell defects are associated with inflammatory monocyte activation. *Brain Behav Immun.* 2016;54:38–44.

14. Snijders G, Schiweck C, Mesman E, et al. A dynamic course of T cell defects in individuals at risk for mood disorders. *Brain Behav Immun.* 2016;58:11–7.

15. Darko DF, Rose J, Gillin JC, Golshan S, Baird SM. Neutrophilia and lymphopenia in major mood disorders. *Psychiatry Res.* 1988;25(3):243–51.

16. Caldwell CL, Irwin M, Lohr J. Reduced natural killer cell cytotoxicity in depression but not in schizophrenia. *Biol Psychiatry.* 1991;30(11):1131–8.

17. Andersson NW, Goodwin RD, Okkels N, et al. Depression and the risk of severe infections: prospective analyses on a nationwide representative sample. *Int J Epidemiol.* 2016;45(1):131–9.

18. Benton T, Staab J, Evans DL. Medical co-morbidity in depressive disorders. *Ann Clin Psychiatry.* 2007;19(4):289–303.

19. Enache D, Pariante CM, Mondelli V. Markers of central inflammation in major depressive disorder: A systematic review and meta-analysis of studies examining cerebrospinal fluid, positron emission tomography and post-mortem brain tissue. *Brain Behav Immun.* 2019;81:24–40.

20. Schleifer SJ, Keller SE, Camerino M, Thornton JC, Stein M. Suppression of lymphocyte stimulation following bereavement. *JAMA.* 1983;250(3):374–7.

21. Kronfol Z, Silva J, Jr., Greden J, et al. Impaired lymphocyte function in depressive illness. *Life Sci.* 1983;33 (3):241–7.

22. Schleifer SJ, Keller SE, Meyerson AT, et al. Lymphocyte function in major depressive disorder. *Arch Gen Psychiatry.* 1984;41 (5):484–6.

23. Schleifer SJ, Keller SE, Siris SG, Davis KL, Stein M. Depression and immunity. Lymphocyte function in ambulatory depressed patients, hospitalized schizophrenic patients, and patients hospitalized for herniorrhaphy. *Arch Gen Psychiatry.* 1985;42(2):129–33.

24. Denman AM. Immunity and depression. *Br Med J (Clin Res Ed).* 1986;293 (6545):464–5.

25. Levy EM, Borrelli DJ, Mirin SM, et al. Biological measures and cellular immunological function in depressed psychiatric inpatients. *Psychiatry Res.* 1991;36(2):157–67.

26. Herbert TB, Cohen S. Depression and immunity: a meta-analytic review. *Psychol Bull.* 1993;113(3):472–86.

27. Hughes MM, Connor TJ, Harkin A. Stress-related immune markers in depression: implications for treatment. *Int J Neuropsychopharmacol.* 2016 Jun;19 (6):pyw001. doi:10.1093/ijnp/pyw001. Epub 2016 Jan 16.

28. Maes M, Stevens W, DeClerck L, et al. Immune disorders in depression: higher T helper/T suppressor-cytotoxic cell ratio. *Acta Psychiatr Scand.* 1992;86(6):423–31.

29. Maes M, Bosmans E, Suy E, et al. Immune disturbances during major depression: upregulated expression of interleukin-2 receptors. *Neuropsychobiology.* 1990;24 (3):115–20.

30. Muller N, Hofschuster E, Ackenheil M, Mempel W, Eckstein R. Investigations of

the cellular immunity during depression and the free interval: evidence for an immune activation in affective psychosis. *Prog Neuropsychopharmacol Biol Psychiatry.* 1993;17(5):713–30.

31. Kubera M, Van Bockstaele D, Maes M. Leukocyte subsets in treatment-resistant major depression. *Pol J Pharmacol.* 1999;51 (6):547–9.

32. Charles G, Machowski R, Brohee D, Wilmotte J, Kennes B. Lymphocyte subsets in major depressive patients. Influence of anxiety and corticoadrenal overdrive. *Neuropsychobiology.* 1992;25(2): 94–8.

33. Scanlan JM, Vitaliano PP, Ochs H, Savage MV, Borson S. CD4 and CD8 counts are associated with interactions of gender and psychosocial stress. *Psychosom Med.* 1998;60(5):644–53.

34. Huang TL, Leu HS, Liu JW. Lymphocyte subsets and viral load in male AIDS patients with major depression: naturalistic study. *Psychiatry Clin Neurosci.* 2006;60 (6):687–92.

35. Manceaux P, Zdanowicz N. Immunity, coping and depression. *Psychiatr Danub.* 2016;28(Suppl-1):165–9.

36. Atanackovic D, Kroger H, Serke S, Deter HC. Immune parameters in patients with anxiety or depression during psychotherapy. *J Affect Disord.* 2004;81 (3):201–9.

37. Muller N, Ackenheil M, Hofschuster E, Mempel W, Eckstein R. Cellular immunity, HLA-class I antigens, and family history of psychiatric disorder in endogenous psychoses. *Psychiatry Res.* 1993;48 (3):201–17.

38. Ellul P, Mariotti-Ferrandiz E, Leboyer M, Klatzmann D. Regulatory T cells as supporters of psychoimmune resilience: toward immunotherapy of major depressive disorder. *Front Neurol.* 2018;9:167.

39. Kohler CA, Freitas TH, Maes M, et al. Peripheral cytokine and chemokine alterations in depression: a meta-analysis of 82 studies. *Acta Psychiatr Scand.* 2017;135(5):373–87.

40. Sowa-Kucma M, Styczen K, Siwek M, et al. Lipid peroxidation and immune biomarkers are associated with major depression and its phenotypes, including treatment-resistant depression and melancholia. *Neurotox Res.* 2018;33 (2):448–60.

41. Patas K, Willing A, Demiralay C, et al. T cell phenotype and T cell receptor repertoire in patients with major depressive disorder. *Front Immunol.* 2018;9:291.

42. Suzuki H, Savitz J, Kent Teague T, et al. Altered populations of natural killer cells, cytotoxic T lymphocytes, and regulatory T cells in major depressive disorder: Association with sleep disturbance. *Brain Behav Immun.* 2017;66:193–200.

43. Slyepchenko A, Maes M, Kohler CA, et al. T helper 17 cells may drive neuroprogression in major depressive disorder: proposal of an integrative model. *Neurosci Biobehav Rev.* 2016;64:83–100.

44. Waisman A, Hauptmann J, Regen T. The role of IL-17 in CNS diseases. *Acta Neuropathol.* 2015;129(5):625–37.

45. Chen Y, Jiang T, Chen P, et al. Emerging tendency towards autoimmune process in major depressive patients: a novel insight from Th17 cells. *Psychiatry Res.* 2011;188 (2):224–30.

46. Poletti S, de Wit H, Mazza E, et al. Th17 cells correlate positively to the structural and functional integrity of the brain in bipolar depression and healthy controls. *Brain Behav Immun.* 2017;61:317–25.

47. Osborne LM, Brar A, Klein SL. The role of Th17 cells in the pathophysiology of pregnancy and perinatal mood and anxiety disorders. *Brain Behav Immun.* 2019;76:7–16.

48. Maes M, Stevens WJ, DeClerck LS, et al. A significantly increased number and percentage of B cells in depressed subjects: results of flow cytometric measurements. *J Affect Disord.* 1992;24(3):127–34.

49. Andreoli AV, Keller SE, Rabaeus M, et al. Depression and immunity: age, severity, and clinical course. *Brain Behav Immun.* 1993;7(4):279–92.

50. Ravindran AV, Griffiths J, Merali Z, Anisman H. Circulating lymphocyte subsets in major depression and dysthymia with typical or atypical features. *Psychosom Med*. 1998;60(3):283–9.

51. Ahmetspahic D, Schwarte K, Ambree O, et al. Altered B cell homeostasis in patients with major depressive disorder and normalization of CD5 surface expression on regulatory B cells in treatment responders. *J Neuroimmune Pharmacol*. 2018;13(1):90–9.

52. Shopsin B, Sathananthan GL, Chan TL, Kravitz H, Gershon S. Antinuclear factor in psychiatric patients. *Biol Psychiatry*. 1973;7(2):81–7.

53. Johnstone EC, Whaley K. Antinuclear antibodies in psychiatric illness: their relationship to diagnosis and drug treatment. *Br Med J*. 1975;2(5973):724–5.

54. Deberdt R, Van Hooren J, Biesbrouck M, Amery W. Antinuclear factor-positive mental depression: a single disease entity? *Biol Psychiatry*. 1976;11(1):69–74.

55. Appleby B. Are anti-nuclear antibodies common in affective disorders? A review of the past 35 years. *Psychosomatics*. 2007;48(4):286–9.

56. Iseme RA, McEvoy M, Kelly B, et al. Autoantibodies and depression: evidence for a causal link? *Neurosci Biobehav Rev*. 2014;40:62–79.

57. Iseme RA, McEvoy M, Kelly B, et al. Autoantibodies are not predictive markers for the development of depressive symptoms in a population-based cohort of older adults. *Eur Psychiatry*. 2015;30(6):694–700.

58. Fjaellegaard K, Kvetny J, Allerup PN, Bech P, Ellervik C. Well-being and depression in individuals with subclinical hypothyroidism and thyroid autoimmunity – a general population study. *Nord J Psychiatry*. 2015;69(1):73–8.

59. Pearlman DM, Najjar S. Meta-analysis of the association between N-methyl-d-aspartate receptor antibodies and schizophrenia, schizoaffective disorder, bipolar disorder, and major depressive disorder. *Schizophr Res*. 2014;157(1–3):249–58.

60. Maes M, Galecki P, Chang YS, Berk M. A review on the oxidative and nitrosative stress (O&NS) pathways in major depression and their possible contribution to the (neuro)degenerative processes in that illness. *Prog Neuropsychopharmacol Biol Psychiatry*. 2011;35(3):676–92.

61. Maes M, Kubera M, Mihaylova I, et al. Increased autoimmune responses against auto-epitopes modified by oxidative and nitrosative damage in depression: implications for the pathways to chronic depression and neuroprogression. *J Affect Disord*. 2013;149(1–3):23–9.

62. Morris G, Berk M, Klein H, et al. Nitrosative stress, hypernitrosylation, and autoimmune responses to nitrosylated proteins: new pathways in neuroprogressive disorders including depression and chronic fatigue syndrome. *Mol Neurobiol*. 2017;54(6):4271–91.

63. White J, Kivimaki M, Jokela M, Batty GD. Association of inflammation with specific symptoms of depression in a general population of older people: the English Longitudinal Study of Ageing. *Brain Behav Immun*. 2017;61:27–30.

64. Jokela M, Virtanen M, Batty GD, Kivimaki M. Inflammation and specific symptoms of depression. *JAMA Psychiatry*. 2016;73(1):87–8.

65. Schleifer SJ, Keller SE, Bartlett JA. Depression and immunity: clinical factors and therapeutic course. *Psychiatry Res*. 1999;85(1):63–9.

66. Jha MK, Miller AH, Minhajuddin A, Trivedi MH. Association of T and non-T cell cytokines with anhedonia: role of gender differences. *Psychoneuroendocrinology*. 2018;95:1–7.

67. Irwin M, Costlow C, Williams H, et al. Cellular immunity to varicella-zoster virus in patients with major depression. *J Infect Dis*. 1998;178(Suppl 1):S104–8.

68. Irwin MR, Levin MJ, Carrillo C, et al. Major depressive disorder and immunity to varicella-zoster virus in the elderly. *Brain Behav Immun*. 2011;25(4):759–66.

69. Irwin MR, Levin MJ, Laudenslager ML, et al. Varicella zoster virus-specific immune responses to a herpes zoster vaccine in elderly recipients with major depression and the impact of antidepressant medications. *Clin Infect Dis.* 2013;56(8):1085–93.

70. Laursen TM, Musliner KL, Benros ME, Vestergaard M, Munk-Olsen T. Mortality and life expectancy in persons with severe unipolar depression. *J Affect Disord.* 2016;193:203–7.

71. Eyre HA, Lavretsky H, Kartika J, Qassim A, Baune BT. Modulatory Effects of Antidepressant Classes on the Innate and Adaptive Immune System in Depression. *Pharmacopsychiatry.* 2016;49(3):85–96.

72. Grosse L, Carvalho LA, Birkenhager TK, et al. Circulating cytotoxic T cells and natural killer cells as potential predictors for antidepressant response in melancholic depression. Restoration of T regulatory cell populations after antidepressant therapy. *Psychopharmacology (Berl).* 2016;233 (9):1679–88.

73. Jha MK, Minhajuddin A, Gadad BS, et al. Interleukin 17 selectively predicts better outcomes with bupropion-SSRI combination: novel T cell biomarker for antidepressant medication selection. *Brain Behav Immun.* 2017;66:103–10.

74. Irwin MR, Cole SW. Reciprocal regulation of the neural and innate immune systems. *Nat Rev Immunol.* 2011;11(9):625–32.

75. Miller AH. Depression and immunity: a role for T cells? *Brain Behav Immun.* 2010;24(1):1–8.

76. Wei J, Zhang M, Zhou J. Myeloid-derived suppressor cells in major depression patients suppress T-cell responses through the production of reactive oxygen species. *Psychiatry Res.* 2015;228(3):695–701.

77. Lewitus GM, Wilf-Yarkoni A, Ziv Y, et al. Vaccination as a novel approach for treating depressive behavior. *Biol Psychiatry.* 2009;65(4):283–8.

78. Sakic B, Szechtman H, Denburg JA. Neurobehavioral alterations in autoimmune mice. *Neurosci Biobehav Rev.* 1997;21(3):327–40.

79. Sakic B, Lacosta S, Denburg JA, Szechtman H. Altered neurotransmission in brains of autoimmune mice: pharmacological and neurochemical evidence. *J Neuroimmunol.* 2002;129 (1–2):84–96.

80. Stock AD, Wen J, Doerner J, et al. Neuropsychiatric systemic lupus erythematosus persists despite attenuation of systemic disease in MRL/lpr mice. *J Neuroinflammation.* 2015;12:205.

81. Cathomas F, Fuertig R, Sigrist H, et al. CD40-TNF activation in mice induces extended sickness behavior syndrome co-incident with but not dependent on activation of the kynurenine pathway. *Brain Behav Immun.* 2015;50: 125–40.

82. Beurel E, Harrington LE, Jope RS. Inflammatory T helper 17 cells promote depression-like behavior in mice. *Biol Psychiatry.* 2013;73(7):622–30.

83. Beurel E, Lowell JA. Th17 cells in depression. *Brain Behav Immun.* 2018;69:28–34.

84. Cheng Y, Desse S, Martinez A, et al. TNFalpha disrupts blood brain barrier integrity to maintain prolonged depressive-like behavior in mice. *Brain Behav Immun.* 2018;69: 556–67.

85. Brachman RA, Lehmann ML, Maric D, Herkenham M. Lymphocytes from chronically stressed mice confer antidepressant-like effects to naive mice. *J Neurosci.* 2015;35(4): 1530–8.

86. Scheinert RB, Haeri MH, Lehmann ML, Herkenham M. Therapeutic effects of stress-programmed lymphocytes transferred to chronically stressed mice. *Prog Neuropsychopharmacol Biol Psychiatry.* 2016;70:1–7.

87. Laumet G, Edralin JD, Chiang AC, et al. Resolution of inflammation-induced depression requires T lymphocytes and endogenous brain interleukin-10 signaling. *Neuropsychopharmacology.* 2018;43 (13):2597–605.

88. Kohler CA, Freitas TH, Stubbs B, et al. Peripheral alterations in cytokine and chemokine levels after antidepressant drug treatment for major depressive disorder: systematic review and meta-analysis. *Mol Neurobiol.* 2018;55 (5):4195–206.

89. Lago SG, Tomasik J, van Rees GF, et al. Exploring the neuropsychiatric spectrum using high-content functional analysis of single-cell signaling networks. *Mol Psychiatry.* 2020 Oct;25(10):2355–72. doi:10.1038/s41380-018-0123-4. Epub 2018 Jul 23.

Transdiagnostic Features of the Immune System in Major Depressive Disorder, Bipolar Disorder and Schizophrenia

Célia Fourrier, Catherine Toben and Bernhard T. Baune

15.1 Introduction

Defining current psychopathology and optimum treatment selection in psychiatry relies solely on clinical symptom assessment but does not consider underlying biological correlates of psychiatric disorders. In particular, dysregulation of neurotransmitter metabolism and function (1,2), neuroendocrine pathways (3,4) and brain plasticity (5, 6) have been consistently reported across psychiatric disorders. Growing evidence points to a significant role of chronic low-grade inflammation in the pathophysiology of neuropsychiatric disorders such as major depressive disorder (MDD), schizophrenia (SCZ) and bipolar disorder (BD) (7–10). This features immune system dysfunctions including alterations in immune cell regulation (10), complement system (11–14), cytokine (15–18) and chemokine (7,8) pathways. As a result, current and conventional therapeutic strategies are not optimally positioned, with low remission and high relapse rates amongst individuals and treatment resistant numbers being high. Hence, the immune system is becoming a suitable target in personalizing treatment of psychiatric disorders. Unclear as yet is whether, unique immunological signatures exist for different psychiatric disorders including MDD, SCZ and BD and how these originate. Clearly a better characterization of the underlying biological aetiology will lead towards a more personalized and targeted approach.

This book chapter reviews, for the first time, evidence linking immune system dysregulation across MDD, SCZ and BD. Evidence for immune cell, complement system, cytokine and chemokine alterations across these psychiatric disorders is used to identify either a specific underlying immune pattern for each psychiatric disorder or a common pattern of immune system dysregulations across conditions.

15.2 Immune Cell Dysregulation across Psychiatric Disorders

15.2.1 Brief Introduction on the Bidirectional Roles of the Innate and Adaptive Immune Cells in Neuroinflammation

The bidirectional link between the brain and immune system might underpin chronic and debilitating psychiatric disorders as characterized by alterations in innate and adaptive cellular and soluble mediators involved in brain plasticity, maintenance of homeostasis and psychopathology (19,20). In the context of psychiatric disorders and in contrast to classical innate immune activation by microbial pathogens, a 'sterile inflammatory' signal including both acute and chronic psychosocial stressors via hypothalamus-pituitary-adrenal (HPA) axis signalling activates innate immune cells such as monocytes/macrophages or innate lymphocytes (natural killer cells (NK)) (21). As the body's 'sentries', innate immune cells rapidly react to stress and danger signals in the central nervous system (CNS) via their conserved pathogen-associated molecular pattern (PAMP) or danger-associated molecular pattern (DAMP) receptors. The resulting signalling cascades stimulate the release of inflammatory mediators which operate via reciprocal receptor networks expressed throughout the CNS and lead to activation of not only the highly specific adaptive immune cells such as T lymphocytes (22) but also CNS cells including glial cells (astrocytes and microglia) and neurons.

Cytokine signalling gradients facilitate innate immune cell entry across tight endothelial cell junctions of the blood-brain-barrier (BBB) and subsequent recruitment of either innate or adaptive immune cells to enhance or resolve the inflammatory process. In the periphery antigen presenting cells (APC) such as dendritic cells (DCs) mediate communication between innate and adaptive immune arms by activating classically defined T helper CD4+ or cytotoxic CD8+T cells and regulating their immune cell function (23). While immune to brain communication involves glial and neuronal cell interactions (24), brain to immune signalling is mediated via noradrenergic innervations of lymphoid organs by the sympathetic nervous system. Neuroimaging studies have defined this physiological link between the brain and peripheral immune system as networks of lymphatic vessels within meninges which drain into deep cervical lymph nodes (25,26). These neuronal and cellular routes enable continued and constitutive surveillance by lymphocytes of the CNS not only for maintenance of brain homeostasis under physiological conditions but also for resolution of neuroinflammation by secretion of cellular signalling mediators such as cytokines and neurotrophic factors.

15.2.2 Circulating Innate Immune Cells in Affective Disorders and SCZ

Underlying pathophysiological conditions as observed within the brain and peripheral immune system of affective disorders and SCZ patients can lead to peripheral monocyte recruitment whereby their interaction with pro-inflammatory or M1 polarized microglia of the brain contributes to either exacerbation or amelioration of the neuroinflammatory response. In the context of stress induced neuroinflammation possibly underlying psychiatric disorders, peripheral myeloid derived monocytes and granulocytes utilize chemokine pathways including (CCL2-CCR2 and CX3CL1-CX3CR1) (27) and vascular adhesion molecules (28) to migrate into specific brain areas. Several studies show an associated peripheral monocytosis in MDD (29,30) and SCZ (31,32) and increased CD16+ (33) or CD14+ monocytes in non-medicated SCZ patients (34) and in particular during acute psychotic episodes also within cerebrospinal fluid (CSF) (35). In contrast, peripherally circulating numbers of intermediate CD14+CD16+ monocytes remained unaltered in euthymic BD (36). Transcriptomic microarray analyses have been instrumental in the identification of distinct and overlapping activated pro-inflammatory monocytic gene expression patterns or 'gene fingerprints' in both SCZ and BD patients. Further cluster analyses albeit in a relatively small case-control study including BD and SCZ (56 BD/27 SCZ with 40 and 32 age/gender matched healthy controls respectively) identified 4 sub clusters characterized by different sets of transcription and/or MAPK regulating factors predominantly linked to inflammatory and chemotactic factor genes to be overlapping for both BD and SCZ but more strongly linked to vascular pathology/metabolic syndrome factors and not motility factors in SCZ (37). Gene expression patterns were influenced by medication as well as disease severity e.g., BD depression vs euthymia but not by age, gender and body mass index (BMI). In contrast in MDD a pro-inflammatory monocyte gene expression signature was found to be significantly associated with increased age i.e., >28 years, in addition to depression severity (38). In BD, this distinct pro-inflammatory transcriptomic signature was also found to be hereditary and a risk factor for later life mood disorders (39). These results support the premise that a high pro-inflammatory set point precedes the onset of the first mood episode and that gene-environmental interactions regulate the distinct clinical phenotype across disorders including environmental factors such as acute and chronic psychosocial stressors and lifestyle factors such as diet.

Separate meta-analytic studies report on decreased CD56+ NK cell number in MDD ($p = 0.01$ fixed effect model, n = 225) (40) while in contrast, in acutely relapsed SCZ inpatients, both absolute CD56+ NK cells (ES = 0.63, 95% CI 0.26–0.99, p <0.01) and percentages (p <0.04) were reported to be increased (41). Further studies on chronic SCZ cohorts report no differences infrequencies of CD56+ NK when compared with controls (42,43), highlighting the contrasting frequencies of NK cells as found within different phases of the disorder. In the meta-anlaytic data for MDD, although a significant decrease was found using the fixed effects model, a non-significant effect was found (p = 0.97) using a random effects model. Caution with meta-analytic data is suggested as it contains limited number of studies, small sample size and between study heterogeneity as well as a general lack of consideration of potential confounding factors. While the fixed effects model is more conservative yielding a lower Type I error rate and wider confidence intervals, the random effects model enables further elaboration of how the effects size varies across studies and thereby supports the significant heterogeneity found between studies being attributable to psychiatric disorders (44). Similarly, meta-analytic findings on NK cell functionality in MDD report a reduced NK cell cytotoxicity (40). Contrary findings exist (45–47) which may be accounted for by the heterogenic clinical course of MDD. Of the few studies which have measured NK cell activity (NKA) in SCZ, it was found to be significantly increased when compared with non-SCZ and healthy controls (SCZ n = 29, non-SCZ (including 4 BD and 4 personality disorder) n = 8, healthy controls n = 31) (48). Dysregulation of NK cell numbers and altered NKA highlight the differing functional roles of either peripheral immune suppression or immune activation across disorders either as state (dependent on disorder activity) or trait markers.

Interestingly a study utilizing computational deconvolution analyses of DNA microarray expression data revealed significant decreases in NK cell counts in SCZ compared with controls but not between BD and controls (49). Furthermore it has been reported that the decrease in NK cell counts post-acute SCZ phase normalized over time (43). This suggests that lower number of NK cells are a state marker as this dysregulation is characteristic of those in remission and in acute relapse. Emerging evidence from infection studies point towards a long lasting 'memory like' functional alteration specific to NK cells, which resembles adaptive immune responses and therefore provides another role for NK cells in bridging the innate and adaptive immune arms (50). Whether this NK cell feature has a role in neuropsychiatric disorders remains to be investigated.

15.2.3 Circulating Adaptive Immune Cells within Affective Disorders and SCZ

Numerous studies have determined dysregulated numbers of circulating lymphocytes (CD3+ T and CD19+ B cells) within SCZ, MDD and BD supporting the 'macrophage T lymphocyte theory'. In the context of MDD an increasing number of reports point towards a continuum tilting the balance towards either a suppressive or stimulative role for T cells (51). Initial studies on minor depression highlighted a dysregulation in T cell subset numbers including an increase in CD7+CD25+ early activated T cells (52) and reductions in CD3+CD4+T helper cells (53) or unaltered numbers concurrent with decreased B lymphocytes (54) while others report an increase in the proportionality of CD4+ (55–57) and thereby an increased CD4/CD8 ratio (58), which was replicated by meta-analytic data (CD4 T cell percentage; p = 9.6E-5 fixed effect only (n = 617)) (40). Furthermore, meta-analytic data reported decreased total number of lymphocytes; p = 0.001 (fixed effect) and percentage of lymphocytes; p =<1.0E-35 fixed effect and random effect p = 0.03. However, the meta-analyses by Zorrilla et al., 2001 (40) reported a significant negative association between the number of lymphocytes (n = 1527) and therefore a lymphopenia associated with MDD (p <1.0E-35), but only for the fixed effect and not the random effects analyses (p = 0.89), which would more accurately account for the heterogeneity associated with MDD. Furthermore, in this meta-analyses, MDD was also significantly associated with a decreased lymphocyte functionality in terms of reduced mitogenic (PHA, n = 1144) lymphocytic proliferative response using fixed (p = 7.0E-10) and random (p = 0.0005) effect modelling.

Similarly, altered lymphocyte numbers and altered CD4/CD8 ratios are reported for SCZ. Involvement of lymphocytes within drug naïve first-episode psychosis (FEP) is supported by meta-analytic data using random effects modelling identifying a significant increase in absolute levels of CD4 T cells (ES = 0.35, 95% CI 0.10–0.61, p <0.01) and thereby increasing the CD4/CD8 T cell ratio (ES = 0.31, 95% CI 0.08–0.54, p <0.06) and considered a state marker (correlate with disease activity). Effect sizes were similar in magnitude and direction in acutely relapsed inpatients compared with controls. While only a trend for absolute CD4 levels (ES = 0.27, 95% CI -0.01–0.56, p <0.01) was determined, a significant increase in CD4% (ES = 0.35, 95% CI 0.10–0.61, p <0.01) was found (41). Caution for this meta-analysis is required with interpretation of results due to small sample size (n = <100–200), heterogeneity between studies and inadequate consideration of potential confounding factors. Importantly, significant alterations in CD4+ T cell number or proportion is associated with clinical status (acute relapse vs FEP) of SCZ. Evidence for adaptive immune cell dysregulation within the CSF and brain is limited and report on increases in activated lymphocytes in CSF of psychosis patients compared with controls (59). Disparate chronic euthymic bipolar studies report unaltered T lymphocytes CD4/CD8 (36) in patients compared with healthy controls aged 18–60 years while results from other BD cohorts >18 years report decreased CD8+ T cells numbers (60) or increased activated CD3+ T cells in both symptomatic and euthymic BD patients compared with healthy controls (61). Few studies have compared circulating T cell subsets between affective disorders and SCZ. To date two separate studies have made direct comparisons between MDD and BD which revealed a deficiency of cytotoxic CD3+CD8+ T cells in MDD and a normal to overactive CD4+ T cell response in BD (62,63).

Disturbances are also found in T cell functionality either as in vivo impairment in MDD (64) or as measured by in vitro mitogenic responses in SCZ as well as BD (65). Furthermore, recent genome-wide association study data report genes involved in T cell adhesion and antigen processing such as CD28 and cytotoxic T lymphocyte antigen-4 (CTLA-4) to be associated with increased susceptibility to SCZ (66) and MDD (67).

A Th1 (pro-inflammatory, cell mediated immunity) predominant immunophenotype has been proposed for MDD (68,69) and in older euthymic BD participants compared to healthy controls (70) while a Th2 (anti-inflammatory, humoral mediated immunity) predominance is considered characteristic for SCZ (41). Importantly this is based on peripheral but not CNS cytokine patterns which may be unreliable surrogate markers due to extra CNS variables not controlled for in the peripheral cytokine pattern studies including age, BMI, psychotropic medication, smoking, stress and circadian fluctuations (71). Interestingly aberrant B lymphocyte numbers have also been reported across the psychiatric disorders. While few studies for MDD report a decrease in CD19+ (early B cell marker) (54) but an increase in CD20+/CD5+ (later stage B cell markers and a subset associated with autoantibody production) (72) these disparate results might point towards a role for autoantibodies and thereby activation of autoimmune pathways in the pathophysiology of MDD. Current meta-analytic data point towards a positive association between depression and the proportion of B cells as measured under fixed but not random effect analyses (40). In SCZ further stratification into those with acute psychosis vs stable forms may impact on an associated increase in CD19+ B cell counts (73) which may underpin the production of autoantibodies and provide further support for a Th2 dominance response hypothesis (74,75). However, this is so far not supported by meta-analyses (41).

The chronic low-grade neuroinflammation present across affective disorders and SCZ may be due to a lack of peripheral regulatory T cells at particular time points across the lifespan. The increase or decrease in regulatory T cells (Treg) cells at particular time points has been found to be particularly relevant in BD studies which report higher numbers of Treg CD4+CD25+FoxP3+ regulatory T cells albeit in patients >18 years of age (60) or <40 years of age (36) or a reduction in those >40 years of age (70). Indeed the same is seen in MDD whereby Treg numbers are reduced in those >28 years of age (68). This suggests age is an important contributing factor to T cell regulation of chronic inflammation. As such the chronic inflammation observed across the aforementioned psychiatric disorders may be characterized by reduced Tregs in conjunction with an increase in the pro-inflammatory Th17 subset as reported in SCZ (76), MDD (77,78) and BD (70,79,80).

15.2.4 Comment on the Overall and Differing Patterns of Cellular Immune Pathways within Affective Disorders and SCZ

Despite differing aetiology, a shared and yet distinct cellular immunoregulatory pathway exists across affective disorders and SCZ. Dysregulation of both innate and adaptive immune cells is observed across disorders including altered concentrations and proportions as well as polarisation and activation status. Preceding altered clinical phenotypes across disorders at the transcriptomic level is an overlapping and yet distinct pro-inflammatory monocytic 'gene fingerprint'. This supports the identification of an at-risk subpopulation preceding onset of first episode and points to epigenomic regulation as being crucial in determining the type and course of disorder (39). Activation of the pro-inflammatory transcriptome is the result of epigenomic regulation and leads to distinct clinical phenotypes. High level evidence for immune cell dysregulation is only available for MDD and SCZ. Interestingly, increased and activated innate and adaptive immune cells are associated with acute phases of the disorders and conversely decreased levels and diminished functionality is associated with remitted or chronic phases. Although high level evidence points towards lymphopenia associated with depression, this has to be viewed under fixed and not random effects modelling, in contrast to increased total lymphocytes (CD3+) but a reduced proportion of T lymphocytes in SCZ. Furthermore the NK cell proportion is decreased in MDD but increased in SCZ patients experiencing acute relapse. After treatment in SCZ, the CD4/CD8 ratio decreased while the proportion of CD56+ cells increased. In both disorders, this points towards an increased CD4/CD8 ratio being a state marker while the CD56 cells are a trait marker. Furthermore an increased level of cells bearing CD25 activation marker was found to be significantly increased in depression under fixed effect analyses but not in SCZ patients with acute relapse or drug naïve FEP. Proportional increases in B cell populations were measured in MDD but not SCZ. Although no higher-level evidence is currently available for Treg or Th17 T cell populations, it is proposed that spontaneous remission across disorders can be achieved through mechanisms including induction of tolerance and immune-regulatory effects mediated by Tregs, which may explain the differences observed between the acute and remitted phases of disorders.

15.3 Complement System across Psychiatric Disorders

The complement system is one of the main components of innate immunity and actively contributes to adaptive immunity (81,82). It includes a number of components that are activated by the classical pathway, the lectin pathway and the alternate pathway. Briefly, C1q is the recognition molecule that activates the classical pathway, mannose binding lectin (MBL) activates the lectin pathway, though activation of the MBL-associated proteases mannose binding lectin serine protease 1 (MASP1) and MASP2 and the alternate pathway is activated by cleavage of the complement factor B. All pathways eventually converge upon generation of C3 convertase, which cleaves complement component C3 into C3a and C3b, participating in the elimination of infectious agents and cellular debris (81,82). Within the brain, complement components regulate synaptic function and dendritic morphological and participate in synapse elimination by microglia (83). Recently, a role of the complement system has been suggested in mood disorders, as reviewed in this entire section (84).

15.3.1 Complement System in MDD

Recent studies reported increased levels of complement proteins in MDD patients. In particular, plasma C4 levels were elevated in MDD patients in comparison to healthy controls, both at the protein and mRNA levels (85,86). In addition, plasma C4-B levels were positively correlated with depressive symptoms in two independent cohorts of patients with MDD (87). However, this finding remains controversial since a more recent study showed no significant correlation of plasma C4 protein levels with the severity of depressive or anxiety symptoms in MDD patients (85). In addition to the association between peripheral C4 levels and MDD diagnosis, C3 levels were increased in the plasma of patients with MDD (86) and levels of C5 protein were significantly elevated in the CSF of patients with MDD in comparison to age-, sex- and ethnicity-matched healthy controls. Complement factor H (CFH) protein may also be associated with MDD. Indeed, MDD patients displayed decreased CFH protein and mRNA levels in comparison to healthy controls. Moreover, the risk allele C of rs1061170 was associated with decreased CFH plasma levels in MDD individuals. It was associated with higher risk for MDD and with age of onset of the disease (86). Altogether, only a few studies have assessed the association between complement system proteins and MDD. Importantly, these studies did not consider disease status (i.e., acute, chronic or remitted MDD). Large-sample studies are lacking to reinforce the findings, which should be followed by systematic reviews and meta-analyses.

15.3.2 Complement System in SCZ

In the last decades, more attention has been given to the association between dysregulations of the complement system and SCZ. The activity of the complement system was found to be higher in SCZ patients than in healthy controls (12), although the results are inconsistent. In particular some studies reported altered concentrations of C3 in SCZ but most studies concluded that there were no alterations or non-significant alterations of peripheral C3 levels in SCZ (12). In spite of small samples size and no replication, one study reported correlations between negative symptoms of paranoid SCZ and serum levels of C3 and C4 (88). Increased activity of the lectin pathway was also reviewed, evidenced by increased MBL MASP-2 activity in SCZ patients when compared to healthy controls (12). More recently, genetic association studies and post-mortem brain studies all suggested that increased mRNA and protein levels of C4A could be a risk factor for SCZ (89). However, meta-analyses and studies evaluating potential differences in complement system dysfunctions across different stages of the disease are lacking.

15.3.3 Complement System in BD

Studies evaluating the association between complement system proteins and BD reported inconsistent results. A recent review described raised peripheral levels of C3a, C5a and C5b-9 in BD patients (90). Similarly, raised levels of C3, C6 and factor B proteins were found in patients with an acute manic episode (91). However, another study reported unaltered plasma levels of C3 and C4 in medication-free manic BD patients compared with healthy controls (92). In agreement with elevated levels of peripheral complement proteins in BD, mRNA expression of C1q, C4 and factor B were significantly higher in peripheral blood mononuclear cells in chronic BD patients than in those of healthy controls, whereas mRNA expression levels of the complement inhibitor CD55 was lower. Interestingly, no difference was found for the expression of these genes between first-episode BD patients and healthy controls, suggesting that peripheral dysregulations of the complement system could be associated with the progression of the disease. In agreement with this assumption, there was an inverse correlation between serum levels of complement factors and disease duration as well as severity of manic symptoms (93). Interestingly CSF levels of C5 protein were similar between healthy controls and BD patients. However, it is noteworthy that more BD patients exhibit high C5 levels than healthy controls (11). It is unknown whether CSF and plasma C5 levels correlate in BD patients. To summarize, more studies are required to validate the association between elevated complement system activation and BD. It is noteworthy that attention should be given to the association between complement system and disease status (i.e., depressive, manic, hypomanic episode or euthymic patients).

15.3.4 Comment on the Overall and Differing Patterns of Complement System Dysfunctions across Psychiatric Disorders

Currently, it is difficult to conclude about potential differences and similarities in the pattern of these alterations between MDD, SCZ and BD. The literature suggests that increased C3 and C4 mRNA and protein levels in peripheral blood are associated with higher risk of psychiatric disease but this hypothesis is not validated yet. Indeed, conclusions are inconsistent between studies and not enough large-samples studies have been conducted so far. In addition, characterization of complement system dysfunctions across disease status in the abovementioned psychiatric conditions is lacking.

15.4 Cytokines across Psychiatric Disorders

Cytokines are small proteins (~5–20 kDa) produced by a diverse range of cells (e.g., macrophages, B and T lymphocytes, fibroblasts) and are pleiotropic in nature, participating in acute and chronic inflammation through activation of their receptors at the periphery as well as in the CNS. Cytokines include interleukins, tumour necrosis factors, interferons, colony-stimulating factors, granulocyte-macrophage colony-stimulating factor and some growth factors. By altering neurotransmitter metabolism and function, neuroendocrine pathways and brain plasticity, cytokines within the CNS can trigger the development of transient 'sickness behaviour', characterized by behavioural changes including reduced appetite, fatigue and lassitude (94). However, sustained production of peripheral and brain cytokines in inflammatory conditions is associated with the induction of neuropsychiatric symptoms (16,95), suggesting that they could participate in the development of such symptoms in psychiatric conditions.

15.4.1 Cytokines in MDD

Numerous studies have evaluated the association between cytokine alterations and MDD and in the last decade, the results have been summarized in several meta-analyses. Meta-analyses controlling for confounders and study quality have consistently reported increased levels of the pro-inflammatory cytokine IL-6 in the plasma or serum of patients with MDD when compared to healthy controls (mean difference (MD) = 1.78 pg/mL, p <0.001/SMD = 0.680, p <0.001/MD = 1.44ng/mL, p <0.001/Z-value = 7.430, p <0.001/ES = 0.621, p <0.001) (96–101). IL-6 levels were increased in either acute (effect size (ES) = 0.76, p <0.01) or chronic (ES = 0.39, p <0.01) MDD patients, suggesting this cytokine is a trait marker of the condition (100). A recent meta-analysis reported similar increased CSF IL-6 levels (ES = 0.40, p = 0.001), although the results are based on independent studies (102). Most studies also reported increased TNF-α protein levels in the plasma or serum (MD = 3.97 pg/mL, p <0.001/SMD = 0.562, p = 0.010/MD = 3.01 ng/mL, p <0.001/Z-value = 3.128, p = 0.002/ES = 0.675, p <0.001), but not in the CSF (CSF: ES = 0.26, p = 0.161), of MDD patients (96–102), although this association is less convincing than the one between IL-6 and MDD (99). It is noteworthy that increased peripheral TNF-α was found to be elevated in acute MDD only (ES = 0.35, p <0.01) and not in chronic MDD (ES = 0.05, p = 0.52) (100). In addition to IL-6 and TNF-α, C-Reactive Protein (CRP) was found to be elevated in patients with MDD compared with healthy controls (Z-value = 4.866, p <0.001/correlation with depressive symptoms: r^2 = 0.046, p <0.001) (99,103) and this association was stronger than the one between IL-6 and MDD (103). However, it is still unclear which cytokine network alterations are dependent on the disease status and could therefore be state markers of the disorder. Association between peripheral cytokine levels and MDD has also been assessed for other cytokines (i.e., IL-1β, IL-4, IL-2, IL-8 and IFN-γ) but the results showed no association or were inconsistent between studies (96–101,104). Similarly, no association was found between IL-1β single nucleotide polymorphisms (SNPs) and MDD (104). Meta-analyses are therefore required to identify whether cytokine SNPs represent potential risk factors for MDD.

15.4.2 Cytokines in SCZ

Recently, a lot of interest has been given to the role of cytokines in the pathogenesis and progression of SCZ. Potvin et al. reported increased IL-1RA (ES = 0.523, p <0.001), IL-6 (ES = 0.465, p <0.001) and sIL-2 R (ES = 0.599, p = 0.0001) in plasma or serum samples of SCZ patients compared to healthy controls (105), although they did not control for disease status (i.e., acute, non-acute or mixed episode). This was however controlled for elsewhere and it is noteworthy that cytokine alterations vary between clinical statuses (106). Indeed, IL-1β, IL-6 and TGF-β appear to be state-related markers as they were increased during acute exacerbations whereas IFN-γ, TNF-α, sIL-2 R and IL-12, may be trait markers since their peripheral levels remained elevated across statuses (100,106). However, peripheral cytokine alterations have been shown to be similar between FEP patients and acutely ill patients with SCZ (100), even after controlling for medication and smoking status, BMI and assay methodology. Recently another meta-analysis (107) found that a reduced variability of IL-1β, IL-4, IL-6, IL-8 and TNF-α but not TGF-β in FEP patients compared with controls does not infer FEP subtypes but instead suggests an inherent dysregulated immune system as a broader feature within psychosis (108).

Cytokines levels in SCZ could also be associated with specific symptoms. For example, elevated plasma and IL-6 levels were positively associated with worse cognitive performance in SCZ patients (109). Wang and Miller recently found that both blood and CSF levels of IL-1β, IL-6 and IL-8 were increased in SCZ patients. By contrast, blood sIL-2 R levels were elevated whereas they were decreased in the CSF (ES = –0.84, p = 0.013), highlighting that changes observed at the periphery do not necessarily reflect brain changes (102). In agreement with this statement, no study reported correlation between blood and CSF levels for any of the cytokines.

In the last decade, meta-analyses have been conducted to evaluate the effect of cytokine polymorphisms on SCZ. In particular, *TNF-α* polymorphisms have drawn attention since the gene coding for TNF-α is located on the chromosome 6, which is a susceptibility locus for schizophrenia (110). Most case-control studies found no overall relationship between SCZ susceptibility and *TNF-α* 308 A/G polymorphism, which might be associated with increased TNF-α transcription (OR = 1.103, p = 0.318/OR = 1.047, p = 0.614/Z-value = 1.39, p = 0.16) (111–113). In addition, no relationship was found between SCZ and *TNF-α* 238 A/G or 857 T/C polymorphisms, which can be associated with lower TNF-α production (111). It is however noteworthy that an association was found between *TNF-α* 1031 C/C and T/T genotype, associated with increased circulating levels of TNF-α, and SCZ in an Asian population only (OR = 1.259, p = 0.0016) (111). Similarly, *IL-10* and *IL-1β* genes are mapped on chromosomes associated with modest risk factor for SCZ (114). A meta-analysis conducted among 11 studies with SCZ patients and healthy controls revealed an association between rs1800872 of *IL-10* and SCZ for genotype A/A, associated with lower IL-10 expression, in both Caucasian and Asian population carrying this genotype (OR = 1.351, p = 2.06E-04) (115). Moreover, no association between rs16944 of *IL-1β* and SCZ suscepti-bility was found in the general population (OR = 1.03) but significant association was found between the minor allele A of rs16944 of *IL-1β*, which facilitates IL-1β production, and SCZ in an East Asian population (OR = 1.08, p = 0.041) (116). These conclusions emphasize the importance of considering ethnic differences when conducting such analyses.

To summarize, meta-analyses have shown consistent alterations in cytokine profile in the blood of SCZ patients, in particular when disease status is controlled for. However, evidence of an association between specific cytokine polymorphism and risk for SCZ is still lacking and requires more attention.

15.4.3 Cytokines in BD

Meta-analyses described cytokine level alterations in patients with BD, although less data is available compared to MDD and SCZ. Concentrations of IL-1β, IL-4, IL-6, IL-10, sIL-2 R, sIL-6 R, TNF-α and sTNFR1 have been reported to be significantly elevated in BD patients compared to healthy controls (p ≤0.01 for each) (100,117,118). Similarly, increased CSF IL-1β levels have been reported in a recent meta-analysis (ES = 0.31, p = 0.020) (102). Interestingly, peripheral levels of IL-6 were not consistently reported to be increased in BD patients compared to healthy controls but subgroups analyses showed that patients with mania displayed elevated IL-6 levels compared with both healthy controls (ES = 0.617, p = 0.014) and depressed patients (ES = 0.346, p = 0.009) (117), suggesting that the cytokine profile could be different across the stages of the disease. In agreement with this hypothesis, TNF-α (SMD = 3.68, p <0.01), sIL-2 R (SMD = 0.85, p <0.01) and sTNFR1 (SMD = 0.87, p <0.01) were found to be elevated in manic BD patients compared to healthy controls whereas sTNFR1 was the only cytokine receptor elevated in euthymic patients compared to healthy controls (SMD = 0.58, p <0.01) (119). However, the significant heterogeneity between studies and the low number of studies evaluating cytokine alterations across disease statuses highlight a need for more studies measuring cytokine levels across phases in BD patients.

15.4.4 Comment on the Overall and Differing Patterns of Cytokines Alterations across Psychiatric Disorders

A cytokine signature has been highlighted for MDD, with IL-6, TNF-α and CRP plasma levels being consistently elevated across studies. Increased blood TNF-α levels are shared between MDD, SCZ and BD, suggesting it could be a common marker of these three psychiatric conditions. Although IL-6 is similarly reported to be elevated in MDD and SCZ patients compared to healthy controls regardless of disease status, it is raised in manic BD patients but not in depressed and euthymic BD patients. IL-6 could hence be a state marker of BD whereas it appears to be a trait marker of MDD and SCZ. It is noteworthy that recent studies highlighted distinct cytokine profiles across stages of the disorders in both SCZ and BD although the results remain inconsistent, suggesting that cytokine network requires more consideration in the future. A meta-analysis comparing cytokine levels between MDD, SCZ or BD patients and healthy controls confirmed that IL-6 and TNF-α levels are elevated in acute phases across the disorders while only IL-6 levels are increased in chronic phases. In addition, sIL-2 R and IL-1β were elevated in SCZ and BD but not in MDD patients (100), suggesting again that MDD could be characterized by a distinct cytokine profile. Hence, although some similarities have been highlighted, there are also distinct immune alterations within disorders, suggesting that specific cytokines could be therapeutic targets in the treatment of psychiatric disorders.

It is noteworthy that most meta-analyses highlighted substantial heterogeneity across studies, suggesting that the relationship between cytokines and psychiatric disorders may be influenced by numerous variables, which must be accounted for. Recently, Horn and colleagues provided a set of recommendations for the field to facilitate replication and reproducibility. These recommendations include controlling for sample collection and assaying procedures, statistical methods and demographic (e.g., age, sex), health (e.g., BMI, medical condition), substance (e.g., nicotine, alcohol), medication, psychosocial (e.g., education) and additional variables (e.g., physical activity) (120). In addition, anti-depressant and antipsychotic medications and mood-stabilizers can alter pro-inflammatory cytokine production, thus highlighting the importance of also considering medication status in future meta-analyses (121–123).

15.5 Chemokines across Psychiatric Disorders

Chemokines, by the nature of their chemotactic function, not only regulate peripheral immune cell migration but can also be involved in the induction of a pro-inflammatory state (124–126). They exert their biological functions by acting on G-protein coupled transmembrane receptors on the surface of their target cells. By participating in the regulation of neurotransmitter and neuroendocrine pathways (127,128), chemokines have a role in neuroimmune processes relevant to psychiatric disorders (8,9). In this section, we review evidence of an association between chemokine network alterations and MDD, SCZ and BD and evaluate potential differences and similarities across these psychiatric conditions. In an attempt to clarify reading, chemokine systematic names are used throughout this section and corresponding historical names are quoted into brackets.

15.5.1 Chemokines in MDD

Two recent meta-analyses reported significantly higher serum or plasma concentration of CCL2 (MCP-1), which regulates migration and infiltration of monocytes and macrophages, in individuals with MDD compared to healthy controls (overall difference: 36.43 pg/mL, p = 0.036/Hedge's g: 1.718, p = 0.045) (7,101). However, this association between CCL2 and MDD was not significant anymore when publication bias was corrected for (mean difference of –8.98, p = 0.548) (7). The CXC chemokine family member CXCL8 (IL-8), whose function it is to promote inflammation and regulate activation and migration of peripheral granulocytes, was not found to be significantly altered in MDD patients when compared with healthy controls (overall difference of –0.58 pg/mL, p = 0.228) (7).

In addition to this meta-analytic, a systematic reviewed published by our group (8) found no difference in CXCL8 serum levels between MDD patients and healthy controls. However, it is noteworthy that serum CXCL8 was positively associated with the severity of depressive symptoms in geriatric patients. Moreover, 251 T/A polymorphism of the *CXCL8* gene (rs4073), related to higher CXCL8 production, was significantly associated with the onset of depression in elderly patients (8). This points to age as being an important factor in affecting the levels of chemokines observed across disorders.

15.5.2 Chemokines in SCZ

Only one meta-analysis has addressed the relationship between chemokines and SCZ compared to healthy controls (129). This study explored whether a brain and/or blood gene expression profile distinguishes SCZ patients from healthy individuals. Among the 13 genes differentially expressed in the same direction in both post-mortem brain samples and blood of SCZ patients, 10 have a role in inflammation, immunity and wound healing. In particular, *CX3CR1* (fractalkine receptor) gene expression was down-regulated in SCZ patients compared to healthy controls (fold change = –1.08; p = 0.025). CX3CR1 is the receptor of the chemoattractant protein CX3CL1 (fractalkine) and can mediate leucocyte migration and adhesion.

It has been reviewed that peripheral levels of CCL2 were increased in both chronic SCZ patients treated with medications and FEP medication-free patients compared to healthy controls (130). In addition, subjects carrying the A/G or G/G genotype for the *CCL2* gene rs1024611, associated with increased CCL2 transcripts levels, had increased susceptibility for SCZ compared to individuals carrying the A/A genotype (130). Hence, this suggests that both protein levels of MCP-1 and *CCL2* genotype can confer susceptibility to SCZ. Although the results for CXCL8 were inconsistent, it was suggested that CXCL8 protein levels and gene expression were increased in the serum and in the brain of SCZ patients, respectively. Because existing results have not been replicated yet and little data is available for other chemokines in SCZ patients, new studies would be helpful.

15.5.3 Chemokines in BD

Only a few studies have evaluated the association between chemokine network and BD so far. Our group reviewed evidence for alterations of chemokines levels in the plasma, serum or post-mortem brain samples of BD patients compared to healthy controls (8). Increased peripheral levels of CXCL8, CCL2 and of the chemoattractant protein CXCL10 (CRG-2) have been described in BD patients compared to healthy controls, along with decreased post-mortem brain levels of CCL3 (MIP-1α), which is involved in leukocyte recruitment. Interestingly, plasma levels of the chemoattractant protein CCL24 (eotaxin-2) were higher in euthymic BD patients than in healthy controls whereas they were similar in manic BD patients and control group, suggesting that CCL24 could be a trait marker of BD (131). Similarly, serum levels of the chemoattractant protein CCL1 (TCA-3) were higher in late-stage BD compared to healthy controls whereas they are similar between early-stage BD patients and healthy individuals, independently of age (132). However, the data linking chemokines and BD obtained so far are insufficient, inconsistent or have not been replicated yet.

More recently, the frequency of G/A and G/G genotypes for the *CCL2* gene rs1024611 was found to be higher in patients with BD compared with healthy individuals. On the contrary, the frequency of A/A genotype was higher in healthy controls and associated with reduced risk for BD (133). This is in agreement with previous studies showing a potential role of *CCL2* polymorphisms in conferring susceptibility to BD (134,135). Especially, *CCL2* polymorphisms were shown to be different between a subgroup of BD patients with manic episode and patients with depressed or mixed episode, suggesting that CCL2 could be associated with BD status rather than with the development of the disease itself (135). BD patients also displayed high frequency of the mutation Δ32 on the *CCR5* gene (resulting in a non-functional receptor) and C138T C+ genotype of *CXCR4*, which might be associated with a gain of function (133). Overall, these findings interestingly suggest an involvement of several chemokine polymorphisms in BD pathogenesis.

15.5.4 Comment on the Overall and Differing Patterns of Chemokine Alterations across Psychiatric Disorders

It is noteworthy that CCL2 and CXCL8 alterations have been reported at both protein and gene level in MDD, BD and SCZ, suggesting that alterations in these two chemokine networks are shared across disorders. However, replication studies are required to confirm inconsistent findings across and within disorders.

15.6 Future Outlook: Transdiagnostic Involvement of the Immune System across Psychiatric Disorders

The current literature as reviewed in this chapter demonstrates significant dysregulation in both innate and adaptive immune system cells and their signalling mediators in association with clinical symptoms of MDD, BD and SCZ as assessed using the Diagnostic Statistical Manual of Mental Disorders (DSM) (Table 15.1). A dysregulated immune system could therefore directly or indirectly alter behaviour due to its ability to impair monoamine levels, activity of the HPA axis, neuroplasticity as well as pathological microglial cell activation and brain structure and function (136).

Initially the research focused solely on the measurement of peripheral cytokine alterations across conditions with the most robust alteration found in an elevation of cytokines of the mononuclear phagocyte system (MPS) including TNF-α and IL-6. Interestingly, cytokine alterations distinguishing SCZ and BD from MDD include elevated levels of sIL-2 R. This supports the premise that T cell and monocyte derived cytokines may induce distinct behavioural abnormalities and that cytokines of the T cell system (IL-2) are elevated independently from cytokines of the MPS/endothelial system (IL-1β, TNF-α and IL-6) (37). Similarly to cytokines, peripheral chemokines levels are found to be altered across MDD, SCZ and BD with the most common pattern being elevations in MCP1 and CXCL8. In addition, complement system factors, in particular C3 and C4, have been shown to be consistently elevated across psychiatric conditions. This is likely to be the result of increased synthesis in the liver in response to elevated pro-inflammatory cytokines levels (i.e., TNF-α and IL-6) contributing to a positive feedback loop and thereby creating a sustained pro-inflammatory state (137). It is noteworthy that most studies in immunopsychiatry focus on mediators only. However, there is evidence for a role of immune-associated intracellular second messengers (e.g., BDNF) and signal transduction cascades in both preclinical models of mood disorders and patients (e.g., NFκB, MAPK) (138–140). This suggests that second messenger/signal transduction abnormalities could also be used as biomarkers to improve diagnoses and further treatment.

Meta-analytic evidence supports relative and total number of immune cell dysregulation across disorders. In particular, MDD exhibits increased immune activation in the form of monocytosis, characteristic of an acute phase response with an impaired NK and T cell number and function. Dysregulation is also observed in the increased proportion of activated CD25+ lymphocytes. In SCZ, distinguishing features between drug naïve FEP and acutely relapsed inpatients demonstrate that episodes of psychosis are associated with elevated inflammatory signatures. These include increased CD4/CD8 ratio. Surprisingly

Table 15.1 Summary of immune system aspects dysregulated across psychiatric disorders

	B Lymphocytes	T Lymphocytes	Microglia (Monocytes/ Macrophages)	Natural Killer Cells	Complement System	Cytokines	Chemokines
MDD	↑ %B cell +++ ↑ CD20/CD5 (NC) ↓CD19 (NC)	↑%CD4 +++ ↑CD4/CD8 ratio + ++ ↓%CD8 ++ ↓Treg +++ ↑%CD25 +++ ↑Th17+	↑CD14 ↑monocytes+++	↓CD56+++ ↓%NK+++	↑C4 + ↑C3 + ↓CFH + ↑C5 +	↑IL-6 +++ ↑TNF-α +++ ↑CRP +++	↑MCP1 +++ ↑CXCL8 (elderly) ++
SCZ (First-Episode Psychosis / Acute)	↑CD19 (NC)	↑CD4 +++ ↑CD4/CD8 ratio + ++ ↓CD3 +++ ↓%CD3 +++ ↑Th17 + ↑%CD4 ++ +(relapsed)	↑ CD14	↑CD16 (NC) ↑%CD56 ++ +(relapsed)	↑C4 + ↑C3 + ↑MBL MASP2 +	↑IL-1β +++ ↑IL-6 +++ ↑TGF-β +++ ↑IL-12 +++ ↑IFN-γ +++ ↑TNF-α +++ ↑sIL-2 R +++ ↑IL1-RA	↑MCP1 ++ ↑CXCL8 ++ ↑CCL2 ++ ↓CX3CR1 + ++
SCZ (Remission / Chronic)	TBC	↓CD4 ↓CD4/CD8 ratio ↑CD4+CD25+foxp3 +Treg	TBC	= CD56 (NC)	TBC	↑IL-12 +++ ↑IFN-γ +++ ↑TNF-α +++ ↑sIL-2 R +++	TBC
BP (Mania)	= CD19 (NC)	= CD4 + ↓CD8 +	= CD14/ ↑CD14/CD16	= CD56(NC)	↑C3 + ↑C5 +	↑IL-4 ↑sIL-2 R +++	↑CXCL8 ++ ↑CCL2 ++

BP (Euthymic / Remitted)	TBC	↑CD4/CD8 ratio + ↓Treg + ↑Th17+	TBC	↑C6 + ↑factor B + ↑C4 + ↑C1 + ↓CD55 +	↑IL-6 R ↑TNF-α ↑sTNF-R1 ↑IL-10	↑CXCL10 ++ ↓CCL3 ++ ↑CCL24 ++
	TBC	TBC	TBC	TBC	↑sTNF-R1 + ++	TBC

NC: not conclusive (due to low number of studies and/or clearly conflicting outcomes), +: low level of evidence from primary source, ++: medium level of evidence from reviews and systematic reviews, +++: high level of evidence from meta-analyses. ↑: increased activity/expression, ↓: decreased activity/expression, =: unaltered number of cells TBC: to be confirmed and in contrast to MDD, no differences in proportions of CD19+ B lymphocytes was observed. While immune cell dysregulation is also observed for BD this remains inconclusive with limited study number. Although the review of the literature indicates BD to be more commonly associated with a monocyte-related immune response (141), each of the disorders has an activated innate immune component. Subsequent adaptive immune activation can lead to further distinction between disorders whereby SCZ appears to be more related to a Th2 type stimulated immune response (142,143) in contrast to a more Th1 type as seen in MDD (144).

There are important limitations in the reviewed studies investigating the relationship between immune system alterations and psychiatric conditions, including small sample size, ethnicity and uncontrolled and underreported confounding factors affecting immune function. For example, increased BMI and age as well as substance abuse including smoking are likely to increase MPS activation and subsequent low-grade inflammation. Furthermore, medication (antipsychotics, anticonvulsants, antidepressants, lithium, anti-inflammatories) are known immune modulators (111,115,116,145,146). It is also important to consider different psychiatric phases as characterized by distinct symptom domains when reporting immune dysfunction. For example the literature indicates that pro-inflammatory cytokines are elevated during the active stage of a disorder such as mania in BD and acute current depression in MDD (147). Furthermore increased peripheral immune cell numbers can represent either an enhancement of adaptive or maladaptive processes. Unfortunately, the current cross-sectional studies represent a limiting factor when trying to discern between the two possibilities. Future longitudinal studies will assist in developing this further to integrate not only new diagnostic stratification of disorders into acute and chronic phases based on biological validity but also personalized prognosis and therapeutic interventions.

The reviewed literature supports the 'inflammation' hypothesis of all three disorders. Furthermore the presence of a pro-inflammatory monocytic gene expression pattern as found within those with BD and SCZ provides the evolutionary bias for a predisposition for chronic low-grade inflammation for certain subpopulations within neuropsychiatric disorders (148). However, manifestation towards psychopathology is a consequence not only of developmental dysregulation but also evolutionary pressures encountered in a rapidly altering modern environment. These alterations promote increased epigenomic changes leading to genomic and microbiome changes as well as inflammation or stress-related dysfunction of the brain and behaviour (149). Therefore, despite differing aetiology, an overlapping and yet distinct cellular and molecular inflammatory response is elucidated by differing gene-environment and gene-gene interactions. Epigenomic regulatory factors (including nutrition, toxicity, psychosocial stressors/trauma, increased gut permeability/microbiome alterations and chronic periodontitis), and not only the gene signature itself, are then instrumental in determining the specific type and magnitude of chronic low-grade neuroinflammation eliciting different disorders and different phases (39).

Induction of the monocytosis as seen in MDD may be due to a more prominent hyperactivation of the HPA axis. Stress has been shown to activate the innate immune response and is associated more often with affective disorders including MDD and BD (most prominently in the manic episode as well as remission) (150) than SCZ (151). Sensitization by first time exposure to either psychosocial or organic stressors can prime response pathways such as HPA axis, which when triggered by re-exposure is likely to lead to an enhanced cellular response. Modulation of subsequent neuroinflammatory cascades involves the differing ratios between the pro- and anti-inflammatory cellular pathways, also leading to the differential induction of a disorder and its distinct phase (152). Although hyperactivation of the HPA axis is a major contributor to immune dysregulation in MDD, comorbidities with autoimmune disorders also point towards autoimmunity as being an aetiological factor. Unclear as yet is whether dysregulation of the immune system or HPA axis are potent activators of autoimmune processes not only within MDD (153) but also other in psychiatric disorders (71). From meta-analytic data, it is apparent that a decrease in Treg and an increase in pro-inflammatory Th17 cells is associated with MDD and BD. In a small case-control study of 40 MDD participants the Th17/Treg ratio and the number of peripheral anti-nuclear autoantibodies were increased compared with healthy controls (154). In contrast, in another small study, the increased Th17/Treg ratio in BD was found to be associated with intact brain white matter, suggesting that the Th17 cells are not destructive under non-autoimmune conditions but could instead confer tropic functions that are essential for mood regulation (79). Future research is required to investigate the risk for and progression of autoimmune pathways across psychiatric disorders. The reviewed literature also determined age to be an important factor with regards to immunoregulatory mechanisms mediated by Tregs and CXCL8. Increasing age sees the decline in naturally occurring and thymus derived Tregs, increasing the risk for comorbid autoimmunity. It is also plausible that an increased IL-2 activity as found in SCZ and BD manic patients might reflect the increased expansion of Tregs as a means of counteracting the pro-inflammatory state of the MPS system and related T cell effector cell activation (37). Another feature of neuroinflammation distinguishing the three disorders and their differing clinical psycho-pathology is the temporal and spatial patterns of neuroinflammation. For example in MDD, core symptoms may be associated with adaptive/maladaptive neuroimmune changes specific to certain brain regions (155,156). The pathophysiology implicating neuroinflammation within affective disorders involves increased microglial number and activation, which may lead to deleterious effects on neuronal plasticity, neurogenesis and apoptosis (157,158). In parallel, SCZ has been hypothesized to be a disorder of excessive synaptic pruning by microglia, which is supported by genetic studies and increased activity of the complement system in SCZ patients (159). These mechanisms could therefore result in altered neuro-transmitter levels as well as structural and functional brain changes (160), therefore promoting the development of psychiatric symptoms. Recent highly powered meta-analytic neuroimaging data provided evidence that subcortical alterations broadly overlap across MDD, SCZ and BD. Reductions in hippocampus, thalamus and amygdala volumes and enlarged lateral ventricles and globus pallidus were reported in both SCZ and BD patients, although the effects were stronger in SCZ than in BD (161,162). Similarly, significant but milder reductions in hippocampal volume were reported in MDD patients (163). This overlap suggests that MDD, SCZ and BD share some common biological mechanisms targeting the medial temporal lobe. Amongst others, actions of inflammation on medial temporal lobe structures in psychiatric patients could underlie the development of core symptoms of the disorders such as somatic and/or cognitive symptoms (164). Part of the neuroinflammatory mechanism could also include recruitment of lymphocytes to meningeal spaces or parenchyma thereby influencing brain plasticity and promoting or impairing cognitive processes dependent on the pro-/anti-inflammatory cell ratio (165).

The dysregulated immune signature in terms of T cell cytokines as found across the disorders may be reflective of an association with core symptoms such as anhedonia in BD or in depression (166). Indeed core features such as cognitive dysfunction are associated with MDD as well as psychosis. This suggests that psychopathology is more dimensional in nature rather than categorical and that certain biological subtypes may exist with the involvement of particular immune system signatures across DSM-V defined categories. Furthermore, co-occurrence of multiple mental disorders may reflect the presence of shared risk factors with similar underlying biological processes resulting in different patterns of symptoms. Becoming apparent is that shared symptom domains across disorders may be accounted for by shared similarities in dysregulated neuroinflammatory pathways. For example a core somatic symptom domain or 'sickness behaviour' is found associated with MDD and as part of an adaptive response leading to dysregulated mood comorbid in BD and SCZ. It signifies the importance of the bidirectionality between the CNS and peripheral immune system (94). Although our review does not directly provide a casual association with core symptom domains and immune signatures within and across disorders, these will in the future further inform the National Institute of Mental Health's Research Domain Criteria (RDoC) (167,168). Ultimately the aim it is to apply a transdiagnostic approach by capturing psychopathology across multiple levels including interactions between symptoms, genetic influences, environmental stressors and time (169). Furthermore, use of this network approach in the future is more synergistic with evolutionary conceptualization of the role of inflammation in human behaviour; e.g., 'sickness behaviour'; and represents the adaptive response to facilitate healing and recovery (170).

To conclude, this chapter substantiates the possible pathogenic role of the immune system within psychiatric disorders. Although the immune response is found to be dysregulated and predominantly of innate immune origin across all three disorders, the interplay of immunogenetic predisposition and environmental factors determine a disorder as classified according to the DSM-V criteria. While BD and SCZ are characterized by predisposition for a pro-inflammatory monocytic gene expression pattern, the combination with environmental stressors such as chronic stress leads to an adaptive immune signature of humoral mediation. In contrast MDD has been found associated with stress susceptibility via the HPA axis dysregulation and a resulting cell mediated immune signature. Clearly, the phenotypic spectrum of innate and adaptive immune cells could become either state or trait markers associated with the episodic nature of the disorder. Conversely peripheral cytokine network signatures, including those as trait and state markers (93,100,106,117,118,131,132), have the potential to be used for diagnostic and prognostic purposes distinguishing between disorders as well as within different phases. Furthermore, reviewed evidence indicates that distinct activation of both the MPS as well as T and B cell systems may play independent roles in the pathophysiology of psychiatric disorders currently defined by clinical evaluation alone. Further investigations are required to determine their exact regulatory mechanisms contributing to the distinct phenotype in MDD, BD and SCZ. These findings are important in the development of new therapeutic strategies. These would be designed to enhance endogenous neuroprotective immune pathways and down-regulate immune pathways that are detrimental, rather than indiscriminately suppress inflammation.

15.7 Acknowledgements

The presented work is supported by the Fay Fuller Foundation. The funders had no role in the design or the content of the presented work or in the decision to publish

References

1. Schur RR, Draisma LW, Wijnen JP, et al. Brain GABA levels across psychiatric disorders: a systematic literature review and meta-analysis of (1) H-MRS studies. *Hum Brain Mapp.* 2016;37(9):3337–52.

2. Allen PJ. Creatine metabolism and psychiatric disorders: does creatine supplementation have therapeutic value? *Neurosci Biobehav Rev.* 2012;36(5):1442–62.

3. Landgraf D, McCarthy MJ, Welsh DK. Circadian clock and stress interactions in the molecular biology of psychiatric disorders. *Curr Psychiatry Rep.* 2014;16(10):483.

4. McEwen BS. Protection and damage from acute and chronic stress: allostasis and allostatic overload and relevance to the pathophysiology of psychiatric disorders. *Ann N Y Acad Sci.* 2004;1032:1–7.

5. Andero R, Choi DC, Ressler KJ. BDNF-TrkB receptor regulation of distributed adult neural plasticity, memory formation, and psychiatric disorders. *Prog Mol Biol Transl Sci.* 2014;122:169–92.

6. Ding Y, Chang LC, Wang X, et al. Molecular and genetic characterization of depression: overlap with other psychiatric disorders and aging. *Mol Neuropsychiatry.* 2015;1(1):1–12.

7. Eyre HA, Air T, Pradhan A, et al. A meta-analysis of chemokines in major depression. *Prog Neuropsychopharmacol Biol Psychiatry.* 2016;68:1–8.

8. Stuart MJ, Baune BT. Chemokines and chemokine receptors in mood disorders, schizophrenia, and cognitive impairment: a systematic review of biomarker studies. *Neurosci Biobehav Rev.* 2014;42:93–115.

9. Stuart MJ, Singhal G, Baune BT. Systematic review of the neurobiological relevance of chemokines to psychiatric disorders. *Front Cell Neurosci.* 2015;9:357.

10. Mazza MG, Lucchi S, Tringali AGM, et al. Neutrophil/lymphocyte ratio and platelet/lymphocyte ratio in mood disorders: a meta-analysis. *Prog Neuropsychopharmacol Biol Psychiatry.* 2018;84(Pt A):229–36.

11. Ishii T, Hattori K, Miyakawa T, et al. Increased cerebrospinal fluid complement C5 levels in major depressive disorder and schizophrenia. *Biochem Biophys Res Commun.* 2018;497(2):683–8.

12. Mayilyan KR, Weinberger DR, Sim RB. The complement system in schizophrenia. *Drug News Perspect.* 2008;21(4):200–10.

13. Rus H, Cudrici C, David S, Niculescu F. The complement system in central nervous system diseases. *Autoimmunity.* 2006;39(5):395–402.

14. Ratajczak MZ, Pedziwiatr D, Cymer M, et al. Sterile Inflammation of Brain, due to Activation of Innate Immunity, as a Culprit in Psychiatric Disorders. *Front Psychiatry.* 2018;9:60.

15. Sayana P, Colpo GD, Simoes LR, et al. A systematic review of evidence for the role of inflammatory biomarkers in bipolar patients. *J Psychiatr Res.* 2017;92:160–82.

16. Capuron L, Lasselin J, Castanon N. Role of adiposity-driven inflammation in depressive morbidity. *Neuropsychopharmacology.* 2017;42(1):115–28.

17. Rodrigues-Amorim D, Rivera-Baltanas T, Spuch C, et al. Cytokines dysregulation in schizophrenia: A systematic review of psychoneuroimmune relationship. *Schizophr Res.* 2018;197:19–33.

18. Suvisaari J, Mantere O. Inflammation theories in psychotic disorders: a critical review. *Infect Disord Drug Targets.* 2013;13(1):59–70.

19. Herkenham M, Kigar SL. Contributions of the adaptive immune system to mood regulation: mechanisms and pathways of neuroimmune interactions. *Progress in Neuro-Psychopharmacology and Biological Psychiatry.* 2017;79:49–57.

20. Haapakoski R, Ebmeier KP, Alenius H, Kivimaki M. Innate and adaptive immunity in the development of depression: an update on current knowledge and technological advances. *Prog Neuropsychopharmacol Biol Psychiatry.* 2016;66:63–72.

21. Kendler KS, Karkowski LM, Prescott CA. Causal relationship between stressful life

events and the onset of major depression. *Am J Psychiatry.* 1999;156(6):837–41.

22. Shastri A, Bonifati DM, Kishore U. Innate immunity and neuroinflammation. *Mediators Inflamm.* 2013;2013:342931.

23. Merad M, Sathe P, Helft J, Miller J, Mortha A. The dendritic cell lineage: ontogeny and function of dendritic cells and their subsets in the steady state and the inflamed setting. *Annu Rev Immunol.* 2013;31:563–604.

24. Tian L, Ma L, Kaarela T, Li Z. Neuroimmune crosstalk in the central nervous system and its significance for neurological diseases. *J Neuroinflammation.* 2012;9:155.

25. Aspelund A, Antila S, Proulx ST, et al. A dural lymphatic vascular system that drains brain interstitial fluid and macromolecules. *The Journal of Experimental Medicine.* 2015;212(7): 991–9.

26. Louveau A, Smirnov I, Keyes TJ, et al. Structural and functional features of central nervous system lymphatic vessels. *Nature.* 2015;523(7560):337–41.

27. Wohleb ES, McKim DB, Shea DT, et al. Re-establishment of anxiety in stress-sensitized mice is caused by monocyte trafficking from the spleen to the brain. *Biol Psychiatry.* 2014;75(12): 970–81.

28. Sawicki CM, McKim DB, Wohleb ES, et al. Social defeat promotes a reactive endothelium in a brain region-dependent manner with increased expression of key adhesion molecules, selectins and chemokines associated with the recruitment of myeloid cells to the brain. *Neuroscience.* 2015;302:151–64.

29. Seidel A, Arolt V, Hunstiger M, et al. Major depressive disorder is associated with elevated monocyte counts. *Acta Psychiatr Scand.* 1996;94(3):198–204.

30. Maes M, Van der Planken M, Stevens WJ, et al. Leukocytosis, monocytosis and neutrophilia: hallmarks of severe depression. *J Psychiatr Res.* 1992;26 (2):125–34.

31. Rothermundt M, Arolt V, Weitzsch C, Eckhoff D, Kirchner H. Immunological dysfunction in schizophrenia: a systematic approach. *Neuropsychobiology.* 1998;37 (4):186–93.

32. Zorrilla EP, Cannon TD, Gur RE, Kessler J. Leukocytes and organ-nonspecific autoantibodies in schizophrenics and their siblings: markers of vulnerability or disease? *Biol Psychiatry.* 1996;40 (9):825–33.

33. Theodoropoulou S, Spanakos G, Baxevanis CN, et al. Cytokine serum levels, autologous mixed lymphocyte reaction and surface marker analysis in never medicated and chronically medicated schizophrenic patients. *Schizophr Res.* 2001;47(1):13–25.

34. Drexhage RC, Hoogenboezem TA, Cohen D, et al. An activated set point of T-cell and monocyte inflammatory networks in recent-onset schizophrenia patients involves both pro- and anti-inflammatory forces. *Int J Neuropsychopharmacol.* 2011;14 (6):746–55.

35. Nikkila HV, Muller K, Ahokas A, et al. Accumulation of macrophages in the CSF of schizophrenic patients during acute psychotic episodes. *Am J Psychiatry.* 1999;156(11):1725–9.

36. Drexhage RC, Hoogenboezem TH, Versnel MA, et al. The activation of monocyte and T cell networks in patients with bipolar disorder. *Brain Behav Immun.* 2011;25(6):1206–13.

37. Drexhage RC, Knijff EM, Padmos RC, et al. The mononuclear phagocyte system and its cytokine inflammatory networks in schizophrenia and bipolar disorder. *Expert Rev Neurother.* 2010;10(1):59–76.

38. Grosse L, Carvalho LA, Wijkhuijs AJ, et al. Clinical characteristics of inflammation-associated depression: monocyte gene expression is age-related in major depressive disorder. *Brain Behav Immun.* 2015;44:48–56.

39. Padmos RC, Hillegers MH, Knijff EM, et al. A discriminating messenger RNA signature for bipolar disorder formed by an aberrant expression of inflammatory genes

in monocytes. *Arch Gen Psychiatry.* 2008;65 (4):395–407.

40. Zorrilla EP, Luborsky L, McKay JR, et al. The relationship of depression and stressors to immunological assays: a meta-analytic review. *Brain Behav Immun.* 2001;15(3):199–226.

41. Miller BJ, Gassama B, Sebastian D, Buckley P, Mellor A. Meta-analysis of lymphocytes in schizophrenia: clinical status and antipsychotic effects. *Biol Psychiatry.* 2013;73(10):993–9.

42. Torres KCL, Souza BR, Miranda DM, et al. The leukocytes expressing DARPP-32 are reduced in patients with schizophrenia and bipolar disorder. *Progress in Neuro-Psychopharmacology and Biological Psychiatry.* 2009;33(2):214–9.

43. Sperner-Unterweger B, Whitworth A, Kemmler G, et al. T-cell subsets in schizophrenia: a comparison between drug-naive first episode patients and chronic schizophrenic patients. *Schizophr Res.* 1999;38(1):61–70.

44. Hunter JE, Schmidt FL. Fixed effects vs. random effects meta-analysis models: implications for cumulative research knowledge. *International Journal of Selection and Assessment.* 2000;8 (4):275–92.

45. Blume J, Douglas SD, Evans DL. Immune suppression and immune activation in depression. 2011;25(2):221–9.

46. Seidel A, Arolt V, Hunstiger M, et al. Increased CD56+ natural killer cells and related cytokines in major depression. *Clin Immunol Immunopathol.* 1996;78(1):83–5.

47. Ravindran AV, Griffiths J, Merali Z, Anisman H. Circulating lymphocyte subsets in major depression and dysthymia with typical or atypical features. *Psychosom Med.* 1998;60(3):283–9.

48. Yovel G, Sirota P, Mazeh D, et al. Higher natural killer cell activity in schizophrenic patients: the impact of serum factors, medication, and smoking. *Brain Behav Immun.* 2000;14(3):153–69.

49. Karpinski P, Frydecka D, Sasiadek MM, Misiak B. Reduced number of peripheral natural killer cells in schizophrenia but not in bipolar disorder. *Brain Behav Immun.* 2016;54:194–200.

50. Rolle A, Pollmann J, Cerwenka A. Memory of infections: an emerging role for natural killer cells. *PLoS Pathog.* 2013;9(9): e1003548.

51. Toben C, Baune BT. An act of balance between adaptive and maladaptive immunity in depression: a role for T lymphocytes. *J Neuroimmune Pharmacol.* 2015;10(4):595–609.

52. Maes M, Stevens WJ, Declerck LS, et al. Significantly increased expression of T-cell activation markers (interleukin-2 and HLA-DR) in depression: further evidence for an inflammatory process during that illness. *Progress in Neuro-Psychopharmacology & Biological Psychiatry.* 1993;17(2):241–55.

53. Miller AH. Depression and immunity: a role for T cells? *Brain Behav Immun.* 2010;24(1):1–8.

54. Pavon L, Sandoval-Lopez G, Eugenia Hernandez M, et al. Th2 cytokine response in major depressive disorder patients before treatment. *Journal of Neuroimmunology.* 2006;172(1–2):156–65.

55. Darko DF, Gillin JC, Risch SC, et al. Mitogen-stimulated lymphocyte proliferation and pituitary hormones in major depression. *Biol Psychiatry.* 1989;26 (2):145–55.

56. Rothermundt M, Arolt V, Fenker J, et al. Different immune patterns in melancholic and non-melancholic major depression. *Eur Arch Psychiatry Clin Neurosci.* 2001;251(2):90–7.

57. Seidel A, Arolt V, Hunstiger M, et al. Major depressive disorder is associated with elevated monocyte counts. *Acta Psychiatrica Scandinavica.* 1996;94 (3):198–204.

58. Maes M, Stevens W, DeClerck L, et al. Immune disorders in depression: higher T helper/T suppressor-cytotoxic cell ratio. *Acta Psychiatr Scand.* 1992;86(6):423–31.

59. Nikkila HV, Muller K, Ahokas A, Rimon R, Andersson LC. Increased frequency of

activated lymphocytes in the cerebrospinal fluid of patients with acute schizophrenia. *Schizophr Res.* 2001;49(1–2):99–105.

60. Barbosa IG, Rocha NP, Assis F, et al. Monocyte and lymphocyte activation in bipolar disorder: a new piece in the puzzle of immune dysfunction in mood disorders. *Int J Neuropsychopharmacol.* 2014;18(1): pyu021.

61. Breunis MN, Kupka RW, Nolen WA, et al. High numbers of circulating activated T cells and raised levels of serum IL-2 receptor in bipolar disorder. *Biol Psychiatry.* 2003;53(2):157–65.

62. Becking K, Haarman BCM, Grosse L, et al. The circulating levels of CD4+ t helper cells are higher in bipolar disorder as compared to major depressive disorder. *Journal of Neuroimmunology.* 2018;319:28–36.

63. Wu W, Zheng YL, Tian LP, et al. Circulating T lymphocyte subsets, cytokines, and immune checkpoint inhibitors in patients with bipolar II or major depression: a preliminary study. *Sci Rep.* 2017;7:40530.

64. Hickie I, Hickie C, Bennett B, et al. Biochemical correlates of in vivo cell-mediated immune dysfunction in patients with depression: a preliminary report. *International Journal of Immunopharmacology.* 1995;17(8):685–90.

65. Pietruczuk K, Lisowska KA, Grabowski K, Landowski J, Witkowski JM. Proliferation and apoptosis of T lymphocytes in patients with bipolar disorder. *Sci Rep.* 2018;8 (1):3327.

66. Frydecka D, Beszlej A, Karabon L, et al. The role of genetic variations of immune system regulatory molecules CD28 and CTLA-4 in schizophrenia. *Psychiatry Res.* 2013;208(2):197–8.

67. Jun TY, Pae CU, Chae JH, Bahk WM, Kim KS. Polymorphism of CTLA-4 gene for major depression in the Korean population. *Psychiatry Clin Neurosci.* 2001;55(5):533–7.

68. Grosse L, Hoogenboezem T, Ambrée O, et al. Deficiencies of the T and natural killer cell system in major depressive disorder: T regulatory cell defects are associated with inflammatory monocyte activation. *Brain, Behavior, and Immunity.* 2016;54:38–44.

69. Mikova O, Yakimova R, Bosmans E, Kenis G, Maes M. Increased serum tumor necrosis factor alpha concentrations in major depression and multiple sclerosis. *Eur Neuropsychopharmacol.* 2001;11 (3):203–8.

70. do Prado CH, Rizzo LB, Wieck A, et al. Reduced regulatory T cells are associated with higher levels of Th1/TH17 cytokines and activated MAPK in type 1 bipolar disorder. *Psychoneuroendocrinology.* 2013;38(5):667–76.

71. Najjar S, Pearlman DM, Alper K, Najjar A, Devinsky O. Neuroinflammation and psychiatric illness. *J Neuroinflammation.* 2013;10:43.

72. Robertson MJ, Schacterle RS, Mackin GA, et al. Lymphocyte subset differences in patients with chronic fatigue syndrome, multiple sclerosis and major depression. *Clin Exp Immunol.* 2005;141(2): 326–32.

73. Steiner J, Jacobs R, Panteli B, et al. Acute schizophrenia is accompanied by reduced T cell and increased B cell immunity. *Eur Arch Psychiatry Clin Neurosci.* 2010;260 (7):509–18.

74. Schwarz MJ, Chiang S, Muller N, Ackenheil M. T-helper-1 and T-helper-2 responses in psychiatric disorders. *Brain Behav Immun.* 2001;15(4):340–70.

75. Schwarz MJ, Muller N, Riedel M, Ackenheil M. The Th2-hypothesis of schizophrenia: a strategy to identify a subgroup of schizophrenia caused by immune mechanisms. *Med Hypotheses.* 2001;56(4):483–6.

76. Debnath M, Berk M. Th17 pathway-mediated immunopathogenesis of schizophrenia: mechanisms and implications. *Schizophr Bull.* 2014;40 (6):1412–21.

77. Slyepchenko A, Maes M, Köhler C, et al. T helper 17 cells may drive neuroprogression in major depressive disorder: proposal of an integrative model. *Neuroscience & Biobehavioral Reviews.* 2016;64:83–100.

78. Beurel E, Lowell JA. Th17 cells in depression. *Brain, Behavior, and Immunity.* 2018;69:28–34.

79. Poletti S, de Wit H, Mazza E, et al. Th17 cells correlate positively to the structural and functional integrity of the brain in bipolar depression and healthy controls. *Brain, Behavior, and Immunity.* 2017;61:317–25.

80. Vogels RJ, Koenders MA, van Rossum EF, Spijker AT, Drexhage HA. T cell deficits and overexpression of hepatocyte growth factor in anti-inflammatory circulating monocytes of middle-aged patients with bipolar disorder characterized by a high prevalence of the metabolic syndrome. *Front Psychiatry.* 2017;8:34.

81. Walport MJ. Complement. Second of two parts. *N Engl J Med.* 2001;344(15):1140–4.

82. Walport MJ. Complement. First of two parts. *N Engl J Med.* 2001;344(14):1058–66.

83. Stephan AH, Barres BA, Stevens B. The complement system: an unexpected role in synaptic pruning during development and disease. *Annu Rev Neurosci.* 2012;35:369–89.

84. Crider A, Feng T, Pandya CD, et al. Complement component 3a receptor deficiency attenuates chronic stress-induced monocyte infiltration and depressive-like behavior. *Brain Behav Immun.* 2018;70:246–56.

85. Wei J, Liu Y, Zhao L, et al. Plasma complement component 4 increases in patients with major depressive disorder. *Neuropsychiatr Dis Treat.* 2018;14:37–41.

86. Zhang C, Zhang DF, Wu ZG, et al. Complement factor H and susceptibility to major depressive disorder in Han Chinese. *Br J Psychiatry.* 2016;208(5):446–52.

87. Stelzhammer V, Haenisch F, Chan MK, et al. Proteomic changes in serum of first onset, antidepressant drug-naive major depression patients. *Int J Neuropsychopharmacol.* 2014;17(10):1599–608.

88. Morera AL, Henry M, Garcia-Hernandez A, Fernandez-Lopez L. Acute phase proteins as biological markers of negative psychopathology in paranoid schizophrenia. *Actas Esp Psiquiatr.* 2007;35(4):249–52.

89. Nimgaonkar VL, Prasad KM, Chowdari KV, Severance EG, Yolken RH. The complement system: a gateway to gene-environment interactions in schizophrenia pathogenesis. *Mol Psychiatry.* 2017;22(11):1554–61.

90. Kucharska-Mazur J, Jablonski M, Misiak B, et al. Adult stem cells in psychiatric disorders – new discoveries in peripheral blood. *Prog Neuropsychopharmacol Biol Psychiatry.* 2018;80(Pt A):23–7.

91. Wadee AA, Kuschke RH, Wood LA, et al. Serological observations in patients suffering from acute manic episodes. *Hum Psychopharmacol.* 2002;17(4):175–9.

92. Maes M, Delange J, Ranjan R, et al. Acute phase proteins in schizophrenia, mania and major depression: modulation by psychotropic drugs. *Psychiatry Res.* 1997;66(1):1–11.

93. Akcan U, Karabulut S, Ismail Kucukali C, Cakir S, Tuzun E. Bipolar disorder patients display reduced serum complement levels and elevated peripheral blood complement expression levels. *Acta Neuropsychiatr.* 2018;30(2):70–8.

94. Dantzer R. Cytokine, sickness behavior, and depression. *Immunol Allergy Clin North Am.* 2009;29(2):247–64.

95. Capuron L, Castanon N. Role of inflammation in the development of neuropsychiatric symptom domains: evidence and mechanisms. *Curr Top Behav Neurosci.* 2017;31:31–44.

96. Dowlati Y, Herrmann N, Swardfager, et al. A meta-analysis of cytokines in major depression. *Biol Psychiatry.* 2010;67(5):446–57.

97. Liu Y, Ho RC, Mak A. Interleukin (IL)-6, tumour necrosis factor alpha (TNF-alpha) and soluble interleukin-2 receptors (sIL-2R) are elevated in patients with major depressive disorder: a meta-analysis and meta-regression. *J Affect Disord.* 2012;139(3):230–9.

98. Jiang M, Qin P, Yang X. Comorbidity between depression and asthma via immune-inflammatory pathways: a meta-analysis. *J Affect Disord.* 2014;166:22–9.

99. Haapakoski R, Mathieu J, Ebmeier KP, Alenius H, Kivimaki M. Cumulative meta-analysis of interleukins 6 and 1beta, tumour necrosis factor alpha and C-reactive protein in patients with major depressive disorder. *Brain Behav Immun.* 2015;49:206–15.

100. Goldsmith DR, Rapaport MH, Miller BJ. A meta-analysis of blood cytokine network alterations in psychiatric patients: comparisons between schizophrenia, bipolar disorder and depression. *Mol Psychiatry.* 2016;21 (12):1696–709.

101. Kohler CA, Freitas TH, Maes M, et al. Peripheral cytokine and chemokine alterations in depression: a meta-analysis of 82 studies. *Acta Psychiatr Scand.* 2017;135(5):373–87.

102. Wang AK, Miller BJ. Meta-analysis of cerebrospinal fluid cytokine and tryptophan catabolite alterations in psychiatric patients: comparisons between schizophrenia, bipolar disorder, and depression. *Schizophr Bull.* 2018;44 (1):75–83.

103. Valkanova V, Ebmeier KP, Allan CL. CRP, IL-6 and depression: a systematic review and meta-analysis of longitudinal studies. *J Affect Disord.* 2013;150 (3):736–44.

104. Ellul P, Boyer L, Groc L, Leboyer M, Fond G. Interleukin-1 beta-targeted treatment strategies in inflammatory depression: toward personalized care. *Acta Psychiatr Scand.* 2016;134(6):469–84.

105. Potvin S, Stip E, Sepehry AA, et al. Inflammatory cytokine alterations in schizophrenia: a systematic quantitative review. *Biol Psychiatry.* 2008;63(8):801–8.

106. Miller BJ, Buckley P, Seabolt W, Mellor A, Kirkpatrick B. Meta-analysis of cytokine alterations in schizophrenia: clinical status and antipsychotic effects. *Biol Psychiatry.* 2011;70(7):663–71.

107. Pillinger T, Osimo EF, Brugger S, et al. A meta-analysis of immune parameters, variability, and assessment of modal distribution in psychosis and test of the immune subgroup hypothesis. *Schizophr Bull.* 2019;45(5):1120–33.

108. Muller N, Weidinger E, Leitner B, Schwarz MJ. The role of inflammation in schizophrenia. *Front Neurosci.* 2015;9:372.

109. Frydecka D, Misiak B, Pawlak-Adamska E, et al. Interleukin-6: the missing element of the neurocognitive deterioration in schizophrenia? The focus on genetic underpinnings, cognitive impairment and clinical manifestation. *Eur Arch Psychiatry Clin Neurosci.* 2015;265 (6):449–59.

110. Shi J, Levinson DF, Duan J, et al. Common variants on chromosome 6p22.1 are associated with schizophrenia. *Nature.* 2009;460(7256):753–7.

111. Lee YH, Song GG. Meta-analysis of associations between tumor necrosis factor-alpha polymorphisms and schizophrenia susceptibility. *Psychiatry Res.* 2015;226(2–3):521–2.

112. Qin H, Zhang L, Xu G, Pan X. Lack of association between TNFalpha rs1800629 polymorphism and schizophrenia risk: a meta-analysis. *Psychiatry Res.* 2013;209 (3):314–9.

113. Sacchetti E, Bocchio-Chiavetto L, Valsecchi P, et al. -G308A tumor necrosis factor alpha functional polymorphism and schizophrenia risk: meta-analysis plus association study. *Brain Behav Immun.* 2007;21(4):450–7.

114. Ripke S, O'Dushlaine C, Chambert K, et al. Genome-wide association analysis identifies 13 new risk loci for schizophrenia. *Nat Genet.* 2013;45 (10):1150–9.

115. Gao L, Li Z, Chang S, Wang J. Association of interleukin-10 polymorphisms with schizophrenia: a meta-analysis. *PLoS One.* 2014;9(3):e90407.

116. Shibuya M, Watanabe Y, Nunokawa A, et al. Interleukin 1 beta gene and risk of schizophrenia: detailed case-control and

family-based studies and an updated meta-analysis. *Hum Psychopharmacol.* 2014;29(1):31–7.

117. Modabbernia A, Taslimi S, Brietzke E, Ashrafi M. Cytokine alterations in bipolar disorder: a meta-analysis of 30 studies. *Biol Psychiatry.* 2013;74(1):15–25.

118. Munkholm K, Brauner JV, Kessing LV, Vinberg M. Cytokines in bipolar disorder vs. healthy control subjects: a systematic review and meta-analysis. *J Psychiatr Res.* 2013;47(9):1119–33.

119. Munkholm K, Vinberg M, Vedel Kessing L. Cytokines in bipolar disorder: a systematic review and meta-analysis. *J Affect Disord.* 2013;144(1–2):16–27.

120. Horn SR, Long MM, Nelson BW, et al. Replication and reproducibility issues in the relationship between C-reactive protein and depression: a systematic review and focused meta-analysis. *Brain Behav Immun.* 2018;73:85–114.

121. van den Ameele S, van Diermen L, Staels W, et al. The effect of mood-stabilizing drugs on cytokine levels in bipolar disorder: a systematic review. *J Affect Disord.* 2016;203:364–73.

122. Capuzzi E, Bartoli F, Crocamo C, Clerici M, Carra G. Acute variations of cytokine levels after antipsychotic treatment in drug-naive subjects with a first-episode psychosis: a meta-analysis. *Neurosci Biobehav Rev.* 2017;77:122–8.

123. Kohler CA, Freitas TH, Stubbs B, et al. Peripheral alterations in cytokine and chemokine levels after antidepressant drug treatment for major depressive disorder: systematic review and meta-analysis. *Mol Neurobiol.* 2018;55 (5):4195–206.

124. Ono SJ, Nakamura T, Miyazaki D, et al. Chemokines: roles in leukocyte development, trafficking, and effector function. *J Allergy Clin Immunol.* 2003 Jun;111(6):1185–99.

125. Le Y, Zhou Y, Iribarren P, Wang J. Chemokines and chemokine receptors: their manifold roles in homeostasis and disease. *Cell Mol Immunol.* 2004;1 (2):95–104.

126. Jo WK, Law AC, Chung SK. The neglected co-star in the dementia drama: the putative roles of astrocytes in the pathogeneses of major neurocognitive disorders. *Mol Psychiatry.* 2014;19 (2):159–67.

127. Rostene W, Buckingham JC. Chemokines as modulators of neuroendocrine functions. *J Mol Endocrinol.* 2007;38 (3):351–3.

128. Rostene W, Kitabgi P, Parsadaniantz SM. Chemokines: a new class of neuromodulator? *Nat Rev Neurosci.* 2007;8(11):895–903.

129. Bergon A, Belzeaux R, Comte M, et al. CX3CR1 is dysregulated in blood and brain from schizophrenia patients. *Schizophr Res.* 2015;168(1–2):434–43.

130. Zakharyan R, Boyajyan A. Inflammatory cytokine network in schizophrenia. *World J Biol Psychiatry.* 2014;15(3):174–87.

131. Barbosa IG, Rocha NP, Bauer ME, et al. Chemokines in bipolar disorder: trait or state? *Eur Arch Psychiatry Clin Neurosci.* 2013;263(2):159–65.

132. Panizzutti B, Gubert C, Schuh AL, et al. Increased serum levels of eotaxin/CCL11 in late-stage patients with bipolar disorder: an accelerated aging biomarker? *J Affect Disord.* 2015;182:64–9.

133. Tokac D, Tuzun E, Gulec H, et al. Chemokine and chemokine receptor polymorphisms in bipolar disorder. *Psychiatry Investig.* 2016;13(5):541–8.

134. Altamura AC, Mundo E, Cattaneo E, et al. The MCP-1 gene (SCYA2) and mood disorders: preliminary results of a case-control association study. *Neuroimmunomodulation.* 2010;17 (2):126–31.

135. Pae CU, Kim JJ, Yu HS, et al. Monocyte chemoattractant protein-1 promoter -2518 polymorphism may have an influence on clinical heterogeneity of bipolar I disorder in the Korean population. *Neuropsychobiology.* 2004;49 (3):111–4.

136. Rosenblat JD, Cha DS, Mansur RB, McIntyre RS. Inflamed moods: a review of

the interactions between inflammation and mood disorders. *Prog Neuropsychopharmacol Biol Psychiatry.* 2014;53:23–34.

137. Robinson MW, Harmon C, O'Farrelly C. Liver immunology and its role in inflammation and homeostasis. *Cell Mol Immunol.* 2016;13(3):267–76.

138. Niciu MJ, Ionescu DF, Mathews DC, Richards EM, Zarate CA, Jr. Second messenger/signal transduction pathways in major mood disorders: moving from membrane to mechanism of action, part I: major depressive disorder. *CNS Spectr.* 2013;18(5):231–41.

139. Niciu MJ, Ionescu DF, Mathews DC, Richards EM, Zarate CA, Jr. Second messenger/signal transduction pathways in major mood disorders: moving from membrane to mechanism of action, part II: bipolar disorder. *CNS Spectr.* 2013;18 (5):242–51.

140. Miklowitz DJ, Portnoff LC, Armstrong CC, et al. Inflammatory cytokines and nuclear factor-kappa B activation in adolescents with bipolar and major depressive disorders. *Psychiatry Res.* 2016;241:315–22.

141. Altamura AC, Buoli M, Pozzoli S. Role of immunological factors in the pathophysiology and diagnosis of bipolar disorder: comparison with schizophrenia. *Psychiatry Clin Neurosci.* 2014;68 (1):21–36.

142. Muller N, Schwarz MJ. Immune system and schizophrenia. *Curr Immunol Rev.* 2010;6(3):213–20.

143. Kubera M, Basta-Kaim A, Wrobel A, Maes M, Dudek D. Increased mitogen-induced lymphocyte proliferation in treatment resistant depression: a preliminary study. *Neuro Endocrinol Lett.* 2004;25(3):207–10.

144. Muller N, Schwarz MJ. The immune-mediated alteration of serotonin and glutamate: towards an integrated view of depression. *Mol Psychiatry.* 2007;12(11):988–1000.

145. Al-Amin MM, Nasir Uddin MM, Mahmud Reza H. Effects of antipsychotics on the inflammatory response system of patients with schizophrenia in peripheral blood mononuclear cell cultures. *Clin Psychopharmacol Neurosci.* 2013;11 (3):144–51.

146. Nazimek K, Strobel S, Bryniarski P, et al. The role of macrophages in anti-inflammatory activity of antidepressant drugs. *Immunobiology.* 2017;222(6):823–30.

147. Brietzke E, Kauer-Sant'Anna M, Teixeira AL, Kapczinski F. Abnormalities in serum chemokine levels in euthymic patients with bipolar disorder. *Brain Behav Immun.* 2009;23(8): 1079–82.

148. Miller AH, Raison CL. The role of inflammation in depression: from evolutionary imperative to modern treatment target. *Nat Rev Immunol.* 2016;16(1):22–34.

149. Fillman SG, Sinclair D, Fung SJ, Webster MJ, Shannon Weickert C. Markers of inflammation and stress distinguish subsets of individuals with schizophrenia and bipolar disorder. *Transl Psychiatry.* 2014;4:e365.

150. Belvederi Murri M, Prestia D, Mondelli V, et al. The HPA axis in bipolar disorder: Systematic review and meta-analysis. *Psychoneuroendocrinology.* 2016;63:327–42.

151. Jacobson L. Hypothalamic-pituitary-adrenocortical axis: neuropsychiatric aspects. *Compr Physiol.* 2014;4(2):715–38.

152. Maes M, Carvalho AF. The compensatory immune-regulatory reflex system (CIRS) in depression and bipolar disorder. *Molecular Neurobiology.* 2018;55 (12):8885–903.

153. Jara LJ, Navarro C, Medina G, Vera-Lastra O, Blanco F. Immune-neuroendocrine interactions and autoimmune diseases. *Clin Dev Immunol.* 2006;13(2–4):109–23.

154. Chen Y, Jiang T, Chen P, et al. Emerging tendency towards autoimmune process in major depressive patients: a novel insight from Th17 cells. *Psychiatry Research.* 2011;188(2):224–30.

155. Steiner J, Bielau H, Brisch R, et al. Immunological aspects in the neurobiology of suicide: elevated microglial density in schizophrenia and depression is associated with suicide. *J Psychiatr Res.* 2008;42(2):151–7.

156. Setiawan E, Wilson AA, Mizrahi R, et al. Role of translocator protein density, a marker of neuroinflammation, in the brain during major depressive episodes. *JAMA Psychiatry.* 2015;72(3):268–75.

157. Wohleb ES, Franklin T, Iwata M, Duman RS. Integrating neuroimmune systems in the neurobiology of depression. *Nat Rev Neurosci.* 2016;17 (8):497–511.

158. Szepesi Z, Manouchehrian O, Bachiller S, Deierborg T. Bidirectional microglia-neuron communication in health and disease. *Front Cell Neurosci.* 2018;12:323.

159. Neniskyte U, Gross CT. Errant gardeners: glial-cell-dependent synaptic pruning and neurodevelopmental disorders. *Nat Rev Neurosci.* 2017;18(11):658–70.

160. Kempton MJ, Salvador Z, Munafo MR, et al. Structural neuroimaging studies in major depressive disorder. Meta-analysis and comparison with bipolar disorder. *Arch Gen Psychiatry.* 2011;68(7):675–90.

161. van Erp TG, Hibar DP, Rasmussen JM, et al. Subcortical brain volume abnormalities in 2028 individuals with schizophrenia and 2540 healthy controls via the ENIGMA consortium. *Mol Psychiatry.* 2016;21(4):585.

162. Hibar DP, Westlye LT, van Erp TG, et al. Subcortical volumetric abnormalities in bipolar disorder. *Mol Psychiatry.* 2016;21 (12):1710–6.

163. Schmaal L, Veltman DJ, van Erp TG, et al. Subcortical brain alterations in major depressive disorder: findings from the ENIGMA Major Depressive Disorder working group. *Mol Psychiatry.* 2016;21 (6):806–12.

164. Harrison NA. Brain structures implicated in inflammation-associated depression. *Curr Top Behav Neurosci.* 2017;31: 221–48.

165. Gemechu JM, Bentivoglio M. T cell recruitment in the brain during normal aging. *Front Cell Neurosci.* 2012;6:38.

166. Jha MK, Miller AH, Minhajuddin A, Trivedi MH. Association of T and non-T cell cytokines with anhedonia: role of gender differences. *Psychoneuroendocrinology.* 2018;95:1–7.

167. Cuthbert BN, Insel TR. Toward new approaches to psychotic disorders: the NIMH Research Domain Criteria project. *Schizophr Bull.* 2010;36(6):1061–2.

168. Sanislow CA, Pine DS, Quinn KJ, et al. Developing constructs for psychopathology research: research domain criteria. *J Abnorm Psychol.* 2010;119(4):631–9.

169. Dooley LN, Kuhlman KR, Robles TF, et al. The role of inflammation in core features of depression: Insights from paradigms using exogenously induced inflammation. *Neuroscience & Biobehavioral Reviews.* 2018;94:219–37.

170. Dantzer R, O'Connor JC, Freund GG, Johnson RW, Kelley KW. From inflammation to sickness and depression: when the immune system subjugates the brain. *Nat Rev Neurosci.* 2008;9(1): 46–56.

Index

Printed in the United States
by Baker & Taylor Publisher Services